The Newborn Child

Peter Johnston FRCP FRCPCH
Honorary Consultant Paediatrician, Dorset County Hospital, Dorchester, UK

Kirstie Flood RN RM DipHE ENB998 ENB405
Senior Staff Nurse, NICU, Royal United Hospital, Bath, UK

Karen Spinks RGN RSCN ENB998 ENB405 ENBR23
Sister, NICU, Royal United Hospital, Bath, UK

NINTH EDITION

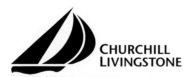
CHURCHILL
LIVINGSTONE

EDINBURGH LONDON NEW YORK OXFORD PHILADELPHIA ST LOUIS SYDNEY TORONTO 2003

CHURCHILL LIVINGSTONE
An imprint of Elsevier Limited

First edition 1961
Second edition 1967
Third edition 1972
Fourth edition 1977
Fifth edition 1982
Sixth edition 1987
Seventh edition 1994
Eighth edition 1998
Ninth edition 2003
   Reprinted 2003, 2004, 2007 (twice)

ISBN 13: 978 0 443 07159 1
ISBN 10: 0 443 07159 4

British Library Cataloguing in Publication Data
A catalogue record for this book is available from the British Library

Library of Congress Cataloging in Publication Data
A catalog record for this book is available from the Library of Congress

Note
Knowledge and best practice in this field are constantly changing. As new research and experience
broaden our knowledge, changes in practice, treatment and drug therapy may become necessary or
appropriate. Readers are advised to check the most current information provided (i) on procedures
featured or (ii) by the manufacturer of each product to be administered, to verify the recommended
dose or formula, the method and duration of administration, and contraindications. It is the
responsibility of the practitioner, relying on their own experience and knowledge of the patient, to
make diagnoses, to determine dosages and the best treatment for each individual patient, and to
take all appropriate safety precautions. To the fullest extent of the law, neither the publisher nor the
author assumes any liability for any injury and/or damage.

The Publisher

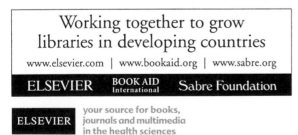

Printed in China
C/05

The
publisher's
policy is to use
**paper manufactured
from sustainable forests**

Contents

Preface   **vii**

1. Introduction   **1**

2. Maternal and fetal health   **13**

3. Resuscitation and respiratory problems of the newborn   **31**

4. Growth and its disorders   **45**

5. Clinical assessment of the newborn baby   **59**

6. Essential care of the newborn baby   **79**

7. Feeding the baby   **91**

8. Preterm infants   **107**

9. Intensive neonatal care   **125**

10. Neurological disorders   **149**

11. Infections   **163**

12. Haematological problems and jaundice   **183**

13. Congenital malformations and genetic disorders   **201**

14. Helping the parents   **239**

15. Neonatal pharmacopoeia   **249**

Index   **255**

Preface

Since 1961, when the first edition of Vulliamy's *The Newborn Child* was published, many aspects of neonatal and perinatal care have advanced – notably, intensive care of preterm infants. Yet the fundamentals of professional care of the newborn remain. With the two new authors for this edition bringing their midwifery and neonatal nursing skills, we have tried to meld the insights of medicine and nursing into a text which gives proper emphasis to both disciplines. We hope it is sufficiently comprehensive for situations where non-specialised care is provided, and, as with previous editions, it remains an introduction to the subject.

Now that the world's medical and nursing research journals are readily accessible through the internet, we believe that all serious students of neonatology should become competent computer-users and learn the skills to discern which papers and abstracts are sufficient for changing practice and which give less complete information. The Cochrane databases and other reviews provide superb analyses of current thinking in some areas of the work and we have given several references to them. We have also included website addresses where we believe readers will find valuable additional information.

Surprisingly, some areas of care, such as care of the umbilical cord, remain under-researched, and our advice on such subjects is based as much on common practice as on research. We hope readers will recognise the relative strengths of our recommendations throughout the book and apply them intelligently.

In this edition we have tried to avoid the duplication of information found in previous editions and have restructured several chapters to reflect the chronology of normal clinical practice. We hope the additional tables and lists of important information we have included will make for easier reading and simpler reference.

We thank the neonatal units in Dorchester and Bath for encouragement and the opportunity to produce this text, and our colleagues, friends and families for their support through its gestation period. If, through reading this book, any are inspired to take up the cause of neonatology, we shall be well pleased.

Peter Johnston
Kirstie Flood
Karen Spinks
2003

Chapter 1
Introduction

CHAPTER CONTENTS

Epidemiology, perinatal statistics and definitions   1
   Definitions   2
General factors influencing perinatal health   4
The causes of perinatal mortality   5
   Treatable predisposing causes of perinatal
   death   6
The quality of survival and prevention of handicap   7
The prevention of ill-health in infancy   8
The psychological dimension of perinatal care   8
The need for special care   9
Ethical aspects of perinatal care   9

EPIDEMIOLOGY, PERINATAL STATISTICS AND DEFINITIONS

Pregnancy and childbirth are usually natural and normal events, and in about two-thirds of healthy mothers no intervention other than the help of a midwife is needed to deliver a healthy child who can be cared for at home with little professional advice. The prospects for the remaining third have also greatly improved in most developed countries through an increasing understanding of the many complications which can affect both the mother and the unborn infant and by learning when and how to intervene appropriately. Despite the wide-held belief that expensive and sophisticated technology has been a major factor in improving the outcome for mothers and babies, in reality its influence has been relatively small, though it has substantially improved the outlook for the minority of infants who are born too small or premature. Many more babies have benefited from attention to the nutrition and health of the mother before the pregnancy, the treatment of pregnancy-related disorders, the reduction of tobacco and alcohol consumption during pregnancy, the prevention and treatment of infections, the active management of prolonged labour and the promotion of breast feeding. The improvements in resuscitation of babies asphyxiated during delivery, the prevention of hypothermia and hypoglycaemia in the hours after birth, and improved nutrition for the newborn infant have had a major impact in reducing the risk to babies in the newborn period and improving their future health and development. Other factors that influence the outcome for the baby include genetic disorders and the socioeconomic circumstances of the family, which may in some cases be amenable to medical or social intervention.

Traditionally, the effectiveness of perinatal care has been measured by monitoring improvements in mortality rates year by year, but the quality of life for the surviving children is equally important, though much more difficult to measure. Major neurological handicaps such as cerebral palsy or severe developmental delay can often be identified within a few months of birth, but minor impairments in development may not show themselves for several years, and it is often difficult to relate them with certainty to complications around the time of birth.

In Britain, mortality rates for both mothers and babies have been progressively falling and are low compared with those in many developing countries. Even so, in 1999, some 5740 babies died before or during birth or in the month after birth, as compared with a total of only 1186 in the rest of the first year and a total of 2971 during the rest of the childhood years. There is, therefore, no room for complacency even in the relative safety of the modern practice of midwifery, obstetrics and neonatology. Saving the life of a baby must be of the greatest importance, but nursing and medical care at this critical time should also aim to prevent permanent disabilities which may be caused by events during childbirth. If the results of perinatal care are to continue to improve, all those involved in the care of the baby must be aware of the effects of complications during the pregnancy on the fetus, the newborn baby and the growing child, and of the impact of their methods of care. Clinical governance now demands that regular local clinical audit meetings and analysis of the annual perinatal statistics, involving clinicians, midwives, pathologists, members of the diagnostic imaging departments and others, should occur. These should enable departments to learn together the aspects of care on which they must focus attention to improve clinical practice. Regional and national audits and research are also attempting to identify perinatal factors that adversely affect the ongoing health of the child. The requirement for the adoption of evidence-based clinical practice is placing more emphasis on clinical research – this should help to increase standards and decrease differences in results which are susceptible to improvement by changes in methods of care. Meta-analysis and regular review of the available literature by the Cochrane Foundation, which is available on the Internet, provides expert analysis of the world literature, bringing the best available valid interpretations of much neonatal research to all concerned in delivering such care.

Definitions

Before discussing perinatal statistics, it is necessary to define the terms used (Tables 1.1 and 1.2).

Live births and stillbirths

All babies born with any signs of life are classified as *live births*.

In Britain, since a change in the legal definition in 1992, a *stillbirth or late fetal death* is any baby

Table 1.1 Perinatal definitions

Live birth	Any signs of life at delivery
Stillbirth	A baby born after 24 weeks of gestation with no sign of life at birth
Low birth weight baby	Any baby weighing 2500 g or less at birth
Preterm baby	A baby born earlier than 37 weeks of gestation
Term baby	A baby born between 37 and 41 weeks of gestation
Post-term baby	A baby born after 42 weeks of gestation
Neonatal period	The first month of life
Infancy	The first year of life

Table 1.2 Perinatal mortality definitions

Perinatal mortality	Stillbirths and first-week deaths per 1000 total births
Neonatal mortality	Deaths of live births in the first month of life per 1000 live births
Infant mortality	Deaths of all live births in the first year of life per 1000 live births
Postneonatal mortality	Deaths of all babies from 1 month to 1 year per 1000 babies alive at 1 month

born after 24 weeks of pregnancy who has no heartbeat, breathing or movement. Babies born before this gestational age are regarded as mid-trimester abortions. This change was a response to the survival of some extreme preterm babies, down to 24 weeks' gestation, with modern neo-natal intensive care.

Categories of babies by birth weight

A baby weighing 2500 g or less at birth is called a *low birth weight baby* whatever his maturity. Babies weighing less than 1500 g at birth are often termed 'very low birth weight'.

Categories by maturity

Babies may be classified as term, preterm or post-term. *A preterm baby* is one born before 37 weeks from the first day of the last menstrual period. A *term baby* is one born between 37 and 41 completed weeks of gestation, and a *post-term baby* is one born after 42 weeks.

The *newborn or neonatal period* is defined as the first month of life, and *infancy* is the whole of the first year.

Mortality statistics

Perinatal deaths include stillbirths and deaths in the first week; *perinatal mortality* statistics thus include both of these categories and are usually quoted as a proportion of 1000 births. *The perinatal mortality rate* per 1000 total births has been taken as a general indication of the standard of health care at this time of life, and the improving trend in England and Wales over the years 1975 to 1999 is shown in Figure 1.1. Though they have differing basic causes, reductions in both still-births and neonatal deaths reflect the continuing improvements in the care both of the mother and of the baby. The small number of fetal deaths between 24 and 28 weeks of gestation were not included before 1992 – the effect of their subsequent inclusion in mortality figures can clearly be seen as an increase in the perinatal mortality data.

The rate of decline in perinatal mortality has varied from country to country, though the rates are very similar in most Western European countries. This downward trend is continuing; however, further reductions in the mortality rates will be much harder to achieve because an increasingly high proportion of the babies dying now

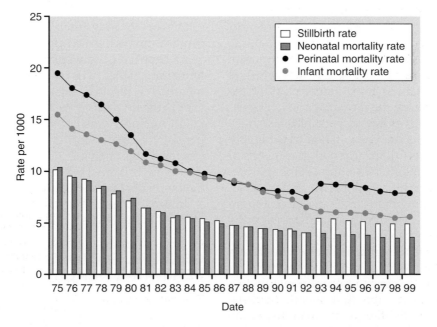

Figure 1.1 Trends in perinatal and infant mortality 1975–1999 in England and Wales.

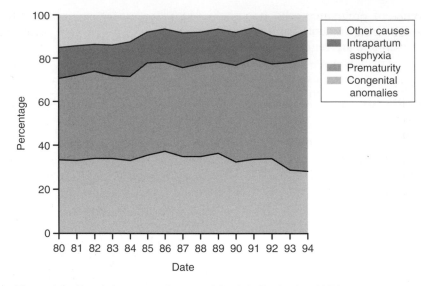

Figure 1.2 Trends in causes of neonatal death in England and Wales 1981–1994.

are too immature to survive with existing methods of care (Fig. 1.2).

The contribution of lethal congenital malformations to perinatal mortality has fallen as more of such cases are being identified prenatally and the pregnancy terminated; if those remaining are excluded from the figures, however, the average perinatal mortality rate drops from approximately 8.2 to about 6 per 1000 births. If all babies of birth weight below 1000 g – of which about two-thirds will survive – are also excluded, the figure comes down to about 5 per 1000. There is, however, still a wide variation between different parts of the country, and in some the mortality rate 'adjusted' in this way reaches as low as 3 per 1000.

First-day deaths have also fallen considerably over the years, yet still nearly half of all neonatal deaths occur in the first 24 hours. Although preterm and low birth weight babies have a much higher risk of dying than larger and more mature babies, around a quarter of neonatal deaths in the UK still occur in babies weighing over 2500 g at birth. Most of these deaths are caused by factors operating before delivery, especially intrapartum asphyxia or a major congenital malformation.

The death rate in the first month (*neonatal mortality*) is only slightly greater than that of the first week, and improvements are the result of advances in assessment and care around the time of birth and in better care of the newborn baby.

Changes in the *infant mortality rate* (deaths in the whole of the first year) are also influenced by reductions in neonatal deaths. However, around two-thirds of deaths occurring between the ages of 1 month and 1 year (*postneonatal mortality*) are due either to the 'sudden infant death syndrome' (SIDS) or to congenital abnormalities. Though deaths from both these causes have fallen in recent years, they have been replaced by some extremely immature babies who survive beyond the first month as a result of intensive care but who die later in the first year. This accounts for the fact that infant mortality was not improving as rapidly as perinatal mortality up to about 1990 (Fig. 1.1). However, the halving of the incidence of cot deaths in Britain consequent to the recommendation that babies should sleep supine – reflecting a similar change in several other countries – has reduced these figures in the last few years (p. 88).

GENERAL FACTORS INFLUENCING PERINATAL HEALTH

The relative impact of different factors on the outcome of pregnancy will vary between one country and another and even between regions of the same country. Where regular antenatal care is not available, the following factors have a major impact on the baby's prognosis:

- eclampsia
- maternal anaemia
- sexually transmitted diseases
- prenatal infection
- prolonged labour.

In contrast, where antenatal services are well developed, these hazards are largely preventable and an adverse outcome for the baby is more likely to be related to:

- low birth weight
- maternal smoking
- alcohol or illicit drug consumption
- socioeconomic factors.

When comparing statistics from one country or region with those of another, it is therefore necessary to obtain more detailed information than the crude mortality rates offer. Since low birth weight (i.e. 1500 g or less) is a major predisposing cause of neonatal death, poor growth in childhood and developmental delay, it is useful to know its prevalence. In Britain, the average rate is about 6% of all births, though it varies widely from one region to another. In certain developing countries, it is much more common and has a major impact on mortality and morbidity rates. Low birth weight is also directly related to adverse socioeconomic conditions, so these have to be taken into account. The incidence of lethal malformations (p. 203) is another variable factor, and termination of pregnancy after antenatal diagnosis of serious fetal abnormalities (p. 20) also lowers the official perinatal mortality figures.

THE CAUSES OF PERINATAL MORTALITY

The immediate cause of a baby's death is not always easy to establish, and an autopsy carried out by a pathologist with specialist knowledge of the newborn is often needed to define it accurately. However, certain maternal and fetal factors are known to predispose the baby to either stillbirth or neonatal death.

A study in Britain indicated that 86% of stillbirths are caused by complications of pregnancy or delivery, including antepartum haemorrhage, abruption or placenta praevia (41%), hypertension (22%), and complications of the umbilical cord such as knots or prolapse (8%). Approximately 32% of the babies suffered lethal intrauterine hypoxia caused by placental malfunction, 5% were already growth retarded and 8% had congenital malformations. In only 14% of cases was there no definable maternal condition.

In neonatal deaths, by contrast, complications of pregnancy presented a significant risk in fewer than 50% of cases, and in 35% of deaths the pregnancy and delivery were normal. Very few neonatal deaths relate closely to complications in labour. Congenital malformations were a major factor in 33% of cases. Nearly half of these were abnormalities of the heart and circulation, some 15% were malformations of the respiratory tract, and less than 10% were defects in the central nervous system (CNS). The proportion of CNS abnormalities, such as spina bifida, has fallen over the years because the affected babies are identified in early pregnancy and a termination is carried out. A small number of babies die from infections but 45% of deaths before 28 days of age follow complications of immaturity, a high proportion of which are due to respiratory disorders such as hyaline membrane disease (p. 131). Around 60% of neonatal deaths and 27% of stillbirths occur in babies of less than 1500 g birthweight and the cause in almost all of these is extreme prematurity. The maternal conditions most commonly contributing to *neonatal deaths* are antepartum haemorrhage, preterm labour and hypertension acting mostly through premature delivery of the baby, and premature rupture of the membranes. Figure 1.2 shows the recent trends in the causes of neonatal deaths and illustrates that prematurity, congenital abnormalities and asphyxia remain the commonest causes, though preterm birth is rising as a proportion of the total as the number of babies born with lethal malformations falls.

Even with modern methods of neonatal intensive care, not all such conditions can be successfully treated at present and further developments in the methods of care will be needed to improve their outlook in future.

Treatable predisposing causes of perinatal death

The factors which increase the chances of a baby dying in the neonatal period and which may be amenable to medical or social intervention during the pregnancy or at the time of birth include:

- socioeconomic disadvantage – acting through inappropriate maternal nutrition, a greater amount of general illness, and inadequate or late antenatal care
- low birth weight – either from early onset of labour or from intrauterine growth failure (especially common in poor social conditions)
- pre-eclampsia
- antepartum haemorrhage
- smoking (more than 5 cigarettes/day) (Pollack 2001)
- excessive alcohol consumption
- illicit drug abuse
- malpresentation (mainly breech)
- disproportion
- post-term birth
- prolonged second stage of labour
- multiple birth
- adverse previous obstetric history (e.g. abortion, stillbirth, eclampsia, premature labour, infertility treatment)
- first pregnancy
- maternal disease (e.g. diabetes, hypertension, urinary infection, serious chronic disease).

Other factors which are not amenable to professional interventions also relate closely to increased perinatal mortality and morbidity. For instance, male infants are at higher risk than females both for stillbirth and neonatal death. Babies of mothers over 40 or under 18 years of age and those born outside marriage are at greater risk, especially when the mother has no partner, and in Britain the incidence of each of these is rising. In some inner-city areas, lone mothers are in the majority, and it is now not uncommon to find a quarter of mothers in an area unmarried and a high proportion without a regular partner.

Although there has been a reduction in perinatal mortality in all social groups over the years, the disparity between the rates in the different categories remains. The more advantaged sections of the population have relatively low rates of perinatal deaths and congenital malformations, whereas the more disadvantaged people have the highest rates. The risk for teenage mothers when delivering at home are some three to four times higher than when delivering in hospital. Lone parenthood, teenage pregnancy, poor housing, unemployment, poor educational attainment at school, and poverty are all associated with higher rates of perinatal mortality and morbidity (Box 1.1). In addition, the risks to the offspring of those mothers who fail to make use of the available antenatal care and health education programmes are increased.

Figure 1.3 shows that there are also variations in mortality rates related to the country of birth of the mother, though in second-generation ethnic

---

Box 1.1 Social factors affecting perinatal death rates

- Lone parenthood
- Teenage pregnancy
- Poor housing
- Unemployment
- Poor school achievement
- Poverty
- Non-attendance at antenatal clinics

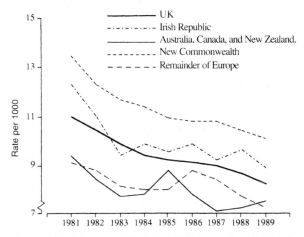

Figure 1.3 Infant mortality in the UK by country of birth of the mother. (By kind permission of the Office of National Statistics.)

minority mothers born in the UK the risks seem to be diminishing. Eight percent of British births are from mothers born in the Indian subcontinent, the Caribbean or Africa. In these infants, there is a higher perinatal mortality rate, which is greatest in the offspring of mothers originating from West and central Africa, the Caribbean and Pakistan. Much of this higher perinatal mortality appears to be due to increased rates of congenital malformations. In parts of the UK where a significant proportion of the population belongs to one of these ethnic groups, the overall perinatal statistics may appear less favourable, and such differences must be interpreted with care.

THE QUALITY OF SURVIVAL AND PREVENTION OF HANDICAP

Although perinatal statistics give valuable information about how many babies live or die, it is equally important to establish the incidence of handicapping conditions and in how many of such cases a potentially preventable perinatal cause can be found.

Most cases of severe learning disability without physical handicap are of genetic origin (e.g. Down's syndrome) or due to some fetal insult at a very early stage of pregnancy (e.g. intrauterine viral infections, prescribed medicines, illicit drugs, genetic disorders), but about 15% result from perinatal difficulties, particularly hypoxic-ischaemic damage associated with placental dysfunction (p. 19) (Box 1.2). Milder forms of learning disability have less connection with events at this time, and hereditary and socioeconomic factors are predominant. Such conditions as fragile X chromosomes (p. 209) and other recognisable syndromes are increasingly being identified in this group.

Cerebral palsy, on the other hand, has many different causes, of which around 50% are attributable to problems occurring before the onset of labour (p. 123) and a significant proportion result from complications occurring during the treatment for extreme prematurity (p. 123) (Badawi 2000). Additional causes include infection or other diseases occurring after birth, but studies now suggest that only a minority of cases are related to factors operating during labour itself. A significant proportion of children who develop cerebral palsy are born after an apparently uncomplicated pregnancy, straightforward birth and a normal neonatal period.

Since extreme preterm birth is known to be associated with cerebral palsy it is reasonable to ask whether keeping increasingly immature babies alive is simply adding to the numbers of damaged babies and children (Fig. 1.4). The fact that the overall incidence of cerebral palsy in very preterm infants remains roughly constant at around 10% suggests that babies who would in the past have been affected are now surviving intact (Marlow 2000). Published reports from the

---

Box 1.2   Organic perinatal origins of learning disability
• Genetic disorders, e.g. Down syndrome, 'fragile X' syndrome • Intrauterine infection • Effects of drugs • Hypoxic-ischaemic brain damage

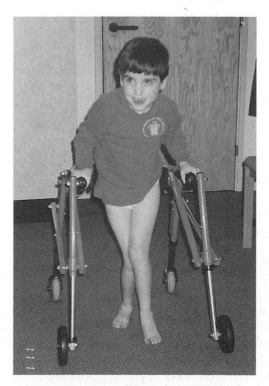

Figure 1.4   Cerebral palsy related to preterm birth.

UK and Australia (Colver et al 2000, Sutton & Bajuk 1999) show that despite overall improvements in perinatal survival there has not been a reduction in such conditions. In the current state of knowledge, it is only a minority of such infants whose handicap could be prevented if every possible modern development in obstetrics and neonatal care were universally available. Other problems which may be related to perinatal events to a much smaller extent include epilepsy, severe deafness and severe visual impairment.

The introduction of antenatal diagnosis for spina bifida with myelomeningocele, Down syndrome, cystic fibrosis and a rapidly increasing number of other genetic disorders (p. 22) has opened up greatly the possibility of termination of the pregnancy if it is acceptable to the parents (p. 241). In families where there is a history of other inherited diseases, genetic tests and counselling are often able to reduce further the incidence of such handicapping conditions (p. 21).

THE PREVENTION OF ILL-HEALTH IN INFANCY

A careful routine examination of all newborn babies (p. 61) in the first few days leads to early diagnosis of many congenital defects, the timely treatment of which can greatly reduce their ill effects. Examples of this are congenital dislocation of the hip, talipes and some forms of congenital heart disease.

The health of normal infants is also affected by maternal factors during the pregnancy and the mother's care of her infant during the first few weeks of life. For example, the infant of a mother who smokes in pregnancy not only is more likely to be growth retarded at birth but also is at greater risk of SIDS (Pollack 2001) or to suffer recurrent wheezing in infancy (Gilliland et al 2001). Positively promoting breast feeding is very important for the health of all babies, but particularly where hygienic preparation of artificial feeds is difficult to achieve. Not only does it provide the best nutrition available for the baby, but also it reduces the likelihood of the baby suffering from respiratory and gastrointestinal infections. Furthermore, it improves the attachment

between the mother and baby, and may as a result reduce the risk of child abuse.

There are many other preventable causes of neonatal or infant ill-health, appropriate professional advice for which can reduce the risk to the growing child. Recent epidemiological research has suggested that low birth weight and fetal malnutrition may cause hypertension, diabetes mellitus and coronary heart disease during middle age (Barker 2001). Thus, there are great responsibilities on those caring for the developing fetus and newborn infant which reach far beyond the first few weeks of life and may result in better physical, emotional and social health for many years to come.

It is no longer sufficient for those caring for mothers and babies to measure their success on the grounds of mortality figures alone. Success in increasing the breast feeding rate (p. 93), reducing the numbers of mothers smoking or drinking alcohol in pregnancy, and teaching parents about diet, clothing and safe sleeping positions for the baby (p. 88) are at least as important.

THE PSYCHOLOGICAL DIMENSION OF PERINATAL CARE

Technological solutions to perinatal problems may also fail if not accompanied by an understanding of wider human needs. The wishes of some women for a return to the practice of home delivery, for example, present a challenge to hospital care which needs to be faced. The selection of mothers for home confinement, for intrapartum care in hospital with immediate transfer to home afterwards or for full hospital care must be balanced with the paramount requirement to keep the mother and infant safe and provide appropriate services for unforeseen emergencies should they arise (p. 40). Making hospital maternity departments more home-like and friendly whilst still maintaining the safety of readily available skills and techniques goes some way to meeting these legitimate requests of mothers but cannot replace the home atmosphere.

The formation of a sound and lasting attachment between mother and child can also be influenced by what happens in a maternity department or special care baby unit. When circumstances interfere with the natural mother–child attachment process during the critical first few hours and days, inadequate 'mothering' is more likely to follow. If adverse social factors are also present, the risks of child abuse and neglect may be increased. The psychological attachment of mother and baby can be greatly enhanced by staff in maternity and neonatal units if they understand its importance and adopt sympathetic attitudes towards the mothers.

THE NEED FOR SPECIAL CARE

Although the great majority of newborn infants will be healthy, about 8–10% will need the attention of the paediatric staff for a medical disorder. Traditionally the response to this has been to admit such infants to a special care baby unit for observation, investigation and treatment. Increasingly, however, such babies are being nursed at their mothers' bedsides or in 'transitional care units' where mother and baby can be kept together under the supervision of trained neonatal nurses until the baby's problem has been resolved. Clearly there is a small number of infants who do need the special skills of highly trained nurses and paediatricians and it is these infants who make up a large part of the work of neonatal units today (p. 126). In some areas of the UK, such units are only available in regional centres a long way from the family home, which only adds to parental concern. In others, intensive care is provided in the majority of district general hospitals in smaller units. The requirements for intensive care are described elsewhere in this book (p. 126). Whatever the additional care the baby requires, it is important for the medical and nursing staff not only to possess skills in the necessary techniques but also to be aware of the broader issues involved. The increasing use of procedures and protocols to guide the care of the mother or baby will not be effective unless these practices are interpreted carefully by those with sound knowledge and experience, with clinical judgement, and with a sensitivity to the needs of the parents. Awareness of these factors will contribute considerably to the baby's future well-being, especially as many parents in this situation have very great anxiety about their infant which adds to the normal emotions of childbirth.

ETHICAL ASPECTS OF PERINATAL CARE

The major developments in perinatal care over the last decade have made it possible to treat increasingly immature infants, and ever more sophisticated antenatal diagnosis has enabled an increasing amount of fetal pathology to be identified earlier in pregnancy. Although these advances have resulted in improved outcomes for many babies, they have also raised complex legal and ethical questions which those caring for the mother and baby will face with increasing regularity. It is necessary in some circumstances to consider not only what can be done but whether it is acceptable or right to do it. In all situations, medical and nursing staff must ensure that parents give adequately informed consent to investigation and treatment of their baby. These dilemmas may relate to life and death issues, such as whether babies of 23 or 24 weeks of gestation should or should not be treated because of the high risk of handicap in the small number of survivors. Others may concern if and when to discontinue life support or whether an infant may be suitable as an organ donor (Doyal & Larcher 2000). It is necessary in these situations to consider how decisions of this type are to be reached, in particular to what extent the parents' views should be involved in solving the dilemma. Occasionally, the courts of law may be needed to judge some of the most difficult dilemmas.

New treatments for newborn infants need evaluation through clinical research which involves subjects who cannot consent to the investigation themselves. Parents will have to decide on behalf of the baby what to do about unexpected abnormalities found on prenatal genetic testing, a situation which may have significant implications for the child's future and often for other family members also. Those who care for neonates are frequently confronted with these and other ethical dilemmas and it is essential for them to listen to the views of others who are involved, including

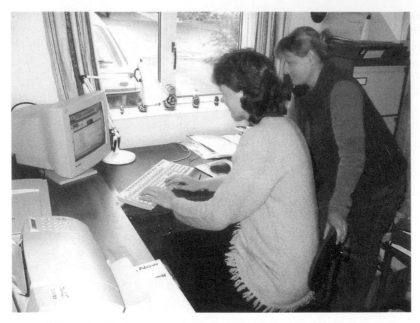

Figure 1.5 Up-to-date information is readily accessible on the Internet.

those with cultural and religious perspectives, and to integrate these opinions into the clinical decision-making process.

Caring for a newborn baby is, for the most part, a rewarding and successful process, and parents will take home the precious new life they had hoped for. However, despite the best efforts of dedicated health care givers, some babies will not have a smooth entry into life and will have an illness requiring immediate treatment, a malformation, be permanently handicapped or even die. The professional care of a mother and baby before, during and after delivery will have a huge impact on the degree of successful outcome for all concerned. The value of practising optimum care founded on research-based evidence cannot be overestimated. Information to guide practitioners, support families and update and increase knowledge is found not only in textbooks and peer-reviewed journals but also increasingly on the Internet (Fig. 1.5). To this end, useful website addresses can be found in the Further Reading sections of some chapters and also in the text. The rest of this book seeks to inform the reader about how best to care for the newborn infant, whether well or ill, and the final chapter is a reminder of the family into which the child is born, and the way the caring team can continue to provide help and support to them when the baby does not progress in the normal way.

REFERENCES

Badawi N 2000 The international consensus statement on cerebral palsy causation. Medical Journal of Australia 172(5):199–200

Barker D J 2001 A new model for the origins of chronic disease. Medical Health Care Philosophy 4(1):31–35

Colver A F, Gibson M, Hey E N et al 2000 Increasing rates of cerebral palsy across the spectrum in northeast England 1964–1993. Archives of Disease in Childhood Fetal and Neonatal Edition 83:F7–F12

Doyal L, Larcher V F 2000 Guidelines for withholding or withdrawing intensive care of the newborn. Archives of Disease in Childhood Fetal and Neonatal Edition 83:F60–F63

Gilliland F D, Li Y F, Peters J M 2001 Effects of maternal smoking during pregnancy and environmental tobacco smoke on asthma and wheezing in children. American Journal of Respiratory and Critical Care Medicine 163(2):429–436

Marlow N 2000 A touch of cerebral palsy. Archives of Disease in Childhood Fetal and Neonatal Edition 84:F4–F5

Office of National Statistics 1993 Birth Statistics series DH3 No 27. HMSO, London

Pollack HA 2001 Sudden infant death syndrome, maternal smoking during pregnancy and the cost effectiveness of smoking cessation intervention. American Journal of Public Health 91(3):432–436

Sutton L, Bajuk B 1999 Population-based study of infants born at less than 28 weeks' gestation in New South Wales, Australia, in 1992–3. New South Wales Neonatal Intensive Care Unit Study Group. Paediatric Perinatal Epidemiology 13(3):288–301

FURTHER READING

Office of National Statistics 1998 Birth Statistics Series DH3 No 31. HMSO, London

Office of National Statistics 1999 Birth Statistics Series DH3 No 32. HMSO, London

Ponsonby A-L, Dwyer T, Kasl S V et al 1995 Correlates of prone infant sleeping position by period of birth. Archives of Disease in Childhood 72:204–208

USEFUL WEBSITES

www.cochrane.org – many reviews and meta-analyses on topics in pregnancy, childbirth and neonatology

www.cesdi.org.uk – reports from the confidential enquiry into stillbirths and deaths in infancy

www.statistics.gov.uk – British Office of National Statistics

www.pedinfo.org – an access database to many other websites in all aspects of neonatal care

Chapter 2

Maternal and fetal health

CHAPTER CONTENTS

Introduction 13
Prenatal factors affecting fetal well-being 13
 Maternal age 14
 Parity 14
 Maternal nutrition 14
 Smoking 15
 Alcohol 16
 Radiation 16
 Social concern during the pregnancy 16
 Drugs of addiction 17
 Pregnancy-related disorders 19
 Acute and chronic illness 19
Assessment of fetal health 20
 Ultrasound 20
 Doppler blood flow studies 21
Prevention and antenatal diagnosis of
fetal disorders 21
 Genetic and chromosomal disorders 22
 Recessively inherited metabolic disorders with
 cell enzyme abnormalities 23
 X-linked diseases 23
 Neural tube defects 23
 Fetal blood sampling 23
 Fetal cardiac monitoring 23
Drugs in pregnancy 23
 Early pregnancy 24
 Late pregnancy 25
Complementary therapy in pregnancy 27
Maternal disease and the fetus 27
 Diabetes mellitus 27
 Epilepsy 27
 Thyrotoxicosis 27
 Parathyroid dysfunction 28
 Myasthenia gravis 28
 Idiopathic thrombocytopenic purpura 28
 Phenylketonuria 28
Maternal infections and the fetus 28
 Dietary factors 28
 Prelabour rupture of the membranes 29
 Maternal HIV infection – AIDS 29
 Maternal hepatitis B and C infection 29
 Maternal genital herpes infection 29
 Syphilis 29

INTRODUCTION

The UK Maternity Advisory Committee (1982) declared that antenatal care should 'ensure as far as possible the health and wellbeing of the woman and her unborn child'. Fertilisation of the ovum occurs some 2 weeks before the first missed period. By the second, much of the differentiation of fetal organs has occurred, and by 12 weeks from conception it is virtually complete. Beyond that time, the fetus grows in size and the organs mature in function until the baby is capable of independent existence. Even some developmental responses such as finger sucking, turning the head towards light, and muscular activity in response to loud sounds occur in the second half of pregnancy (Table 2.1).

Fetal medicine has advanced and much can be done to affect the health and development of the unborn baby. Medical and nursing responsibilities start before pregnancy has been confirmed and, at times, even before conception. It is therefore increasingly important for all those involved in the care of mother and baby to be aware of advances in fetal medicine so as to advise the mother appropriately.

PRENATAL FACTORS AFFECTING FETAL WELL-BEING

From the time the fertilised ovum implants in the endometrium onwards, the fetus depends on the placenta to maintain growth and development. The placenta is a large and complex organ where the fetal and maternal blood come into close proximity, separated only by a thin membrane. Across this, the mother provides appropriate nutrition

Table 2.1   The development of the fetus

0–12 Weeks	12–24 Weeks	24–40 Weeks
Conception to 4 weeks: • Early central nervous system develops • Heart forms and beats • Limb buds form	12–16 weeks: • Skeletal development • Nasal septum and palate fuse • Meconium is present in gut	24–28 weeks: • Eyelids reopen • Respiration movements practised

4–8 weeks:
• Early organ development
• Head and facial features form
• External genitalia develop
  (sex not distinguishable)
	16–20 weeks:
	• Fingernails appear
	
	20–24 weeks:
	• Fetus becomes viable
	• Most organs can now function
	• Fetus experiences periods
	  of sleep and activity
		28–32 weeks:
		• Fat and iron stored in body
		• Testes descend into scrotum
		
		32–36 weeks:
		• Ear cartilage soft
		• Plantar crease visible

8–12 weeks: • Eyelids fuse • Kidneys function; urine is excreted • Fetal circulation functions • Sucking and swallowing is practised		36–40 weeks: • Skull firm

From Bennett & Brown 1993

for the fetus and adequate oxygenation of the fetal blood, and ensures the excretion of carbon dioxide, urea, hydrogen ions and other waste products of metabolism. The unborn child is also protected from infection both by the physical barrier of the fetal membranes and by the immune mechanisms of the mother.

There are many factors which adversely influence this complex interaction between mother and fetus or increase the risk during labour, delivery or in the neonatal period. Preventive or curative treatment during the pregnancy can, in some cases, reduce the harm to the infant. The effect of poor socioeconomic circumstances (p. 16), on the other hand, cannot be influenced by medical means alone.

Maternal age

The safest maternal age for the baby is between 18 and 30 years. Complications of pregnancy and labour are rather more likely above and below these ages (Fig. 2.1), whilst certain congenital abnormalities such as Down syndrome have an increased incidence in older mothers (p. 208). Younger teenage mothers have significantly more low birth weight babies both because of an increased risk of premature labour and from fetal growth retardation, which is only partly explained by their poorer socioeconomic circumstances and

a lower use of antenatal care than older mothers (Smith & Pell 2001).

Parity

Some problems occur more frequently in the first pregnancy than in later ones – for example, pre-eclampsia, breech presentation and low birth weight. In multiparity, the risks appear to increase independently of maternal age after the second pregnancy, until in the fifth they are as high as in the first; however, other social factors associated with larger families account for much of this increase.

Maternal nutrition

Maternal nutrition in industrialised populations seems to have only a small effect on placental function and birth weights. Other possible determinants of fetal and placental growth should be investigated if there is a problem (p. 21) (Mathews et al 1999). Studies from developing countries confirm that periods of serious undernutrition during pregnancy can reduce the birth weight of the baby by 300 g and that giving dietary energy supplements to chronically malnourished mothers can increase birth weight significantly.

A diet that is relatively high in protein and low in carbohydrate, consisting of meat, vegetables,

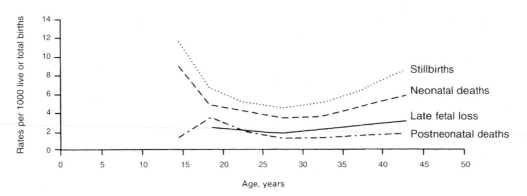

Figure 2.1 Incidence of perinatal deaths by the age of the mother. (By kind permission of the Office of National Statistics.)

milk, cereals and fruit, which enables the mother to put on 10–12 kg of weight during the pregnancy, should provide the fetus with all the necessary nutrition. A vegetarian diet carries no disadvantage so long as an adequate protein intake is achieved from eggs, cheese, beans and pulses. Women with conditions such as coeliac disease, where significant dietary modification is required, should receive advice from a dietician. The very few people who keep to extremely limited diets, such as vegans, will need dietetic advice to ensure the fetus is adequately supplied with nutrients.

Short maternal stature, though frequently genetic, may result from chronic dietary insufficiency in childhood and can reduce fetal size more than a poor diet in pregnancy. Inadequate maternal diet is commonly related to low socioeconomic status but also to poor supervision in pregnancy and a failure to make use of antenatal education classes. A contracted pelvis caused by rickets secondary to vitamin D deficiency in childhood is occasionally seen in some ethnic minority groups in Britain and may cause obstructed labour from disproportion.

In the absence of clinical or pathological evidence of deficiency of specific dietary components, few mothers require prescribed dietary supplements other than folic acid for the prevention of neural tube defects (p. 230). A physiological anaemia develops during normal pregnancy due to haemodilution. The fetus is at no risk from a lack of oxygen until the mother's haemoglobin falls below 10.5 g/dl, and maternal iron supplements are only needed below this level. Studies have shown that British Asian women are particulary likely to need prescribed iron (Cuervo & Mahomed 2001).

Vitamin D deficiency is also relatively more common in pregnancy in women of Asian origin in Britain, though it is rare in other ethnic groups. Hypocalcaemia may occur in the newborn infant if the deficiency is not corrected, so it is wise to investigate such women and prescribe vitamin D if needed.

Vitamin C and folic acid are heat labile and foods containing them should not be overcooked. These include potatoes and green vegetables. However, since many foods are now fortified with folic acid (Wald & Bower 1995) and vitamin C is present in citrus fruits, there is little risk of deficiency.

Smoking

Smoking in pregnancy is the major avoidable cause of perinatal and infant morbidity and should be strongly discouraged (Bonellie 2001, Chung et al 2000). In general, the more cigarettes the mother smokes, the higher the risk to the infant. Nicotine, carbon monoxide and other toxic constituents of tobacco smoke cross the placenta, having a direct effect on the supply of oxygen and nutrients to the fetus by reducing placental blood flow. This diminishes fetal growth, causing a reduction, on average, of about 300 g in birth weight. There is an increase in the incidence of babies who are small for gestational age and thus more susceptible to perinatal asphyxia and neonatal hypoglycaemia (p. 54). Increased rates of placental abruption and antepartum haemorrhage also add to the risk of intrapartum asphyxia in the fetus. Although there is also an increase in preterm delivery, the incidence of respiratory distress syndrome is lower than expected, which is likely to be the result of stress to the infant from prolonged placental insufficiency (p. 19). The incidence of cleft lip or palate in the offspring of mothers who smoked during pregnancy is greater than that in babies born to non-smokers (Chung et al 2000). In infancy, the risk of sudden unexpected death is increased and the incidence of recurrent wheezing is much greater, even if the baby is not exposed to cigarette smoke after birth; furthermore, there is an overall reduction in their educational attainment as they grow older (Table 2.2).

Alcohol

Maternal alcohol ingestion in excessive amounts occasionally causes fetal alcohol syndrome. The characteristics of this include fetal growth retardation and a recognisable facies, the child remaining small throughout childhood and having at least moderate learning difficulties. There is also a small increase in the incidence of congenital heart disease and renal anomalies. Withdrawal

symptoms may be apparent in the infant and include:

- hyperactivity/poor sleeping patterns
- irritability/tremors and, occasionally, fits
- poor suck reflex but suffers from hyperphagia.

There is no clear information about how much alcohol is safe in pregnancy. The UK Department of Health (1993) recommends that pregnant women should not drink more than 1–2 units of alcohol once or twice a week and should avoid episodes of intoxication. However, the Royal College of Obstetricians and Gynaecologists (2000) guidelines state that there is no conclusive evidence of adverse effects in either growth or IQ at levels below 15 units/week. Nonetheless, they recommend that women limit intake to no more than one standard drink per day.

Radiation

Down syndrome, and possibly other malformations, seem to occur more frequently during periods of increased environmental ionising radiation. This effect seems to afflict all ages of mothers, though it may be greater in older women and it only accounts for a small proportion of cases of the condition. Irradiation of the ovaries for medical purposes may also have a similar effect.

Social concern during the pregnancy

It is important to realise that psychosocial factors may affect the baby adversely before and after birth. During some pregnancies the family circumstances may suggest that social work support is needed to ensure that the baby will receive proper care during pregnancy and after birth. Such situations may include:

- serious or terminal illness in a parent
- a family member with a serious disability
- where the baby is to be placed for adoption
- a concealed or late-presenting pregnancy
- where one or both parents abuse drugs or alcohol
- a parent with a psychiatric disorder

Table 2.2 Effects of smoking and alcohol on the baby

Smoking	Alcohol
Decreased placental function	Fetal alcohol syndrome
Intrauterine growth retardation	Fetal growth retardation
Fetal and birth asphyxia	Withdrawal symptoms
Antepartum haemorrhage	after birth
Increased risk of preterm birth	Growth failure in childhood
Increased incidence of	Learning difficulties
cleft lip and palate	
Higher risk of cot death	
More likely to wheeze	
in infancy	
Reduced educational	
achievements	

- a history of family violence
- child abuse or neglect in another child
- when one parent has a conviction for offences against children
- a very young mother with poor family support.

In many such cases, the social worker can provide sufficient support to ensure the child will receive suitable care. However, where there is a history of child abuse or neglect, a case conference may be held under the local child protection procedures before the baby is born to agree a plan, including court action if necessary, to protect the child from abuse.

Drugs of addiction

There are numerous addictive drugs which can have a serious effect on the child before and after birth. The types of drugs and their effects are listed in Table 2.3 and Box 2.1, respectively. However, around 25% of women addicted to substances take more than one drug (polydrug misuse) and many more smoke cigarettes and drink alcohol as well. Socioeconomic disadvantages may also prevent them from making use of the available antenatal care (Ahluwalia et al 2000). Some intravenous drug users become infected by hepatitis B virus or human immunodeficiency virus (HIV) (p. 180) from either shared needles or unsafe sexual activity. Unsterile injections may cause septicaemia and there is a higher risk of other sexually transmitted diseases in this group of mothers, which may put the fetus at risk or affect the mode of delivery (see p. 179) (Faden & Graubard 2000).

Sudden withdrawal of drugs during the pregnancy can result in intrauterine death since the drugs cross the placenta, and if the mother experiences withdrawal, so does the addicted fetus (Table 2.4). Fetal withdrawal manifests itself with fetal hyperactivity and persisting tachycardia. This movement demands increased oxygen consumption, and if it is not available because of placental insufficiency, fetal asphyxia and sometimes death may result (Lissauer et al 1994, Klonoff-Cohen & Lam-Kruglick 2001). There is also a risk

Table 2.3 Types of drugs of abuse

Group	Examples
Opiates	Morphine, diamorphine (heroin), methadone
Stimulants	Amphetamines, cocaine
Tranquillisers	Benzodiazepines, e.g. diazepam, temazepam
Sedatives	Barbiturates, dichloralphenazone
Solvents	Acetone, butane, trichloroethylene
Cannabis	
Nicotine	
Alcohol	

Box 2.1 Risks to the fetus from drugs of abuse

- Addiction
- Fetal withdrawal symptoms
- Diminished placental function
    Growth retardation
    Fetal asphyxia
    Intrauterine death
- Increased incidence of congenital malformations
- Increased risk of preterm birth
- Neonatal withdrawal symptoms
- Increased risk of sudden infant death syndrome
- Social consequences
    Social disadvantage
    Developmental delay
    Increased exposure to sexually transmitted disease, e.g. HIV, hepatitis B
- Additional exposure to cigarette smoking and alcohol

---

of preterm delivery, as withdrawal also causes uterine muscle spasms and premature labour.

However, if the drugs can be withdrawn progressively from early pregnancy and the mother abstains completely for 4–6 weeks before the birth, withdrawal symptoms in the baby are unlikely. In some centres, regularly decreasing doses of methadone are prescribed as an alternative to the stronger opiates where abstinence cannot be achieved; the lower the dose the mother is taking by the time of delivery, the less severe are the baby's withdrawal symptoms.

Social management of drug abuse in pregnancy

In view of the risk from the abused substances to which the baby is exposed before and after birth, the chaotic lifestyle and the social disadvantage of many drug-abusing families, a full

Table 2.4   Symptoms of neonatal abstinence syndrome

System affected	Timing	Symptoms
Central nervous system	Appear within 24–72 hours	Hyperactivity and inability to sleep Irritability and hypertonia Cerebral cry, tremors or convulsions
Gastrointestinal system	Approximately 4 days	Regurgitation or vomiting Poor feeding or disorganized suck Loose stools and weight loss
Autonomic, metabolic and respiratory systems	Approximately 24–72 hours	Sweating and fever Nasal stuffiness or sneezing Yawning Mottling of the skin Nasal flaring, tachypnoea and recession

multidisciplinary case conference should be held during the pregnancy under the local child protection procedures. This should ensure the safety of the child through the pregnancy and after birth, and establish what professional social support will be needed. This may include court action to obtain one of the care or specific issues orders available under the Children Act 1989 when it is considered that the safety of the child cannot be adequately secured by professional care alone.

Problems for the infant after birth

Opiate addiction   Opiates, including morphine, heroin and methadone, are powerful respiratory depressants. The baby should not be given naloxone at birth even if her respiratory efforts are diminished, since it causes the rapid onset of a pattern of withdrawal symptoms, sometimes referred to as neonatal abstinence syndrome. Respiratory support including ventilation may be necessary if breathing is inadequate. In many hospitals, such infants are admitted to the neonatal unit for up to 10 days for close observation and active management of the neonatal withdrawal syndrome. Many units monitor the severity of the baby's withdrawal symptoms 4-hourly against a recognised scoring system such as that devised by Finnegan et al (1975), which enables the baby's progress to be evaluated accurately.

Symptoms can come on at any time within the first week of life and are managed by giving the infant small and decreasing doses of opiates, or a sedative such as chlorpromazine, until the symptoms resolve.

Anticonvulsants may be needed for fits. Both hepatitis B immunoglobulin and vaccination should be given to the infant to prevent infection if the mother is known to carry the virus antigen (p. 180). Once the withdrawal programme is complete, the baby usually remains healthy, though there is an increased incidence of sudden infant death syndrome in these children.

Cocaine and crack cocaine addiction   Cocaine addiction is becoming more common and has serious consequences for the unborn baby. Spontaneous abortion is common in abusing mothers, as are placental abruption and preterm delivery, which carry their own risks for the newborn baby (pp. 19 and 107). Cocaine is a powerful vasoconstrictor and this results in a threefold increase in congenital malformations and a higher risk of intrauterine growth retardation (see p. 50). Affected infants have diminished respiratory reflexes in the neonatal period and may require assisted ventilation. Some have cardiac arrhythmias. The drug is also excreted freely in the mother's milk. Later follow-up shows an increased incidence of delay in language development, and brain growth is often diminished. However, since addicted mothers usually smoke cigarettes and drink alcohol, these too may contribute to the adverse neurological outcome for such children. There is also an increased risk of sudden infant death during the first year of life.

Marijuana Smoking cannabis may slightly increase the risk of preterm delivery but does not appear to add significantly to the effects of cigarette and alcohol use, young maternal age and the socioeconomic disadvantage which affect many marijuana users. The resin appears in breast milk in sufficient concentration to cause significant effects including constipation in the infant (Kozer & Koren 2001).

Since most of these drugs pass to some extent into breast milk, it is necessary to balance the disadvantages to the infant of formula feeding (p. 94) against the risk from the drugs. In many instances it may be best to allow breast feeding and monitor the progress of the baby closely, though it is not always successful.

Nursing care of infants

Infants who are suffering from drug withdrawal are very challenging babies to care for as they are irritable, excessively wakeful and feed poorly. Nursing the infants in darkened, quiet rooms to reduce extra stimuli, swaddling them or using other calming measures all help to relax the infant. The parents also need support, advice and reassurance that they are capable of caring for their baby.

Pregnancy-related disorders

Pregnancy-induced hypertension and pre-eclampsia

Pregnancy-induced hypertension – usually defined as the onset of hypertension during pregnancy with a sustained diastolic pressure over 90 mmHg – is a common condition and carries little risk for the mother or fetus. However, if proteinuria and evidence of liver or renal dysfunction accompanies it, there is a significant risk of placental insufficiency, which may result in fetal growth retardation, asphyxia, placental abruption or even fetal death. This condition, known as pre-eclampsia, has an unknown cause, but the predisposing factors are: primigravidae, multiple

pregnancy, a new sexual partner, diabetes and rhesus isoimmunisation. The severity of placental dysfunction does not always correspond to the degree of hypertension, and hypotensive therapy seems to have little beneficial effect on the fetus. Beta-adrenoreceptor antagonists such as atenolol and labetalol which are used to lower blood pressure may sometimes add to fetal growth impairment and should only be used – and then with caution – in the third trimester. Outpatient hospital observation is the mainstay of treatment, with a careful watch on fetal growth and the mother's health in order to pick the optimal time to deliver the baby. Factors which help in deciding this are a progression to severe hypertension and the occurrence of maternal renal, hepatic and haematological impairment, which carry a risk for the mother, and the results of fetal assessment. The latter should include evaluation of fetal heart rate patterns by cardiotocography, ultrasound scanning for growth, and Doppler blood flow studies of the fetal circulation.

Placenta praevia

If the placenta implants itself in the lower part of the uterus and obstructs the cervical opening to the vagina, it is known as placenta praevia. The condition is associated with scarred endometrium, multiple pregnancy, multiparity, previous caesarean section and large placentas. It is easily diagnosed by ultrasound scanning. In this condition, repeated placental haemorrhage can reduce placental function, causing fetal growth retardation, hypoxia and, occasionally, death. In the latter weeks of pregnancy, observation in hospital will be needed since severe bleeding, the onset of labour, or dilatation of the cervix are all indications for expediting the inevitable caesarean section.

Acute and chronic illness

Any acute severe illness or accident causing significant trauma may affect the pregnancy by precipitating a miscarriage or causing preterm labour and delivery, or may affect the infant by compromising the placental function. In addition, certain infective agents may also cross the placenta and cause fetal infection (p. 164).

Chronic illnesses of many sorts can affect placental function and cause a degree of intrauterine growth retardation. These include urinary tract infection, renal failure, cystic fibrosis, malnutrition, ulcerative colitis and Crohn's disease. Other disorders which have more specific effects on the infant are discussed later in this chapter. It should also be remembered that the course of such conditions as cystic fibrosis, chronic renal failure, congenital heart disease and cancer is sometimes adversely affected by the pregnancy and this may occasionally justify a therapeutic termination.

ASSESSMENT OF FETAL HEALTH

The maternity team needs as much information about the health of the fetus as possible to assess whether intervention is needed and to time the delivery of the infant most appropriately. Though early antenatal assessment is desirable, parents' attitudes to antenatal screening and intervention vary greatly. Some women choose not to accept certain screening procedures for abnormalities on moral or religious grounds, and would continue with the pregnancy regardless of the findings. Such attitudes should be respected. Language and socioeconomic difficulties may also affect the uptake of antenatal care.

Since many of the available methods of assessment do not clearly distinguish between the growth, maturity and well-being of the fetus, it is reasonable to consider them together. A full clinical evaluation forms the basis of the assessment of fetal health. Practices vary but the evaluation should include some of the following: date of the last period, measurement of uterine size using a tape measure, maternal weight gain, and assessment of general health. Reductions of fetal movements and 'kick counts' can give an indication of fetal distress. Normally, 10 kicks should be felt in a 12-hour period, and research suggests that fetal movement often stops 12 hours prior to death. This is a very non-specific test and must be supplemented with one or more of the following fetal health tests (Table 2.5).

Table 2.5 Current methods of assessment of the fetus during pregnancy

Method	What it can assess
Ultrasound	Fetal maturity Fetal growth (serial measurements) Malformations of the fetus Placental position Liquor volume
Maternal plasma alpha-fetoprotein	Screening for neural tube defects
Amniotic fluid analysis – cytogenetic – biochemical or DNA analysis	Chromosome pattern in fetus Fetal sexing Rare enzyme defects
Chorionic villus sampling	Chromosome pattern in fetus DNA analysis
Doppler blood flow studies	Fetal arterial blood flow
External cardiotocography	Fetal cardiac arrhythmias Fetal asphyxia
Fetal umbilical blood sampling	Rhesus isoimmunisation Exclusion of haemoglobinopathies Rare enzyme defects

Ultrasound

Ultrasound (Fig. 2.2A) is the most accurate method of assessing the gestational age and growth of the fetus. The presence of a fetus can be confirmed and multiple pregnancy diagnosed at about 6 weeks by vaginal ultrasound scanning. Gestational age is best established in early pregnancy by measurement of the crown–rump length, which predicts the date of delivery more accurately than measuring the biparietal diameter of the head. At 12 weeks of pregnancy, the gestational age can be estimated to within a week either way, and at 18 weeks, to within 14 days.

Repeated ultrasound measurements can also identify some fetuses which are failing to grow at the appropriate rate. Doppler ultrasound studies of the fetal circulation may be needed in these babies.

Structural abnormalities

Ultrasound can identify polyhydramnios or oligohydramnios, the site of the placenta, and an increasing number of congenital abnormalities (Table 2.6) (Carrera et al 1995, Whiteman & Reece

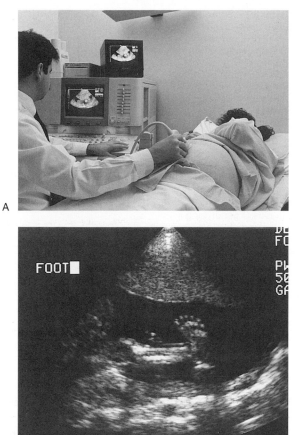

Figure 2.2 A: Prenatal ultrasound screening.
B: Talipes of the foot shown on prenatal sonography.
(By kind permission of Dr Jo Fairhurst.)

Table 2.6 Examples of fetal conditions diagnosed by ultrasound

Condition	Ultrasound abnormality
Hydrocephalus	Dilated cerebral ventricles
Anencephaly	Absence of the brain
Spina bifida	Widened spinal canal
Renal tract anomalies	Dilated pelvis of the kidney; tumour
Talipes	Abnormal foot posture
Limb deformities	Absent or deformed bones
Congenital heart disease	Single ventricle; absent septum
Cardiac arrhythmias	Irregularity of the heart rhythm
Diaphragmatic hernia	Gut in the chest
Duodenal atresia	Dilated stomach and duodenum

Doppler blood flow studies

Prolonged fetal asphyxia secondary to placental insufficiency causes changes in blood flow waveforms in the major fetal blood vessels. These can be visualised and blood flow rates measured using Doppler ultrasound. A rising resistance index in the umbilical artery or descending aorta is indicative of a poor blood flow from fetus to placenta resulting from increasing placental insufficiency. Diminished cerebral blood flow can be deduced by changes in the carotid artery waveforms. The technique is used to indicate when early delivery is needed to prevent significant cerebral ischaemia in growth-retarded fetuses.

PREVENTION AND ANTENATAL DIAGNOSIS OF FETAL DISORDERS

Since the cause of most abnormalities of fetal development is still uncertain and a clear hereditary pattern exceptional, intervention to prevent fetal malformations is currently possible in only a minority of cases. The best known examples are the rubella immunisation programme for all infants (p. 176) and the dietary supplementation with folate to prevent neural tube defects (p. 230). A careful family history taken in early pregnancy may reveal an inherited disorder. Genetic counselling plays an important role in reducing the incidence of such diseases, particularly when a mother has already had a baby with a specific disorder known to follow a clear pattern

1994). Intrauterine treatment of obstructive uropathy and other fetal anomalies is occasionally carried out in specialist centres. Choroid plexus cysts may be seen in the developing cerebral ventricles, and cystic hygromas identified in early screening ultrasound examinations. They often resolve spontaneously and only occasionally persist after birth. Dilatation of the renal pelves is common, but only in a minority of cases does it indicate significant bladder or kidney disease after birth. Increased thickness of the tissues at the nape of the neck, known as the nuchal translucency, occurs in Down syndrome, and in some other abnormalities, but it is not specific enough for screening purposes and is not commonly used.

of inheritance or familial incidence, e.g. cystic fibrosis (Scotet et al 2000), mucopolysaccharidosis, phenylketonuria, Duchenne muscular dystrophy and many others.

Diagnosis for a rapidly increasing number of such disorders is now possible from about 8 weeks of pregnancy by biochemical investigation of amniotic fluid or analysis of fetal cells obtained at amniocentesis or chorionic villus sampling. Examination of the chromosomes in the cell nucleus or the genes contained in them ensures that cytogenetic or DNA-based diagnoses are available at a time when termination of the pregnancy is possible. Ultrasonography localises the placenta accurately, which reduces the risks, but in all invasive investigations of the fetus in early pregnancy there is a small risk of producing a placental bleed or abortion which, in a Rhesus-negative mother, may stimulate the formation of Rh antibodies (p. 191). This can be prevented by routinely offering the Rh-negative mother an injection of anti-D globulin after the procedure. The woman should be informed that anti-D is a blood product, to enable her to make an informed decision about the accompanying risks of blood-borne infections such as hepatitis B and C, HIV and cytomegalovirus, though all such products are tested to minimise the risk of infection (p. 185).

Genetic and chromosomal disorders

Examples of the types of abnormalities which can be identified by chromosomal or gene analysis of samples taken at amniocentesis or chorionic villus biopsy are listed in Table 2.7. The subject is discussed in more detail in Chapter 13 (p. 205).

Down syndrome

This condition, in which the baby inherits an additional number 21 chromosome, needs special mention, as a biochemical screening test has been developed to try to identify the condition prenatally. Although the incidence of this condition increases with advancing maternal age (p. 208) and rises steeply after 35 years, age alone is not an adequate criterion to screen for the

Table 2.7 Some conditions identifiable by cytogenetic and DNA analysis of fetal cells

1. Cytogenetic analysis

Condition	Cytogenetic pattern
Down syndrome	47 XY (or XX)[a] + 21
Klinefelter's syndrome	47 XXY
Turner's syndrome	45 XO[b]
Trisomy 18	47 XY (or XX)[a] + 18
Trisomy 13	47 XY (or XX)[a] + 13

2. DNA analysis
Cystic fibrosis
Duchenne muscular dystrophy
Huntingdon's disease
Myotonic dystrophy
Fragile X syndrome
Rhesus D genotyping in
 Rh-incompatible pregnancies
Spinal muscular atrophy
X-linked retinitis pigmentosa
Neurofibromatosis
Haemophilia
Sickle cell disease
Thalassaemia

[a] XY in boys, XX in girls
[b] XO indicates the absence of a second X chromosome

anomaly since the majority of Down babies are born to younger mothers. It is calculated that offering amniocentesis and chromosome analysis on the amniotic fluid to all mothers over the age of 35 would detect only 25% of the total number of babies with Down syndrome, mainly because pregnancies in that age group are so much in the minority.

Biochemical testing of the mother's blood in early pregnancy can be used to assess the likelihood of a baby having Down syndrome. This triple test measures the level of alpha-fetoprotein (which is low in Down syndrome), beta-human chorionic gonadotrophin (which is high) and oestriol (which is low). From these results, the probability of the baby having the condition is calculated. Where the risk is high, amniocentesis is needed to obtain the fetal cells needed to make a full diagnosis. Even if all those mothers identified as being at high risk had cytogenetic studies on amniotic fluid, it is estimated that only 66% of Down babies would be identified. No system provides complete identification of affected infants but, provided that a full explanation is given and personal views are respected, the introduction of such a policy is justifiable.

Recessively inherited metabolic disorders with cell enzyme abnormalities

These are relatively rare diseases in which the enzyme abnormality may be identified by complex histochemical techniques on fetal cells. The best known examples in this group are the gangliosidoses (e.g. Tay–Sachs disease), glycogen storage disease (Pompe's disease), the mucopolysaccharidoses, metachromatic leukodystrophy and galactosaemia. Such disorders are increasingly being detected by DNA analysis as their genes are identified.

X-linked diseases

In these conditions, half of all male fetuses will be affected and sexing of the fetus can be obtained by amnioscopy or chromosomal studies. Some X-linked conditions can be identified from biochemical analysis of fetal blood samples, including Duchenne muscular dystrophy and haemophilia. In these and many other such conditions, the abnormal gene has been identified and gene analysis of chorionic villus samples can identify affected fetuses.

Neural tube defects

Raised levels of alpha-fetoprotein in maternal blood at 16–18 weeks of gestation identify most mothers carrying a baby with spina bifida (p. 230). One in 20 women with raised levels will actually be bearing an affected child. An ultrasound examination of those with a positive blood test will normally identify an open myelomeningocele (Fig. 2.3) if present, though in a minority it may be necessary to confirm the diagnosis by testing the amniotic fluid for an acetylcholinesterase specific for neural tissue, as a raised alpha-fetoprotein level on its own may also be found in conditions such as gastroschisis and exomphalos (p. 219).

The following methods may be used to identify certain other abnormalities.

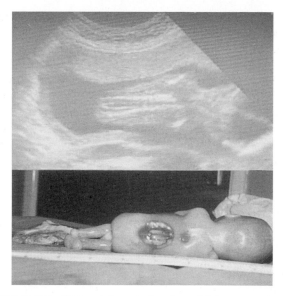

Figure 2.3 Open meningomyelocele on fetal sonography and after termination of pregnancy.

Fetal blood sampling

Haematological disorders such as thalassaemia may be identified by analysis of fetal blood samples obtained by cordocentesis under ultrasound guidance or at amnioscopy, and these techniques open the way to the early identification of many more conditions affecting the blood.

Fetal cardiac monitoring

Fetal cardiac monitoring by means of an external cardiotocograph can sometimes identify cardiac arrhythmias and has also been used to confirm the tachycardia of fetal thyrotoxicosis (p. 27). The response of the fetal heart pattern to vibroacoustic stimulation may reduce the incidence of non-reactive recordings, but its impact on the outcome for the baby has not yet been evaluated.

DRUGS IN PREGNANCY

Great care must be taken over prescribing in the first trimester of pregnancy. Some drugs may cause congenital malformations by influencing the development of the fetus in the first 3 months of the pregnancy, whilst others are known to have an affect on the newborn infant when taken in later pregnancy. Consequently, in general, it is better for the mother to avoid taking drugs, though the risk to the fetus must be balanced against the need to provide proper treatment for maternal conditions. The British National Formulary provides regularly updated information about the suitablility of drugs for use in pregnancy, and the reader should consult the latest edition for further information or visit its website.

Early pregnancy

In early pregnancy, the outstanding drugs which have been associated with developmental malformations are:

Cytotoxic drugs

Cytotoxic drugs for treatment of neoplastic disease, e.g. chlorambucil and methotrexate, are known to be teratogenic.

Anticonvulsants

Babies of epileptic mothers have a two to three times increased incidence of congenital malformations (p. 27).

Antibiotics

Streptomycin and neomycin have been known to cause eighth-nerve deafness. Tetracycline chelates with teeth and bone, causing yellow staining and possibly enamel hypoplasia, and the use of chloroquine phosphate may result in retinal damage or deafness. Repeated doses of fluconazole have been associated with birth defects. Fusidic acid may cause kernicterus (p. 190) in babies of up to 1 month of age, due to the displacement of bilirubin from plasma albumin, and should be avoided in the last month of pregnancy.

Steroids

Some progestogens given in the past to prevent premature labour may cause masculinisation of the female fetus. Danazol, a drug which raises the level of fetal plasma testosterone, also has a similar effect. Certain preparations containing oestrogen and progestogens were used in the early detection of pregnancy, but an association with congenital malformations led to their withdrawal. Synthetic glucocorticoids, e.g. prednisolone, can occasionally suppress fetal growth when given throughout pregnancy and may increase susceptibility to infection after birth. However, when given to the mother for 48 hours to accelerate surfactant production in the unborn preterm infant's lungs to reduce the risk of respiratory distress syndrome, the benefits greatly outweigh any potential harm.

Hypotensive agents

Methyldopa has been used for many years and has not been shown to have any adverse effect on the unborn baby. Propranolol and labetolol are able to cause not only fetal growth suppression but also respiratory depression and bradycardia in a small proportion of cases, which can reduce the ability of the infant to respond to resuscitation at birth. There is also an increased risk of neonatal hypoglycaemia in the infant. Angiotensin-coverting enzyme inhibitors such as captopril or lisinopril should be avoided as they may cause intrauterine growth retardation, fetal renal failure and oligohydramnios. Nifedipine appears to be a safe alternative, though such calcium channel blockers carry the potential to produce fetal hypoxia associated with maternal hypotension. Intravenous hydralazine may cause fetal distress and fetal arrhythmia in the third trimester.

Anticoagulants

Warfarin is a potent teratogen in the first 3 months of pregnancy and may give rise to stunting of growth with abnormalities of the eyes and skeleton in up to a quarter of cases. It also carries the increased risk of abortion. If it is given to the mother in the last month of pregnancy, the baby may be born with a serious lack of vitamin K-dependent clotting factors. In these circumstances, the newborn infant should be given vitamin K intravenously and the clotting status checked to confirm that the defect has been corrected.

Heparin may be used in pregnancy since it does not cross the placenta and has no direct effect on the infant. It is, however, associated with a higher rate of preterm labour, which may leave the infant at risk of the complications of prematurity.

Late pregnancy

Drugs given to the mother in late pregnancy may often cause problems to the baby immediately after birth. A few known examples are given in Table 2.8.

Psychotropic drugs

Antidepressants Lithium, which may be used to treat manic depressive psychosis, can cause

malformation of the tricuspid valve in the heart, and also may depress fetal thyroid and renal function when used in later pregnancy. Phenothiazines such as chlorpromazine do not cause malformations, but a syndrome of tremor, hypertonia and hyperreflexia lasting for some months may affect the baby if the drug is taken near term. Similar withdrawal symptoms have been seen in babies whose mothers have taken fluoxetine ('Prozac') or paroxetine during pregnancy (Stiskal et al 2001).

Tricyclic drugs such as imipramine and amitriptyline are generally safe in pregnancy, though occasional neonates may have a mild withdrawal syndrome.

Sedatives and tranquillisers The increasing use of these drugs is a cause for concern because of

Table 2.8 Some problems caused by drugs in late pregnancy

Drugs	Possible effects on the infant
Antimicrobials	
tetracycline	Staining of deciduous teeth
chloramphenicol	Inhibits protein synthesis
streptomycin	Damage to the eighth cranial nerve
co-trimoxazole	Severe neonatal jaundice by competing for albumin-binding sites
isoniazid	Fits from pyridoxine deficiency
quinine	Bleeding from thrombocytopenia
chloroquine phosphate	Retinal damage
nitrofurantoin	Haemolysis
Anticonvulsant drugs, e.g. phenobarbital and phenytoin	Blood coagulation defects (relieved by vitamin K)
Anticoagulants, e.g. phenindione and warfarin	Bleeding at delivery
Analgesics	
salicylates (aspirin) in large doses	Jaundice, by competing with albumin binding sites, and bleeding from decreased platelet function; premature closure of the ductus arteriosus
indometacin	Premature closure of the ductus arteriosus
Oral antidiabetic drugs, e.g. tolbutamide	Hypoglycaemia, thrombocytopenia
Antithyroid drugs	Goitre and hypothyroidism
Antihypertensive drugs	
reserpine	Hypotonia, lethargy, excessive nasal mucus
propranolol	Respiratory depression, bradycardia, hypoglycaemia
Psychotropic drugs	
chlorpromazine	Tremor, hypertonia, hyperreflexia
lithium	Thyroid and renal dysfunction
imipramine	Mild withdrawal symptoms
amitriptyline	
diazepam	Hypotonia
fluoxetine and paroxetine	Mild withdrawal symptoms
Diuretics	Electrolyte disturbances
thiazides	Bleeding from thrombocytopenia
caffeine	Jaundice
Vitamins	
K (water-soluble forms)	Jaundice and kernicterus
D (in excess)	Hypercalcaemia
Oxytocin	Jaundice, hyponatraemia
Ritodrine	Tachycardia and hyperglycaemia

their possible effects on the baby after delivery. Most of them are capable of causing sufficient central nervous system depression to affect the onset of breathing at birth and cause general lethargy in the first 24 hours or more. The benzodiazepines, e.g. diazepam, can enhance the effect of other depressant drugs and, besides lethargy and muscular hypotonia, can cause defective control of body temperature and thus hypothermia in the infant. If the drugs have been used regularly or frequently by the mother, withdrawal symptoms may occur (p. 18).

Tocolytic agents

Ritodrine and other beta-2 stimulants are commonly given to the mother to suppress uterine contractions in preterm labour in order to prolong the pregnancy until the fetus is more mature. If used for long periods, these drugs can cause neonatal tachycardia and hypokalaemia, and may sometimes accentuate neonatal hypoglycaemia.

Non-steroidal anti-inflammatory drugs

Drugs such as aspirin, ibuprofen and other non-steroidal anti-inflammatory agents inhibit prostaglandin synthesis. When given in late pregnancy, they may cause closure of the fetal ductus arterious, fetal renal impairment, inhibition of platelet aggregation and a delay in labour and birth. There is some evidence to suggest that there is an increased risk of miscarriage (Nielson et al 2001).

Anaesthetics and analgesics used in obstetrics

When a drug is given to the mother in labour, the extent of its effect on the baby depends on several variable factors. The blood level of the drug may remain higher for a longer time if the maternal liver or renal function is impaired, the drug thus passing more readily to the fetus. If the maternal serum protein level is low, any drug which normally binds to protein reaches the fetus in greater amounts. The reduction of blood flow to the placenta during contractions may partially protect the fetus from large doses of a drug such as an anaesthetic agent, but the depression of maternal respiration caused by any such drug may contribute significantly to fetal hypoxia.

Anaesthetics by inhalation Used for analgesia or light anaesthesia, nitrous oxide has no measurable effect on the baby at birth. Deeper anaesthesia for caesarean section or forceps delivery requires other agents such as halothane and enfluorane. All anaesthetic agents cross the placenta and depress the baby's respiratory mechanisms to some extent and can delay the onset of respiration at birth. The effect is minimised by using the lowest effective concentration of the drug for the shortest possible time and ensuring a paediatrician is present at delivery to resuscitate the baby if necessary.

Morphine and pethidine Morphine and pethidine given to the mother as intrapartum analgesics both cause central nervous system depression and are contributory causes of neonatal asphyxia (p. 38). The duration of the effect is longer with pethidine than with morphine and is maximal when given about 3 hours before delivery. Since pethidine crosses the placenta, the baby may be sleepy initially and this may lead to a delay in establishing breast feeding. Pethidine is also excreted in breast milk for up to 2 days post delivery (Rajan 1994).

Local anaesthesia The use of epidural anaesthesia in labour has increased considerably in Britain. A local anaesthetic agent which is injected into the mother's lumbar and sacral epidural space abolishes the pain of labour and can even enable a caesarean section to be performed without a general anaesthetic. Consequently, the risk of respiratory depression often seen in the baby at birth after the use of either opiates or general anaesthesia is significantly reduced. The drug most commonly used for this purpose is bupivacaine, which appears to have relatively little effect on the infant, though respiratory depression and reduced activity may be seen for up to 24 hours after birth. Lidocaine (lignocaine), which passes rapidly across the placenta and may cause fetal central nervous system depression and bradycardia, is mainly used for pudendal blocks.

COMPLEMENTARY THERAPY IN PREGNANCY

Complementary therapies are increasingly used for many conditions, pregnancy among them. Few have been tested scientifically, so their value is not established. Acupuncture is reported to help the mother with certain pregnancy symptoms, but no information is available on the consequences for the baby. Prescribed homeopathic remedies are not known to harm the fetus and should normally be safe.

On the other hand, certain aromatherapy oils may cause uterine bleeding in pregnancy (Tiran 1996), though scientific evidence is incomplete. Most oils used are classified as safe food additives, and for massage the quantities applied are small.

MATERNAL DISEASE AND THE FETUS

Almost any disease in the mother is capable of affecting the progress of the fetus to some degree, if only indirectly through impaired nutrition. In some maternal diseases, specific effects may occur which are potentially serious for the infant, and these merit a separate description.

Diabetes mellitus

The outlook for a baby of a mother with diabetes mellitus that is well controlled in pregnancy is good. However, if the control is poor, one or more of the following complications may occur:

- excessive fetal growth
- placental vasculitis and vascular infarcts
- increased incidence of congenital malformations
- increased risk of preterm delivery
- Sudden unexpected fetal death.

Diabetic mothers should be regarded as having high-risk pregnancies and monitored closely. Frequent adjustment of diet and insulin doses to keep the maternal blood glucose levels well within the physiological range minimises the risks for the baby and enables many pregnancies to go to term and deliver vaginally. If control is poor, elective early delivery by caesarean section may be considered in order to avoid a prolonged and difficult birth which carries the risk of trauma to the oversized baby and the possibility of fetal death. These risks must be carefully weighed up against the consequences of preterm birth. To reduce the likelihood of respiratory distress syndrome (p. 131), a 48-hour course of dexamethasone may be needed if delivery before 34 weeks is contemplated, though this can cause serious temporary instability of the mother's diabetic control.

The management of the infant of a diabetic mother is discussed on page 52.

Epilepsy

Around one pregnancy in 200 occurs in women taking anticonvulsants for recurrent fits. An episode of status epilepticus during pregnancy is associated with a significant fetal mortality, but in controlled epilepsy the pregnancy is usually uneventful and the baby healthy. Occasionally, fetal growth is diminished, though this appears not to affect the infant's later development. Congenital malformations occur two to three times more frequently than in the general population. Neural tube defects (p. 230) occur in 1–2% of infants exposed to sodium valproate or carbamazepine; cleft lip and palate occur with increased frequency with phenytoin or phenobarbital. A combination of unusual facial features and abnormalities of the fingers may also occur in over 5% of infants. The drugs may affect blood clotting in the newborn infant and all should receive vitamin K intramuscularly after birth. An occasional infant may be irritable or have a fit from 'withdrawal' of the drugs.

Thyrotoxicosis

Maternal thyrotoxicosis can very occasionally cause fetal hyperthyroidism through the overstimulation of the baby's thyroid gland by a maternal IgG immunoglobulin known as long-acting thyroid stimulator, which crosses the placenta into the fetal circulation. Persistent fetal tachycardia is the cardinal sign of this condition, which may be treated by giving the mother antithyroid drugs such as carbimazole to suppress the fetal thyroid gland. More frequently, though, the baby will develop thyrotoxicosis in the few days after birth, when he may become alarmingly ill, with the rapid onset of hyperactivity, tachycardia and exophthalmos, and may even go into cardiac failure. The condition usually responds to treatment with carbimazole, with or without propranolol, which should continue for about 6 weeks.

If the mother's thyrotoxicosis is treated in pregnancy with antithyroid drugs and her thyroid function is monitored carefully, the baby is usually unaffected; however, the infant may be born with a goitre if the treatment is too vigorous. The goitre results from the effect of thyroid-stimulating hormone, which is secreted in excess by the pituitary gland as a reaction to inhibition of the baby's own thyroid hormone synthesis.

Parathyroid dysfunction

Maternal hypoparathyroidism can affect the fetus by producing secondary increased fetal parathyroid hormone secretion, which may cause demineralisation of the baby's bones at birth. Conversely, maternal hyperparathyroidism may cause neonatal hypocalcaemia and tetany (p. 157) by suppression of fetal parathormone production.

Myasthenia gravis

About one-third of the babies born to mothers with myasthenia gravis show a temporary form of the disease, presenting a few hours after birth with severe muscular hypotonia and weakness. This may extend to the muscles of respiration and swallowing and thus threaten life. Confirmation of the diagnosis can be obtained by the response to an injection of edrophonium chloride 100–200 µg/kg intramuscularly. The condition is self-limiting and is usually over in 2 days, though it can occasionally last up to a month.

Idiopathic thrombocytopenic purpura

In this condition, the maternal IgG antiplatelet antibodies responsible for destroying her own platelets cross the placenta and cause neonatal thrombocytopenia. It is most frequently transient, but the platelet count may remain low for several weeks until the baby loses the maternal antibodies. Corticosteroids are usually ineffective in increasing the platelet count when given either to the mother in pregnancy or to the baby after birth, and their prolonged use may result in neonatal adrenal insufficiency when they are withdrawn. Treatment of the mother with intravenous immunoglobulin infusions prior to delivery will frequently raise her platelet count and that of the fetus to a level at which the risk of bleeding is minimal and which will allow a normal delivery to proceed safely. When the infant's platelet count remains below $50 \times 10^9/L$, there is a risk of serious bleeding and the baby should be treated with intravenous immunoglobulin.

Phenylketonuria

There is an increasing number of girls now reaching adult life with normal development, having been treated for this disorder in childhood. Experience has shown that unless they return to a diet which keeps the serum phenylalanine level within or near the normal range before conception and continue it through the pregnancy, there is a greatly increased risk of damage to the fetus, causing malformation and resulting in developmental delay (p. 211).

MATERNAL INFECTIONS AND THE FETUS

Many maternal infections can affect the fetus and newborn baby, and these are discussed in Chapter 11. The purpose of this section is to describe those situations where action is needed during the pregnancy or at delivery to prevent or treat infection of the baby.

Dietary factors

Certain foods such as soft cheeses and pâtés contain the bacterium *Listeria monocytogenes*, which can infect the fetus or cause neonatal infection (p. 169). These should be avoided during pregnancy. Eggs and chicken should be cooked well to destroy the salmonella bacteria which can infect them. Undercooked meat can transfer the organism that causes toxoplasmosis (p. 177).

Prelabour rupture of the membranes

Infection of the amnion surrounding the fetus may occur as a result of prolonged prelabour rupture of the membranes, and the organisms may spread to the baby through the infected amniotic fluid before delivery. Contamination of the infant by pathogenic organisms colonising the birth canal may also occur during labour.

If the membranes rupture before the onset of labour and a *group B beta-haemolytic streptococcus* has been isolated from the mother's genital tract, it is possible to reduce significantly the risk of infection in the baby by treating the mother with erythromycin or ampicillin during labour. However, without routine culture of vaginal swabs it is difficult to tell which mothers carry the organism, and it is not yet clear whether antibiotic treatment of a carrier during a normal pregnancy affects the risk of infection in the infant after birth.

Maternal HIV infection – AIDS

The acquired immune deficiency syndrome (AIDS) is a fatal infectious disease caused by the human immunodeficiency virus (HIV). Pregnancy appears to reactivate the virus, and in around 25% of HIV-positive mothers, the baby will be infected. The intrapartum and early postnatal periods are the most common at-risk periods for the infant to contract HIV infection (UNAIDS 2000). Though it does not cause apparent fetal or neonatal disease, a high proportion of infected babies will develop the full syndrome and die in infancy. The subject is discussed in detail on page 178.

Since 1999, an HIV test has been offered to every pregnant woman in Britain at antenatal screening clinics. The following measures could then be recommended to women to reduce the risk of contracting the infection or transmitting it to the fetus (UNAIDS 1999):

- reduction in the frequency of unprotected sexual intercourse during pregnancy
- reduction in the number of sexual partners in pregnancy
- treatment of the infected woman during the pregnancy with antiretroviral drugs
- treatment of additional sexually transmitted infections.

In addition, recommendations regarding the management of infected women at and after delivery include:

- avoidance of invasive tests, for example the insertion of scalp electrodes
- caesarean section delivery
- avoidance of breast feeding
- heat treatment of expressed breast milk.

Maternal hepatitis B and C infection

Both these infections are blood borne and the same precautions should be taken at delivery as for HIV infection. Delivery by caesarean section is the usual mode of delivery but the neonate will need immunisation and hepatitis immunoglobulin after birth to prevent hepatitis B infection (p. 180).

Maternal genital herpes infection

This is most commonly caused by herpes simplex type II virus. If active genital herpes is present at the time of labour, delivery by caesarean section will normally prevent infection in the baby.

Syphilis

Though uncommon in Britain, syphilis is very prevalent in many other parts of the world. Confirmation of the infection with a Veneral Disease Research Laboratory (VDRL) test in very early pregnancy allows for treatment with penicillin, which in most cases prevents congenital infection (p. 181).

REFERENCES

Ahluwalia I B, Merrit R, Beck L F et al 2000 Multiple lifestyle and psychosocial risks and delivery of small for gestational age infants. Obstetrics and Gynecology 97(5):649–656

Bennett V, Brown L 1993 Myles textbook for midwives, 12th edn. Churchill Livingstone, London

Bonellie S R 2001 Effect of maternal age, smoking and deprivation on birthweight. Paediatric and Perinatal Epidemiology 15(1):19–26

Carrera J M, Torrents M, Mortera C et al 1995 Routine prenatal ultrasound screening for fetal abnormalities: 22 years experience. Ultrasound in Obstetrics and Gynecology 5:174–179

Chung K C, Kowalski C P, Kim H M et al 2000 Maternal cigarette smoking during pregnancy and the risk of having a child with cleft lip/palate. Plastic and Reconstructive Surgery 105(2):485–491

Cuervo L G, Mahomed K 2001 Treatments for iron deficiency anaemia in pregnancy (Cochrane Review). Cochrane Database of Systematic Reviews 2:CD003094

Dallaire L, Lortie G, Des-Rochers M et al 1995 Parental reaction and adaptability to the prenatal diagnosis of fetal defect or genetic disease leading to pregnancy interruption. Prenatal Diagnosis 15:249–259

Department of Health 1993 Sensible drinking: the report of an inter-departmental working group. HMSO, London, p 34

Faden V B, Graubard B I 2000 Maternal substance abuse during pregnancy and developmental outcome at age three. Journal of Substance Abuse 12(4):329–340

Finnegan L P, Connaughton J F Jr, Kron R E, Emich J P 1975 Neonatal abstinence syndrome: assessment and management. Addictive Disorders 2(1–2):141–158

Kozer E, Koren G 2001 Effects of prenatal exposure to marijuana. Canadian Family Physician 47:263–264

Klonoff-Cohen H, Lam-Kruglick P 2001 Maternal and paternal recreational drug use and sudden infant death syndrome. Archives of Pediatrics and Adolescent Medicine 155(7):765–770

Lissauer T, Ghaus K, Rivers R 1994 Maternal drug abuse – effects on the child. Current Paediatrics 4:235–239

Maternity Services Advisory Committee 1982 Maternity care in action Part 1- Antenatal care. HMSO, London

Mathews F, Yudkin P, Neil A 1999 Influence of maternal nutrition on outcome of pregnancy. British Medical Journal 317:339–343

Nielson G, Sorensen H, Larsen H et al 2001 Risk of adverse birth outcome and miscarriage in pregnant users of non-steroidal anti-inflammatory drugs: population based observational study and case control study. British Medical Journal 322:266–270

Smith G C, Pell J P 2001 Teenage pregnancy and risk of adverse outcomes associated with first and second births: population based retrospective cohort study. British Medical Journal 323(7311):476–481

Rajan L 1994 The impact of obstetric procedures and analgesia/anaesthesia during labour and delivery on breastfeeding. Midwifery 10:87–103

Royal College of Obstetricians and Gynaecologists 2000 Alcohol consumption in pregnancy. RCOG, London

Scotet V, de Braeckeleer M, Roussey M et al 2000 Neonatal screening for cystic fibrosis in Brittany, France: assessment of 10 years' experience and impact on prenatal diagnosis. Lancet 356(9232):789–794

Stiskal J A, Kulin N, Koren G et al 2001 Neonatal paroxetine withdrawal syndrome. Archives of Disease in Childhood Fetal and Neonatal Edition 84:F134–F135

Tiran D 1996 Aromatherapy in midwifery: benefits and risks. Complementary Therapies in Nursing and Midwifery 2:88–92

UNAIDS 1999 HIV in pregnancy: a review Occasional Paper 2. Joint United Nations Programme on HIV/AIDS, Geneva

UNAIDS 2000 Report on global HIV/AIDS epidemic. Joint United Nations Programme on HIV/AIDS, Geneva

Wald N J, Bower C 1995 Folic acid and the prevention of neural tube defects. British Medical Journal 310:1019–1020

Whiteman V E, Reece E A 1994 Prenatal diagnosis of major congenital malformations. Current Opinion in Obstetrics and Gynecology 6:459–467

FURTHER READING

NHS Executive 1999 Reducing mother to baby transmission of HIV. Health Service Circular 183

Russell J 1982 Early teenage pregnancy. Churchill Livingstone, Edinburgh

Chapter 3

Resuscitation and respiratory problems of the newborn

CHAPTER CONTENTS

Birth and adaptation to independent life   31
   The onset of respiration   32
Perinatal asphyxia   33
   Factors predisposing to birth asphyxia   33
   Recognition of the asphyxiated
   fetus – fetal distress   33
Resuscitation of the newborn baby   34
   Predicting the need for resuscitation   34
   Apparatus required for neonatal resuscitation   35
   Assessment at birth   36
   Resuscitation of the asphyxiated infant   36
   Resuscitation in special circumstances   40
   Ethical dilemmas in the resuscitation room   40
   Care of the baby after resuscitation   41
Breathing and respiratory disorders   41
   Normal breathing   41
   Babies with respiratory distress   41

BIRTH AND ADAPTATION TO INDEPENDENT LIFE

During intrauterine life, the fetus depends for oxygen and carbon dioxide exchange on the placenta. The lungs play no role before birth, and little blood flows through the pulmonary arteries. However, the heart and circulation are specially adapted to enable the major change from placental to pulmonary respiration to occur at birth. To understand the respiratory problems from which some newborn infants suffer, it is important to know of the fetal circulation and the changes which occur at birth (Fig. 3.1).

Around half of the cardiac output passes down the fetal aorta and umbilical arteries to the placenta, and oxygenated blood returns via the inferior vena cava to the right atrium. This blood flows through the flap-valve foramen ovale in the interatrial septum to the left atrium. It passes to the left ventricle, which pumps it to the developing brain through the carotid arteries. This blood returns depleted of oxygen to the right atrium, where it flows past the oxygenated stream into the right ventricle. The right ventricle is hypertrophied and the pressure it achieves on contraction is equal to that of the left ventricle. Blood cannot flow through the pulmonary arteries, which are constricted, so it passes from the main pulmonary artery to the descending aorta through the ductus arteriosus, where it joins the remaining left ventricle output of blood along the aorta and umbilical vessels to the placenta.

At birth, the following events occur:

1. The placental blood flow ceases as the cord is cut. As a result, the right atrial

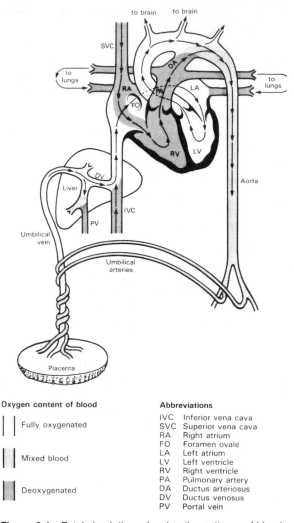

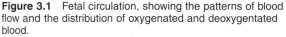

Oxygen content of blood

| | Fully oxygenated |

| | Mixed blood |

| | Deoxygenated |

Abbreviations

IVC   Inferior vena cava
SVC Superior vena cava
RA   Right atrium
FO   Foramen ovale
LA   Left atrium
LV   Left ventricle
RV   Right ventricle
PA   Pulmonary artery
DA   Ductus arteriosus
DV   Ductus venosus
PV   Portal vein

Figure 3.1 Fetal circulation, showing the patterns of blood flow and the distribution of oxygenated and deoxygentated blood.

flow diminishes and the pressure in it drops.

2. The lungs expand with air. This causes a marked drop in the vascular resistance in the pulmonary arteries and a substantial increase in the blood flow through them. The right ventricular pressure falls as its work rapidly decreases.

3. A substantial increase occurs in the blood flow from the lungs to the left atrium, which raises the left atrial pressure. The pressure difference which therefore develops between

the atria then closes the foramen ovale and prevents mixing of blood between them.

4. The oxygen saturation in the pulmonary venous and systemic arterial blood rises from 3–4 kPa to 10–11 kPa. This triggers the contraction and closure of the ductus arteriosus, thus preventing flow between the pulmonary artery and aorta.

These changes create the separate pulmonary and systemic circulations, but during episodes of hypoxia from respiratory or cardiac disorders in the first few weeks of life, the ductus arteriosus or foramen ovale can open up again. Under normal circumstances, however, the change from fetal to neonatal circulation is so efficient that arterial blood oxygen saturation reaches 90% within an hour of delivery.

The onset of respiration

Precisely how breathing is initiated is imperfectly understood. During fetal life, the lungs are fluid filled. Breathing movements develop during fetal life but diminish towards term. They are probably initiated in the respiratory centre in the brain stem, since fetal asphyxia increases the depth of the movements. During a normal vaginal delivery, the thorax is compressed, expelling some of the lung fluid before the first inspiration of air is taken. So long as the brain has not been impaired by intrapartum asphyxia, the respiratory centre responds to the mild acidosis and increased CO_2 level through the chemoreceptors in the aorta and carotid arteries by initiating an inspiratory gasp followed by strong breathing movements. Reflex responses by the baby to the sudden exposure to bright light, loud sounds, the relative cold of the ambient air, the unfamiliarity of being handled, feeling weight and touching new surfaces probably also contribute.

The negative pressure in the thorax required to take the first few breaths to expand and fill the alveoli is greater than that needed later, due to surface tension produced by the film of intra-alveolar fluid. Sometimes this pressure can be as high as 60 cmH$_2$O, but is usually between 20 and 30 cmH$_2$O. Phospholipid substances lining the alveoli reduce this tension and prevent them from collapsing completely between each expansion. The negative pressure required for breathing after the first few minutes is smaller – in the region of 5 cmH$_2$O.

During intrauterine life, little oxygen is expended except on growth, basal metabolic activity and functioning of the brain, heart and kidneys. After delivery, the addition of muscular activity, the production of heat to maintain the body temperature, and the metabolic activity in the gut to enable enteral feeding all increase very substantially the infant's oxygen requirement. Thus, so crucial is the transition from placental to pulmonary respiration for the baby's survival and health that anything which prevents the baby from breathing adequately immediately is a neonatal emergency. Although, in most cases, the minor degree of asphyxia temporarily caused by the normal diminution of gas exchange during each contraction of labour has no effect on the baby's brain, it can do so in some circumstances. More profound degrees of asphyxia before or during labour can leave permanent brain damage and it is this risk which makes an understanding of asphyxia and its management so crucial (Perlmann & Risser 1993). The impact of asphyxia on the infant is described in detail in Chapter 10 (p. 151). This chapter describes the circumstances predisposing to asphyxia and the necessary responses to it.

PERINATAL ASPHYXIA
Factors predisposing to birth asphyxia

When there has been a period of oxygen deprivation during the birth, the resultant asphyxia can render the infant acidaemic and his brain less responsive to the stimuli which normally initiate breathing. After minor degrees of asphyxia during labour, the baby may be born apnoeic but recover rapidly with relatively little resuscitation ('primary apnoea'). Greater degrees of asphyxia are followed by irregular slow gasping breaths or a state of 'terminal apnoea' in which none of the ordinary stimuli are effective, and a progressive

acidosis develops from which only vigorous resuscitation can rescue the infant.

An occasional baby fails to breathe without apparent cause, but the great majority of infants requiring resuscitation are born after a complicated labour or delivery. Known predisposing causes before labour are:

- placental dysfunction from pre-eclampsia or smoking
- growth retardation of the fetus
- prolongation of pregnancy
- retroplacental haemorrhage
- congenital abnormalities
- congenital infections.

During labour they are:

- prolongation of the second stage
- prolapse of the umbilical cord
- excessive maternal analgesia
- malpresentation (especially breech)
- cerebral injury.

These risks are greatly increased if the fetus is preterm, has suffered from prolonged partial asphyxia or is growth retarded from chronic intrauterine malnutrition, especially if unfavourable patterns of fetal blood flow have been found on Doppler ultrasound studies.

Recognition of the asphyxiated fetus – fetal distress

Several clinical and biochemical features may indicate that the fetus is asphyxiated during labour. Meconium staining of the liquor often, but not always, results from fetal hypoxia, but not all asphyxiated babies pass meconium before birth. A more consistent finding is a fetal bradycardia of less than 120 beats per minute or a tachycardia of more than 160 beats per minute. This has led to the practice of fetal heart monitoring, which can be done by a direct electrocardiographic recording from a fetal scalp electrode or more commonly from external cardiotocography in which a sensitive microphone, placed over the mother's abdomen, picks up the fetal heart sounds whilst a pressure transducer records uterine contractions. The apparatus identifies

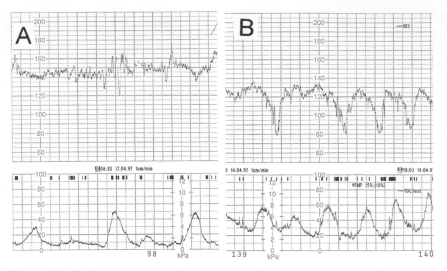

Figure 3.2 Cardiotochography. A: Normal trace. B: Fetal heart rate decelerations progressing beyond the uterine contraction, with slow return to the baseline level (Type II dips), indicating fetal asphyxia. (By kind permission of Mr Michael Dooley.)

patterns of change in heart rate with contractions, and records them on moving paper. A recording in which the heart rate varies with activity within a range of 110–160 beats per minute, and there is good beat-to-beat variation, usually excludes asphyxia (Fig. 3.2A). During uterine contractions, there is often a fall of the fetal heart rate, which returns to the resting level immediately the contraction is over (type 1 deceleration). This is usually of no significance, but a delay in the recovery of the heart rate to the resting level (type 2 deceleration; Fig. 3.2B) is considered particularly indicative of asphyxia. Other patterns that may signify fetal distress are a drop in the heart rate which continues after the height of the uterine contraction, profound deceleration to a rate of less than 80 beats per minute, and a loss of the normal beat-to-beat variation in the heart rate. A persistent fetal bradycardia of less than 100 beats per minute is almost always associated with a poor fetal cerebral circulation and demands urgent delivery of the baby.

During episodes of hypoxia, the fetus derives its energy from the breakdown of glycogen stores by anaerobic metabolism, which is relatively inefficient. The consequent accumulation of lactic acid and other acidic products of this metabolism lowers the fetal blood pH. Repeated sampling of capillary blood from the fetal scalp through the dilating cervix and measurement of its pH provides a direct measure of the degree of fetal acidosis and gives the clearest indication of the state of the baby's health. A pH of 7.2 or less indicates severe asphyxia. However, this method should not be used in mothers infected with HIV or hepatitis B virus, to prevent infection of the baby (p. 179). If asphyxia is clearly demonstrated on clinical or instrumental evidence, steps must be taken to deliver the baby as rapidly and safely as possible, and this may mean an emergency caesarean section, forceps or Ventouse assisted delivery.

RESUSCITATION OF THE NEWBORN BABY
Predicting the need for resuscitation

A large study in Sweden (Palme-Kilander 1993) has demonstrated that only 1% of babies of greater than 2500 g birth weight and 0.2% of babies born at more than 32 weeks of gestation after an apparently normal delivery needed any resuscitation. Of those who did require assistance, between 80% and 90% responded to bag and mask resuscitation alone. For term babies born after an uncomplicated pregnancy and delivery, therefore, advanced resuscitation is required in only about 1% of cases.

It is imperative that health professionals involved in the care of the newborn are proficient in resuscitation techniques. The type of education varies from hospital to hospital, some providing in-service training, others accessing national courses. The Resuscitation Council (UK) runs a newborn life support course in centres around the country, covering all aspects of newborn resuscitation. The UK Resuscitation website (www.resus.org.uk) has very useful information on training and all matters relating to neonatal resuscitation.

The majority of babies who require resuscitation at birth are born after a complicated pregnancy or delivery. The following circumstances require the presence of a professional who is competent at assessment and resuscitation of the newborn even though many babies in these categories will establish normal breathing spontaneously:

- preterm babies under 36 weeks of gestation (p. 113)
- fetal distress or meconium staining of the liquor (p. 40)
- prenatal diagnosis of fetal growth retardation (p. 21)
- prenatal diagnosis of a congenital abnormality
- multiple pregnancy
- breech presentation
- caesarean section
- instrumental delivery other than lift-out forceps
- rhesus haemolytic disease (p. 193)
- prolapsed cord
- where a perinatal complication has occurred in a previous delivery.

Apparatus required for neonatal resuscitation

Since only about 80% of babies needing resuscitation will be identified before birth, it is essential for a resuscitation service to be available for all

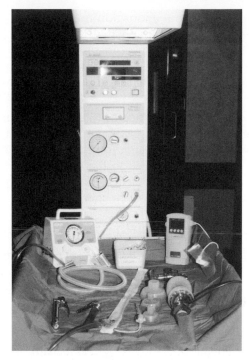

Figure 3.3 Equipment required for resuscitation of newborn babies.

deliveries. A trained midwife or doctor should be present or immediately available solely to resuscitate the infant. The room itself should be well illuminated, draught-free and be warmed to at least 25°C; warm towels are required to dry the infant and maintain his temperature, a suitable padded surface at table height is needed and there should be a telephone or emergency call system to summon more assistance. Ideally, the equipment required (Fig. 3.3) includes:

- overhead radiant heater
- a clock with a sweep second hand
- mechanical suction apparatus with suction catheters with side holes
- oxygen supply with facilities to regulate the pressure and flow rate
- face masks
- self-inflating bag
- laryngoscope with infant blades
- endotracheal tubes sizes 2.5, 3.0 and 3.5 mm
- syringes and needles
- umbilical venous catheterisation set
- infant oral airways of several sizes

- drugs for intravenous administration:
  - —adrenaline (epinephrine) 1:10 000 (may also be given by tracheal instillation)
  - —naloxone
  - —sodium bicarbonate 4.2%
  - —10% dextrose.

There must be rapid access to emergency group O-negative blood for neonatal use. For preterm deliveries, surfactant should be available (p. 133). This will often be taken to the delivery room by the attending neonatal team. All the above equipment and supplies must be checked regularly.

Assessment at birth

At birth, the state of the baby depends on the duration and degree of asphyxia before and during delivery. The healthy baby who has not suffered any asphyxia will emerge as an active, pink infant who cries immediately after birth. A mild degree of asphyxia will cause the baby to be cyanosed and apnoeic, though he remains responsive to skin stimulation and has good muscle tone and a heart rate above 100 beats per minute. More prolonged asphyxia results in the onset of circulatory failure in which the baby becomes a pale grey-blue colour, is limp, unresponsive to skin stimulation and has a heart rate below 100 beats per minute.

A quantitative and objective clinical evaluation of the state of the baby directly after delivery is desirable because it serves as an immediate indicator of whether resuscitation is required and, if so, what form it should take. The most widely used scoring system is that devised by Apgar (Table 3.1) in which each of five features is given a score of 0, 1 or 2. The higher the total, the less likely is it that resuscitation will be required. The evaluation is made 1 minute and 5 minutes after birth, but can be repeated every 5 minutes if the baby has not responded adequately. Although some infants with an Apgar score of 5 or more have inadequate breathing, a score of 4 or less at 1 minute suggests a degree of asphyxia for which immediate active resuscitation should be implemented; low values persisting after 5 or 10 minutes suggest that asphyxia has been prolonged and resuscitation should continue. Unfortunately, the scoring system predicts less than half of the babies with a significant degree of acidosis from intrapartum asphyxia, and there is little correlation between Apgar scores and long-term neurological outcome.

Resuscitation of the asphyxiated infant

When respiration does not immediately start, or when, after a preliminary gasp, it fails to become established, the action taken depends on the condition of the baby, evaluated as described above. The following scheme gives an idea of how to proceed. The actions required are summarised in the Resuscitation Council algorithm (Table 3.2). The paper by Harling and Yoxall (1999) also discusses neonatal resuscitation well.

Initial step

In all cases, the first step is to note the time and start the clock on the resuscitation trolley. The baby should be placed supine under the radiant heater, quickly dried and placed on a warm

Table 3.1 Apgar method of scoring in the evaluation of asphyxia in newborn infants

	Score		
	0	1	2
Sign			
Heart rate	Absent	Under 100 beats/min	Over 100 beats/min
Respiratory effort	Absent	Weak, irregular	Strong, regular
Reflex response to stimulation of the feet	None	Weak movement	Cry
Colour	Blue or pale	Body pink, extremities blue	Completely pink
Muscle tone	Limp	Partial flexion	Active movement

Table 3.2 Resuscitation Council of the UK algorithm for resuscitation of the newborn

Dry the baby, remove any wet cloth and cover

↓

Initial assessment at birth:
Start the clock and assess colour, tone, breathing and heart rate

↓

If not breathing...

↓

Control the airway
Hold the head in a neutral position

↓

Support the breathing
If not breathing, give five inflation breaths with a bag and mask
Confirm the response – increase in heart rate or visible chest movement

↓

If there is no response:
a. Check the head position and apply jaw thrust
b. Confirm the response again

↓

If there is still no response:
a. Get help with airway control and repeat inflation breaths
b. Inspect the oropharynx and give suction if needed. Repeat inflation breaths
c. Insert oropharyngeal airway and repeat inflation breaths
d. Consider intubation if heart rate not increasing or chest not moving

↓

When the chest is moving:
Continue ventilation breaths until spontaneous breathing occurs

↓

Check the heart rate
If heart rate is not detectable or slow (<60 beats/min) and not increasing

↓

Start chest compressions
First confirm chest movement – if not moving, check airway again
3 chest compressions to 1 breath for 30 seconds

↓

Reassess heart rate
If improving, stop chest compressions and continue ventilating
If heart rate still slow, continue ventilating and chest compressions
Consider venous access and drugs at this stage

dry towel. This act of drying the baby acts as a good respiratory stimulant and allows for the assessment of the baby's colour, tone and respiratory status. The baby's airway must be patent to enable a safe transition to extrauterine life. The head should be placed in the neutral position or with slight extension, and gentle suction applied, if necessary, to clear the oro-pharynx and nasal passages of mucus, liquor and blood. Care must be taken to avoid vigorous deep suctioning as this can cause laryngospasm and bradycardia through stimulation of the vagus nerve. If at this point the baby is vigorous, centrally pink, breathing spontaneously and the heart rate is over 100 beats per minute, he can be wrapped and handed to the parents. A less vigorous baby may require facial oxygen until his colour improves. Since mouth breathing is not possible at this age, the clearing of the nasal passages is vital if respiratory efforts are being made but are obviously failing to inflate the lungs.

The baby with mild asphyxia

If the baby has good muscle tone, makes some movement in response to stimulation, and the heart rate is over 100 beats per minute yet breathing is inadequate (Apgar score 5 or more), stimulation of the skin may be adequate to initiate breathing. If breathing fails to start after 60–90 seconds, the baby will need to be ventilated with a bag and mask. The technique of bag and mask ventilation is easy to learn, safe and almost free of complications. Everyone involved in the care of a baby at birth should become proficient in the method and be prepared to use it as and when needed (Fig. 3.4).

Generally, the baby's respiratory effort and heart rate will improve after a short period of adequate ventilation. In order to efficiently administer bag and mask ventilation, the following must be achieved:

- The baby's head must be in a neutral position or slightly extended. Over-extension or flexion of the neck should be avoided.
- An appropriately sized face mask must be used. The mask should cover the nose and mouth

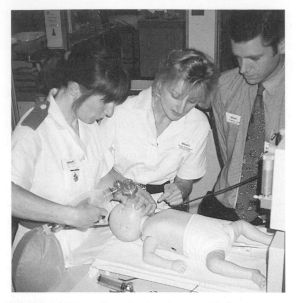

Figure 3.4 Bag and mask resuscitation – the importance of both good technique and adequate training.

without pressing on the eyes or overhanging the chin.

• A good seal must be ensured between the baby's skin and the mask by using a flexible mask and applying reasonable pressure. This is best achieved by using the thumb and forefinger to press down the mask while the other fingers elevate the chin to open the airway.

• The first five breaths need to be given at higher pressures and with a longer inspiratory time than subsequent breaths, to overcome the initial resistance of the previously fluid-filled unexpanded lungs. For premature babies, inspiratory pressures of up to $30\,cmH_2O$ may be required, and up to $50\,cmH_2O$ for term babies, for these initial 'inflation' or 'rescue' breaths.

• The inflation rate should be 30–40 breaths per minute.

• The chest wall must move adequately.

• The heart rate and respiratory status must be reassessed every 30 seconds.

• Traditionally, 100% oxygen has been used for resuscitation. There are theoretical risks that pure oxygen may cause brain damage as a result of free radical production, but there is little research evidence to back up these concerns.

Most modern resuscitation equipment has the facility to give air/oxygen mixtures.

• If pethidine has been given to the mother within the 4 hours prior to delivery, naloxone hydrochloride 10–30 μg/kg should be given intravenously or 70 μg/kg intramuscularly, to reverse the respiratory depressant effect of the drug, but this is not an alternative to adequate ventilation of the lungs. Naloxone should not be given to the babies of drug-dependent mothers as it can induce apnoea.

Most babies will respond to bag and mask ventilation. It should be discontinued once adequate, spontaneous respirations are established.

Failure of the baby to respond to bag and mask ventilation may indicate a more compromised baby or, more likely, a failure to adequately inflate the lungs. The following possibilities should be considered:

• the neck may be too extended
• the seal around the mask may be leaking
• too low a pressure may be being used to inflate the lungs
• whether an oral airway would help to keep the airway open
• the airway may be obstructed by mucus.

The severely asphyxiated infant

A baby who fails to respond to bag and mask ventilation despite adequate chest movement, should have an endotracheal tube inserted to enable more effective inflation of the lungs.

Endotracheal intubation and ventilation With the infant lying on his back and the neck slightly extended, the baby laryngoscope is inserted to the back of the tongue so that the tip of the blade elevates the epiglottis, and the vocal cords can be seen through the oval glottis. After clearing the pharynx of accumulated mucus by gentle suction, the endotracheal tube is inserted 1–2 cm through the opening. A finer catheter may then be quickly passed through the tube and suction applied to clear the trachea. The tube is then connected to either a self-inflating bag or a pressure-regulated air/oxygen supply. Intermittent positive pressure ventilation can then be given

Table 3.3 Drugs used in neonatal resuscitation

Drug	Dose	Actions	Comments
Adrenaline (epinephrine) 1 in 10 000	0.1–0.3 mL/kg i.v. 1 mL/kg via ETT	Increases heart rate, myocardial contractility and blood pressure	If no response, repeat dose or increase i.v. dose up to 1 mL/kg; 1 in 1000 solution can be used
Sodium bicarbonate 4.2%	2–4 mL/kg of 4.2%	A blood buffer which counteracts acidosis	Do not give rapidly Baby must be adequately ventilated to counteract a rise in carbon dioxide
10% Dextrose	2.5 mL/kg i.v.	Raises blood glucose levels	
Volume expanders: 0.9% NaCl 4.5% albumin	10–20 mL/kg i.v.	Restores circulatory volume; increases perfusion and cardiac output	Do not volume overload as it may cause cardiac failure If there is severe blood loss, give O-negative blood

using either the bag or a Y-connector operated with the thumb. Resuscitation equipment has a gauge to indicate the pressure being applied and a valve which limits the maximum pressure to a level set by the operator. This will normally be no more than 30 cmH$_2$O, since higher pressures can cause lung damage. Inflation pressures can be altered according to the movements of the chest wall, and pressures above 10–15 cmH$_2$O are not normally needed to achieve this. If the lungs are not distending adequately, the endotracheal tube may have dislodged into the oesophagus or may not be large enough to deliver sufficient air into the lungs. As soon as the baby starts to breathe spontaneously, is pink and has a heart rate above 100 beats per minute, the endotracheal tube may be withdrawn.

External cardiac massage External cardiac massage is indicated if the heart rate remains below 60 beats per minute despite adequate ventilation by either bag and mask or endotracheal tube. Compressions should be given over the lower third of the sternum, approximately one finger breadth below an imaginary line joining the nipples. Either the tips of two fingers of one hand can be used or the thumbs of both hands while the fingers encircle the baby's chest. The chest must be compressed between a third and a half of the depth of the chest. Broken ribs may be a consequence of this necessary chest wall deformation, but less adequate cardiac massage will not have a good outcome for the child. Compressions should be given at a rate of between

100 and 120 per minute or a ratio of three compressions to one lung inflation. The baby's heart rate should be assessed every 30 seconds using a stethoscope on the chest wall or by palpating the base of the umbilical cord. Trying to feel for peripheral pulses is difficult in this situation. Effective cardiac massage is imperative in providing adequate circulation to the brain and major organs. Once the heart rate has risen over 80 beats per minute, cardiac massage can stop. In the unlikely event of the baby not responding to these measures, emergency drugs will need to be used (Table 3.3). Those most commonly used are:

- adrenaline (epinephrine) 1:10 000
- sodium bicarbonate 4.2%
- 10% dextrose
- volume expanders such as saline or colloid solutions.

Venous access for drug administration is best gained by cannulating the umbilical vein.

A baby who fails to respond to the above measures despite adequate performance of the equipment and the operator, may have another underlying cause such as:

- cyanotic congenital heart disease
- diaphragmatic hernia
- pneumothorax
- severe anaemia
- neurological disorder
- depression of the respiratory centre by drugs or asphyxia.

In these circumstances, immediate action is required to exclude remediable causes. A chest X-ray should identify a diaphragmatic hernia (p. 220). A pneumothorax is more rapidly identified by cold light transillumination, and often improvement can be obtained by briefly inserting a small needle to allow air under pressure to escape, but a pleural drain will be needed if the situation recurs. Pallor, hypotension and tachycardia are the clinical signs of severe blood loss and they require immediate restoration of the blood volume with colloid if necessary until a blood transfusion is given to replace both the lost volume and red cells (p. 184).

Resuscitation in special circumstances

Preterm infants

Endotracheal intubation and positive pressure ventilation as a first step immediately after delivery is recommended for all preterm infants under 34 weeks of gestation who do not cry vigorously at birth, in order to reduce the incidence and severity of respiratory distress syndrome (p. 131).

This approach may also be needed when a baby (usually after caesarean birth) breathes immediately but then becomes apnoeic.

Meconium in the liquor

Meconium can cause considerable inflammation in the bronchi if aspirated into the lungs during or after labour. Light meconium staining of liquor usually causes few problems and, apart from clearing the mouth and pharynx of liquor, little help is usually needed.

If thick meconium is present, it may indicate that the baby has been asphyxiated or that meconium has been inhaled into the lungs, and both meconium aspiration syndrome and the consequences of asphyxia are common (Ziadeh & Sunna 2000). Correct handling of this condition is important, and the following is a guide to its management, though it may not prevent meconium aspiration syndrome (Yoder 1994):

- After delivery of the head, the meconium should be aspirated from the mouth, nose and pharynx before the thorax has been delivered, using a mechanical sucker with a large suction tube.
- If the baby is vigorous and cries, no further action is normally needed after birth.
- If the respiratory effort is poor, the larynx and trachea should be sucked out under direct vision with a laryngoscope using a large suction tube.
- The baby should be kept well oxygenated, using bag and mask or endotracheal resuscitation if needed, as described above.

Resuscitation at home deliveries

Since most home births will be low-risk deliveries, resuscitation will only occasionally be needed (p. 34). A second midwife or a doctor trained in bag and mask resuscitation should be present at the birth and must have available a portable resuscitation kit including an oxygen supply with a flow regulator, suction equipment and a suitable neonatal bag and mask. Immediate access to a telephone is essential to summon more expert help if required. Only rarely will intervention be needed beyond the bag and mask technique except in such emergencies as precipitate preterm delivery. Even in these circumstances, adequate ventilation can usually be maintained with a bag and mask until a paediatrician with advanced resuscitation skills arrives.

Ethical dilemmas in the resuscitation room

Midwives and doctors may be faced with difficult ethical decisions in the delivery room. These decisions will include whether to resuscitate extremely premature babies at the limit of viability, those with multiple abnormalities, and unexpected fresh stillbirths. It is sometimes possible to anticipate these in the first two situations, to discuss them with the parents beforehand and agree a policy with them. Unexpected stillbirth occurs in 0.5:1000 births over 24 weeks gestation (Casalaz 1998) and a small number of these can be successfully resuscitated and survive without adverse consequences. The degree of the prenatal insult will determine the outcome, and asystole beyond 10 minutes or continued apnoea beyond 20 minutes after birth is correlated with a high risk of severe disability or death of the infant.

Care of the baby after resuscitation

The majority of infants requiring resuscitation respond rapidly, becoming active and starting to cry. Once it is clear that the baby's condition is stable, the infant should be wrapped in a warm towel and given to the parents. Since very few of these babies develop hypoxic-ischaemic encephalopathy (p. 151) as a complication of their transient asphyxia, the infant should normally stay with the mother, only being admitted to the neonatal unit if there is another reason to do so (p. 60).

BREATHING AND RESPIRATORY DISORDERS
Normal breathing

Once respiration is established, the baby's breathing is usually regular and rhythmic at about 30–50 breaths per minute, but irregular breathing at rates from 15 to 100 breaths per minute are not uncommon. Respiration rates consistently above 60 breaths per minute may be caused by lung disease, metabolic acidosis or congenital heart disease, and should always be investigated. Decreased rates may be caused by suppression of the respiratory centre by drugs or cerebral asphyxia. If the mother received an opiate analgesic in labour, depression of the infant's respiration can persist for up to 48 hours and administration of naloxone 70 μg/kg i.m. should reverse the effect.

Occasionally, during sleep a healthy baby will have a brief self-limiting apnoeic spell caused by relative immaturity of the respiratory centre in the midbrain. These may last up to about 12 seconds and they resolve spontaneously as the carbon dioxide rises in the blood and stimulates breathing again. So long as they are not accompanied by cyanosis or bradycardia, they do no harm and cease within a few weeks.

The volume of air taken with each breath (the tidal volume) is 6 mL/kg of body weight and this ensures that the baby receives the 6 mL/kg/min of oxygen required to keep the blood gases within the normal range (p. 77). Control of the depth and rate of breathing is achieved by the respiratory centre in the medulla of the brain, which is fully mature in most term infants and responds to changes of the carbon dioxide and oxygen levels in the blood and its pH.

Babies with respiratory distress

Many respiratory conditions present in the same way in the newborn infant and they cannot often be distinguished clinically. Respiratory symptoms such as dyspnoea, tachypnoea, grunting respirations and indrawing of the lower sternum or ribs on inspiration (costal and subcostal recession) should always be investigated by a chest X-ray. Grunting alone can be a feature of hypothermia or septicaemia, which should be urgently investigated and treated (p. 168). Persistent cyanosis suggests complex congenital heart disease or a very serious pulmonary disorder, including congenital diaphragmatic hernia (Fig. 3.5). Box 3.1 shows causes of neonatal respiratory distress.

Since respiratory distress is the presenting feature of many different lung and heart disorders whose treatment will be different, it is essential to make a correct early diagnosis. Even a chest X-ray appearance may not be diagnostic, similar appearances occurring in respiratory distress syndrome, transient tachypnoea and pneumonia. A blood culture should be performed to exclude septicaemic pneumonia (p. 171), and blood gases measured to ascertain the impact of the disease on the acid–base status of the baby. If cyanosis is the most prominent feature, congenital heart disease should be excluded by clinical examination, an ECG and a nitrogen washout test (p. 222). In cyanotic congenital heart disease, serious acidosis can occur rapidly and the advice of a specialist paediatric cardiac unit may be urgently required.

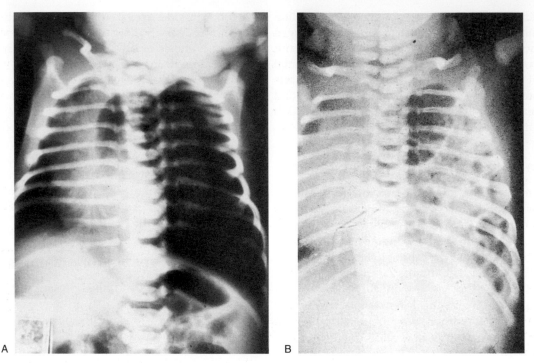

Figure 3.5 X-ray appearances in (A) tension pneumothorax and (B) diaphragmatic hernia.

> **Box 3.1** Causes of neonatal respiratory distress
>
> Atelectasis
> Aspiration of:
>   liquor
>   meconium
> Pneumonia (p. 171)
> Pneumothorax
> Diaphragmatic hernia (p. 220)
> Hypoplastic lungs (p. 220)
> Respiratory distress syndrome (p. 131)
> Choanal atresia (p. 219)
> Heart failure (p. 226)
> Persistent metabolic acidosis
> Transient tachypnoea of the newborn

Atelectasis

The failure of portions of the lungs to expand with the first few breaths or collapse of part of the lung secondary to inhalation of fluid or mucus is described as atelectasis. In this situation, the respiratory distress is at its maximum immediately after delivery, and in the case of primary atelectasis it eases off over the first 24 hours. Fine crepitations and diminished air entry may be detectable clinically, but the collapse is difficult to localise accurately.

Pneumothorax

Occasionally, especially after over-vigorous resuscitation, a baby will develop a pneumothorax from rupture of a distended alveolus into the pleural space. So long as only a small amount of air is present and the pressure does not rise, many of these events cause little respiratory distress and will resolve without treatment. In some instances, administering oxygen will accelerate the recovery.

If the hole is valvular, gradually more air will collect in the pleural space and the rising pressure will push the mediastinal contents to the opposite side (Fig. 3.5). The clinical signs are respiratory distress, the absence of breath sounds over the affected lung, and a shift of the heart sounds away from the side of the collecting air. Known as a tension pneumothorax, this condition can cause serious cardiorespiratory embarrassment, and urgent treatment with an indwelling pleural drain is essential (p. 139). It is a not uncommon accompaniment of ventilation of the preterm infant (p. 139).

The meconium aspiration syndrome

The inhalation of meconium occurs when the fetus has passed meconium into the liquor before birth. This usually follows fetal asphyxia and is commoner in the baby who has suffered intrauterine malnutrition. There may be evidence of inhaled meconium when suction from the pharynx is undertaken at birth, but tracheal suction does not necessarily prevent lung disease from developing (Yoder 1994). The symptoms vary from mild to very severe and may progress rapidly over the first day. X-rays show scattered opacities in both lungs, with intervening areas of overinflation, and depression of the diaphragm caused by airways obstruction. A pneumothorax may result from the rupture of an emphysematous bulla.

In mild cases, maintaining the baby's oxygen saturation with supplementary inhaled oxygen may be all that is needed until recovery occurs. Unless there is evidence of additional infection, antibiotics are not usually necessary. In more severe cases, particularly where oxygen saturation cannot be maintained, mechanical ventilation may be required with the full accompaniments of neonatal intensive care. A pnuemothorax will require insertion of an intercostal pleural drain connected to an underwater seal to re-expand the lung (p. 139). Very occasionally, all this cannot sustain the infant and transfer to one of the specialist centres for extra-corporeal membrane oxygenation (ECMO) may be required (p. 137).

Persistent metabolic acidosis

If an infant develops a persistent metabolic acidosis, a compensatory increase in respiration rate and depth occurs to reduce the CO_2 level and thus restore the pH of the blood. This overbreathing may occasionally be mistaken for cardiac or pulmonary disease, but it can be distinguished by a low pCO_2 in the arterial blood gas values. Further investigation of the cause of the acidosis is required before deciding on treatment.

Transient neonatal tachypnoea

'Transient neonatal tachypnoea' occurs in about 2% of babies and presents as respiratory distress on the first day. It is normally mild and resolves without treatment in a few days. It is usually attributed to delayed absorption of the fetal lung fluid and in the first day or two it mimics respiratory distress syndrome. It occurs more frequently in male infants born at term, particularly after fetal asphyxia, and occurs in around 9% of infants born by elective caesarean section. X-rays show no atelectasis or pneumonia and, so long as sepsis can be confidently excluded, no specific treatment is needed, though oxygen supplementation may be required if the oxygen saturation is low.

Congenital laryngeal stridor

An inspiratory crowing noise noticeable in the first few days of life, louder at some times than others and especially with crying, is almost always due to a 'floppy larynx' or laryngomalacia. The noise is probably caused by a valvular closure of the glottis on inspiration, due to softness of its supporting structures. Most cases resolve spontaneously and gradually before the age of 2 years. It is alarming to the parents but appears to do no harm to the infant, and reassuring the parents is usually all the treatment that is needed.

Very rare causes of congenital stridor include abnormalities of the larynx, such as obstructing webs, and combined oesophageal and tracheal compression from a vascular ring. A barium swallow reveals a characteristic indentation in the oesophagus.

REFERENCES

Casalaz D M, Marlow N, Speidel B D 1998 Outcome of resuscitation following unexpected apparent stillbirth. Archives of Disease in Childhood Fetal and Neonatal Edition 78(2):F112–F115

Harling E, Yoxall B 1999 Resuscitation of babies at birth. Journal of Neonatal Nursing 5(4):centre insert

Palme-Kilander C 1993 Methods of resuscitation in low-Apgar score newborn infants – a national survey. Acta Paediatrica 81:739–744

Perlmann J, Risser R 1993 Severe fetal acidemia: neonatal neurological features and short term outcome. Pediatric Neurology 9:277–282

Yoder B A 1994 Meconium-stained amniotic fluid and respiratory complications: impact of selective tracheal suction. Obstetrics and Gynecology 83(1):77–84

Ziadeh S M, Sunna E 2000 Obstetric and perinatal outcome of pregnancies with term labour and meconium-stained amniotic fluid. Archives of Gynecology and Obstetrics 264(2):84–87

FURTHER READING

American Heart Association 2000 Emergency Cardiovascular Care Committee Guidelines. Neonatal resuscitation. Circulation 102 (suppl 1):343–356

Handbook on resuscitation of babies at birth 1997 College of Paediatrics and Child Health, London

Milner A D 1998 Resuscitation at birth. European Journal of Paediatrics 157:524–527

Milner A D 1999 Resuscitation at birth: consensus and controversy. Journal of Neonatal Nursing 5(6):15–18.

Resuscitation Council (UK) 2001 Newborn life support provider manual. Resuscitation Council (UK), London

Yu V Y H (ed) 1995 Clinical paediatrics: pulmonary problems in the perinatal period and their sequelae. Baillière Tindall, London

USEFUL WEBSITES

www.rcpch.ac.uk – Royal College of Paediatrics and Child Health

www.resus.org.uk – Resuscitation Council of the UK

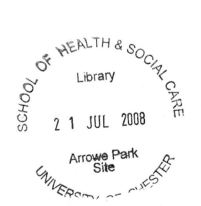

Chapter 4
Growth and its disorders

CHAPTER CONTENTS

Introduction   45
Growth in weight, length and head circumference   45
   Weight   45
   Length   46
   Head circumference   47
   Growth charts   48
Disorders of intrauterine growth   49
   Low birth weight babies   49
   The light for dates infant   49
   The post-term infant   52
   Infants of diabetic mothers   52
   Hypoglycaemia   54
   The heavy for dates infant   56
   Twins and higher-order births   56

INTRODUCTION

Those who work with the newborn soon come to realise that no two infants are alike and that there is a wide range of size, proportion, nutritional state and patterns of growth among healthy 'normal' infants. It is by learning how to recognise the range of variation of the normal infant and the characteristics of the various disorders of growth that it is possible to assess which infants have a problem that requires assessment or treatment and which are more likely to be normal.

GROWTH IN WEIGHT, LENGTH AND HEAD CIRCUMFERENCE
Weight

The average term infant in Britain weighs 3500 g at birth, and 95% are between 2500 g and 4250 g. Approximately 80% of all babies grow normally during fetal life and are born within the range of 2500 to 3800 g birth weight and between 37 and 41 weeks of completed gestation. They are referred to as 'appropriately grown for their gestational age' (Fig. 4.1). Most of these infants will be entirely healthy and have an uncomplicated neonatal course. The weight at birth is influenced by many factors in addition to the length of gestation. Maternal disease, such as pre-eclampsia, which affects placental function, reduces the size of the baby, whereas inadequately controlled diabetes mellitus results in excessive fetal growth. Mothers of shorter stature usually have small babies, though taller women do not necessarily have big infants. Extreme maternal malnutrition may

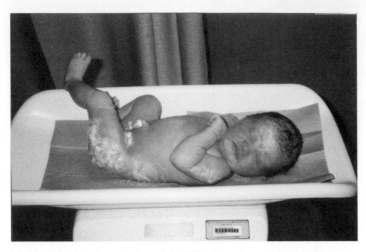

Figure 4.1 A well-grown term infant. The importance of accurate weighing at birth.

restrict fetal growth. Ethnic differences also occur. British-born babies of mothers of West Indian origin tend to be larger than ethnic white babies. A higher percentage of births in Britain to mothers of Asian origin are below the 10th percentile, but in the second generation their birth weights seem to be rising. The average boy at term weighs nearly 250 g more than the average girl. Birth weight of appropriately grown healthy babies bears some relation to size in later childhood, mainly through the common factor of parental height, but the connection is less clear in those infants towards the extremes of the centile ranges. Lifestyle habits such as smoking and alcohol restrict growth significantly (Ahluwalia et al 2000, Bonellie 2001). However, caffeine intake appears not to have a significant impact on the growth of the infant (Grosso et al 2001).

During the first 3 to 5 days of life, infants usually lose between 5% and 10% of their birth weight as the kidneys excrete the small physiological excess of body fluid which is present at birth. Thereafter, adequate feeding ensures sufficient protein and calories to promote real growth, and the birth weight is often reached or exceeded by the 10th day. In the following month, weight gain is usually between 180 and 210 g each week, but it is often not an even rise; days of slow progress are followed by days of compensatory gain. Plotting the weight of the baby about once or twice a week on a chart such as the one shown in Figure 4.2 is a valuable guide to growth and progress, and the majority of infants grow along their birth centile. Provided that the baby's health is not judged on this alone, consistent growth usually indicates a healthy infant; however, one whose weight centile continues to fall, a condition referred to as 'failure to thrive', may either be receiving inadequate nutrition or have some medical condition preventing growth. Such babies must be evaluated carefully for the underlying reason for the poor weight gain. A baby whose growth was restricted by diminished placental function may show catch-up growth, the weight rising through the centiles on a growth chart (p. 52).

Length

The average length of a term baby is 51 cm, and 95% measure between 46 and 56 cm. Increase in length gives an indication of skeletal growth, but it is much more difficult to measure accurately than weight even if special apparatus is used. Little useful information is gained from measurement of length at intervals of less than 3 months. Measurements can vary by several centimetres depending on the techniques employed, so they have little value in predicting the future height of the child.

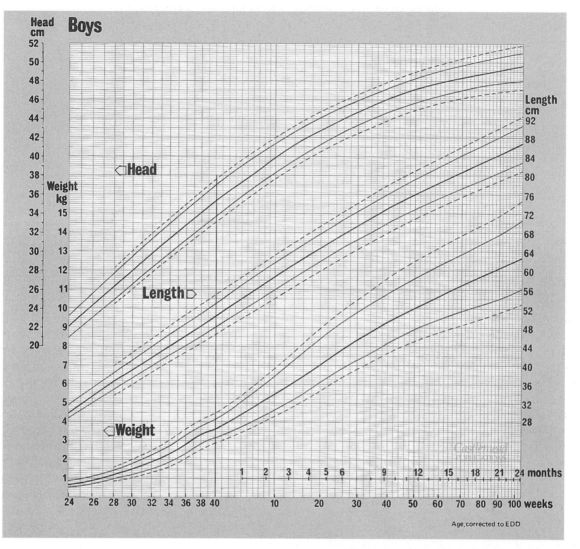

Figure 4.2   Growth chart showing the 3rd, 10th, 50th, 90th and 97th centiles for weight, length and head circumference from 24 weeks of gestation to 2 years of age. (By kind permission of Castlemead Publications.)

Length should be measured as carefully and accurately as possible at birth, to serve as a baseline against which to judge future growth. This should be done with the infant in the supine position, with the head held straight by one person and the legs held fully extended by another. The distance is measured between the topmost point of the head and the heels, with the feet held at a right angle to the table. A simple apparatus consists of a flat measuring mat with two end-plates at right angles to the base, one fixed at the end while the other slides along its length (Fig. 4.3). Simple tape measurements are very inaccurate, and measuring around the curves of the baby from crown to heel has no scientific validity and should not be performed.

Head circumference

The head circumference is the greatest measurement around the forehead and the occiput (the occipitofrontal circumference) and should be

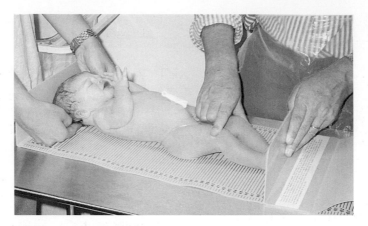

Figure 4.3 Simple apparatus for measurement of length at birth.

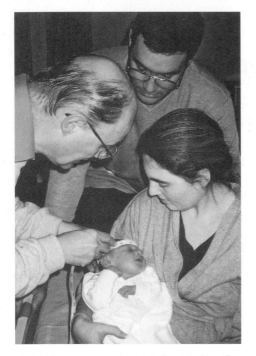

Figure 4.4 Measurement of occipitofrontal circumference after birth.

recorded 2 to 4 days after birth, when the effects of moulding during delivery have resolved (Fig. 4.4). The circumference normally lies between 33 and 37 cm, with an average of 35 cm, the head circumference centile being similar to those for weight and length. During the first month of life, the head circumference normally grows by about

0.5 cm per week. Abnormally rapid head growth may be seen from weekly charting of the head circumference, and, if accompanied by widened cranial sutures and increased tension of the anterior fontanelle, it may indicate raised intracranial pressure (p. 231). Too small a head may mean that the brain has not grown adequately and is a cardinal sign of microcephaly (p. 232). A head circumference within the normal range, however, is not a guarantee of normal development.

Table 4.1 shows average dimensions of babies at different gestational periods, and the growth chart in Figure 4.2 gives a guide to the changes in length, weight and head circumference usually seen in healthy infants from birth to 2 years of age, indicating the 3rd, 10th, 50th, 90th and 97th percentiles.

Growth charts

Several different charts have been devised which reflect the range of weight, length and head circumference of newborn babies at different gestational ages. The mean represents the centre of the range, with 1 and 2 standard deviations (SD) above and below it including the majority of measurements. Another way of plotting the figures is to indicate what percentage of babies fall below the defined line. In this method, the 50th centile line shows the figure below which half of the babies fall. Only 2% are below the 2nd centile line and only 2% are above the 98th centile. The further

Table 4.1 Average dimensions at different periods of gestation

Weeks of gestation	Weight g (±2 SD)	Length cm (±2 SD)	Head circumference cm (±2 SD)
24	700 (±200)	32 (±4)	22 (±2)
28	1200 (±350)	37 (±4)	26 (±2)
32	1800 (±500)	43 (±5)	30 (±2)
36	2700 (±800)	49 (±5)	33 (±2)
40	3600 (±750)	53 (±6)	35 (±2)

outside these extreme centiles a baby's measurement fall, the more likely is the infant to be abnormal or require investigation, but such variations from the commoner values must be interpreted in the light of many other factors.

Some guidance on the use of information from growth charts may be given as follows:

1. Those measurements more than 2.5 SD from the mean or beyond the 2nd to 98th centiles should be investigated.
2. It is unusual for weight, length and head circumference centiles at birth to be very different from one another.
3. The method of measurement – especially of length – can make a major difference to the centile value obtained.
4. Maternal short stature restricts the intrauterine growth of the fetus, while the offspring of larger mothers have a much greater range of sizes.
5. It is important to chart birth figures at the correct gestational age if it falls outside the range of 37 to 41 weeks. For convenience, it is appropriate for all healthy term infants to be charted at 40 weeks.

DISORDERS OF INTRAUTERINE GROWTH

Many babies are affected by one or more factors which alter fetal growth and leave them more vulnerable in the first few days of life to the consequences of the abnormal growth or its causes. The baby may be heavier or lighter than expected and may be assigned to one of several groups which are defined according to specific criteria.

Each group has its own causes and problems, which will be described.

Low birth weight babies

The birth weight of between 6% and 9% of babies born in Britain is below 2500 g and these babies are called 'low birth weight' (LBW) babies. Only about 1% of infants have a birth weight below 1500 g. Low birth weight is a major contributor to perinatal and neonatal mortality, with around 60% of perinatal deaths occurring in this group of infants. Its incidence rises to 10–12% in UK babies of mothers of Afro-Caribbean and Asian origin, which partly explains the higher perinatal mortality figures in these groups (p. 6) (Office of National Statistics 1999). Approximately half of all low birth weight babies have grown well for their period of gestation but are born before term (preterm babies), and, in general, the lower the birth weight in this group, the more preterm the infant is likely to be. The other half are more mature but have not grown as well as expected before birth. These are called light (or small) for dates babies (LFD or SFD). Although most perinatal statistics classify infants according to birth weight categories (Fig. 4.5), and the smaller the babies the higher the perinatal mortality and morbidity, preterm and light for dates babies have very different origins, problems and outcomes and thus are described separately. The effects of preterm birth are described in Chapters 8 and 9; however, those infants who have reached term but have suffered restricted intrauterine growth have the problems of light for dates infants and are discussed here.

The light for dates infant

Those babies whose weight, when plotted on a growth chart, lies below the 10th percentile for their gestational age are called light for dates infants. Such a baby may be preterm (less than 37 weeks of gestation), term (37–41 weeks) or post-term (more than 41 weeks). It is therefore necessary to assess the gestational age of an infant in order to put her into one of these categories, and the way this is done is described on page 108.

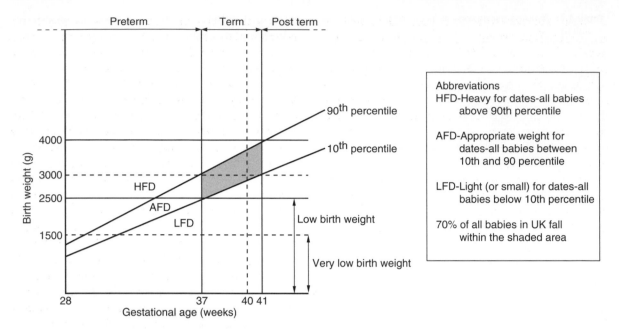

Figure 4.5 Categories of babies according to weight and maturity.

Intrauterine growth retardation is a clinical description of a state in which the infant at birth is malnourished or appears to have lost weight during the latter stages of the pregnancy.

There are several known factors which may cause an infant to be of unexpectedly low birth weight for the gestation period, and in some mothers more than one may apply (Ahluwalia et al 2001). These include:

- placental insufficiency, often associated with pre-eclampsia (p. 19)
- maternal chronic illness (p. 20)
- extreme maternal malnutrition
- maternal heavy smoking (p. 15) (Bonellie 2001)
- excess alcohol consumption in pregnancy (p. 16)
- congenital abnormalities
- maternal drug abuse (p. 17)
- congenital infections (p. 176)
- normal small babies from small mothers.

Congenital malformations and intrauterine infections (p. 176) can largely be excluded by clinical examination. In most light for dates infants, placental function will have been reduced often for several weeks, progressively preventing the transfer of adequate nutrients and oxygen to the fetus and impairing the excretion of waste products and CO_2. During labour and delivery, such babies are at increased risk of certain problems which may affect them in the neonatal period or impair their developmental progress later.

During uterine contractions, placental function ceases as blood flow to the organ is restricted. The reduction in transfer of oxygen may cause significant fetal hypoxia in labour, which may be associated with signs of fetal distress (p. 33). Birth asphyxia, the need for cardiorespiratory resuscitation at birth, prenatal passage of meconium into the liquor and meconium aspiration pneumonia are all more common in light for dates babies than in the well-grown infant, though none of these complications occurs frequently. Intrapartum asphyxia may also result in neonatal hypoxic-ischaemic encephalopathy. Fortunately, the majority of the infants will be well, and will behave and feed normally for their gestation, and hence will need little additional attention.

Because these babies are small, heat loss from the skin at birth is increased, and this can result in hypothermia and hypoglycaemia (p. 54).

These babies are often more polycythaemic than well-nourished infants since the mild chronic hypoxia which results from placental insufficiency causes a compensatory increase in red cell production before birth (p. 183). Occasionally, the blood is so viscous from the excessive number of red cells that the circulation becomes sluggish. In these circumstances, removal of some blood and replacement with human albumin improves the blood flow to vital organs (p. 184).

Some of these infants will also be preterm and they may need additional treatment for any of its complications (p. 120). However, the physiological stress of intrauterine growth retardation frequently accelerates the maturation of the lungs, and hyaline membrane disease is often less severe as a result.

Clinical features

A mature light for dates infant is shown in Plate 1. There is an appearance of wasting of soft tissues and a lack of subcutaneous fat, which are features of inadequate intrauterine nutrition. The skin is loose and rather dry, often peeling and discoloured, and there is little vernix. The ribs are easily seen and the abdomen may be hollowed, a feature sometimes identifiable by ultrasound examination before birth to demonstrate poor fetal growth. Scalp hair is sparse and the skull bones feel relatively hard. The head often appears large when compared with the size of the body, and the head circumference is on a higher percentile line on the growth chart than is the weight. The length centile is often comparable with the head circumference centile unless growth retardation has been particularly prolonged. The umbilical cord is thin and often yellowish-brown.

When over 1800 g, most of these infants are vigorous and active, with good muscle tone and a flexed posture at rest, since they are more mature, and they are often particularly hungry feeders.

Management after birth

During the first day or two of life, the light for dates infant is particularly prone to the closely related problems of hypothermia and hypoglycaemia.

A small thin baby will lose heat rapidly at birth. To counteract the potential fall of body temperature, such infants raise their heat production by increasing the rate of glucose metabolism. Blood glucose is used up in this process and, as the diminished liver glycogen stores in these infants are insufficient to replenish it, the baby becomes hypoglycaemic. Particular attention therefore should be paid to keeping the baby warm at birth and it may be necessary to nurse such infants in an incubator until their temperature is stable and they are feeding well (p. 80). Breast feeding should start as soon as possible after birth, feeds being given at least every 3–4 hours initially. Regular measurement of capillary blood glucose using a calibrated digital glucose meter should be done at 4-hourly intervals for the first day, then 8-hourly until 48 hours. A level below 2.5 mmol/L (35 mg/100 mL) at any time should be regarded as potentially hazardous and treated accordingly (see p. 54).

Feeding the light for dates infant

On average, an appropriately grown newborn requires 150–180 mL/kg/day (105–115 kcal/kg/day) of milk to thrive and grow. Malnourished light for dates infants require a calorie intake above this to enable their weight to catch up, and often such term infants are hungry feeders. If these infants are breast fed but do not seem satisfied with the quantities taken, they should be given additional formula milk by cup feeding after the breast feed, allowing them to determine the amount they take. The fully formula-fed baby should be offered an amount appropriate for a baby whose weight is somewhere nearer the average for the gestational age rather than using the baby's actual weight for the calculation. For example, a 38-week baby of only 2.4 kg birth weight (−2SD) might be fed with volumes calculated for a 2.8 kg baby (−1SD). A similarly increased intake can be achieved by feeding 70 mL/kg on the first day, rising to 200–220 mL/kg by day 5. These regimens will give the infant around 120–130 kcal/kg/day. Either of these modifications to the normal feeding schedule will enable the baby to make up for the calorie deprivation suffered before birth, but an occasional infant will not tolerate these increased amounts.

In most cases the modified regimen results in a period of accelerated weight gain which levels off when the baby nears her genetic centile on the growth chart.

Despite these measures, blood glucose values commonly fall to levels of 2 mmol/L (35 mg/100 mL) or below in the first 2 days. If clinical signs of hypoglycaemia, such as apnoeic attacks, lethargy, jitteriness, cyanosis or fits, appear, they must be treated immediately and vigorously to prevent brain damage (p. 158).

Prognosis

Whereas the mildly malnourished baby normally suffers no adverse long-term consequences, the very light for dates baby (less than the 5th percentile weight for gestation period) who has suffered significant malnutrition or hypoxia in the third trimester of pregnancy may grow slowly and remain small throughout childhood. Although severe neurological handicap or frank cerebral palsy is unlikely unless the infant was also very immature at birth, there is a greater chance of the individual developing mild learning difficulties in childhood and of the emergence of epilepsy. Other neurological disorders such as hyperactive or impulsive behaviour, dyspraxia and specific learning difficulties (e.g. dyslexia) are also more common. The development of adult chronic diseases such as hypertension, coronary artery disease, diabetes and obesity may all be longer-term consequences of intrauterine malnutrition (Eriksson et al 2000, Barker 2001).

The post-term infant

Prolongation of pregnancy beyond 41 weeks can sometimes be due to a variation in the feto-maternal physiology and result in a perfectly normal baby. On the other hand, it is also clear that the impairment of placental function which tends to take place after about 40 weeks' gestation results, in the most severe cases, in intrauterine death from malnutrition and asphyxia, or, in less serious cases, the delivery of a sick newborn infant. During labour there is a much higher risk of fetal distress (p. 33) and meconium staining, and the need for resuscitation is significantly greater in such babies. The baby presents a recognisable clinical picture. They are much thinner than normal; the skin is parchment-like, cracked and peeling, and, in severe cases, there is yellowish-green discoloration of the nails and umbilical stump. The thin face bears a worried expression. If she has not suffered the consequences of intrapartum asphyxia (p. 34), the baby appears unusually alert, restless and hungry for feeds. The haemoglobin content of the blood is relatively high, as a compensation for intrauterine hypoxia in the previous weeks. Hypoglycaemia, hypoxic-ischaemic encephalopathy from intrapartum asphyxia, and meconium aspiration pneumonia are common hazards after birth.

Antenatal ultrasound measurements can sometimes identify these infants, and the complications can be prevented by induction of labour at the optimal time. Where the gestation period is accurately known, induction of labour is usually undertaken before 42 weeks. More accurate methods for the assessment of fetal distress in the early stages have also helped to reduce the mortality from this cause (p. 33). Hypoglycaemia is the main immediate hazard and the baby should be treated along the same lines as the light for dates baby with intrauterine malnutrition. They require similarly increased nutrition (p. 51) and too show catch-up growth.

Infants of diabetic mothers

Although in the past the risk to the infant of a diabetic mother was high, the careful control of the condition before conception and during the pregnancy can bring down the risk to little more than that seen in normal infants of healthy mothers (Jensen et al 2000, Walkinshaw 2000). When the mother has been able to keep her blood glucose values within the normal range throughout most of the pregnancy, the baby will look quite normal at birth, but with higher average blood glucose values the infant will develop a characteristic physical appearance. The baby is often larger and heavier than the period of gestation would suggest, the umbilical cord is thickened and the appearance of the baby with its bulging cheeks, plethoric complexion and hirsuitism is reminiscent of Cushing's syndrome (Plate 2). The excess weight is due to a real increase in growth of the skeleton and internal organs, including the heart, as well as generalised excess fat deposition and fluid retention. It is sometimes possible to diagnose the pre-diabetic state in mothers who have borne babies of successively increasing birth weight.

Hazards to the infant are listed in Table 4.2, the main ones being as follows:

- Trauma during delivery can occur, particularly if the baby is of large size. This can be a fracture of the clavicle, which is often asymptomatic and found incidentally when a lump is noticed on the bone. More serious is damage to the cervical nerve roots which can occur during delivery of the neck if there is shoulder dystocia. The consequent Erb's palsy can take many months to abate and in some cases improvement is incomplete (p. 159).
- There is an increased incidence of congenital malformations, particularly of the heart (p. 221) and, much more rarely, sacral agenesis.
- Hypoglycaemia commonly occurs in the first few hours of life, resulting from overproduction of insulin by the baby's islets of Langerhans, which have hypertrophied because of maternal – and therefore fetal – hyperglycaemia. It has by far the most serious consequences of the neonatal complications of maternal diabetes and its prevention is paramount. It is common even if the mother's diabetes has been well controlled during the pregnancy (Agrawal et al 2000).
- Respiratory distress syndrome with all the clinical features seen in the preterm baby (p. 131) may occur.
- Polycythaemia is common and a dilution exchange may be required if the haematocrit rises above 70% (p. 184).
- Occasionally, hypocalcaemia may occur.
- Weight gain after birth is often less than normal and the infant's growth chart shows a falling weight centile. This is usually a natural adjustment to the child's genetic size, and so long as the infant is well and apparently feeding to her own satisfaction, there is usually no reason to intervene.

Table 4.2 Problems of the infant of a diabetic mother

System	Problems encountered
General	Birth trauma
	Macrosomia
	Heavy for dates birth weight
	Preterm birth
Congenital malformations	Doubled risk – especially in the heart
Respiratory	Respiratory distress syndrome
Heart	Cardiomegaly
	Transient hypertrophic cardiomyopathy
CNS	Seizures
	Hypotonia
	Lethargy
Metabolic	Hypoglycaemia
	Hypocalcaemia
Blood	Polycythaemia
Growth	Lag down growth

Management to prevent hypoglycaemia

Because of the high circulating insulin levels, the baby's blood glucose falls rapidly to a minimum value some 2 to 6 hours from the time of delivery. During this time, the baby should be cared for and monitored at the mother's bedside provided specialised neonatal care is immediately available if symptoms of hypoglycaemia appear. Breast or formula milk feeding should be started before 1 hour of age and continued at no more than 3-hourly intervals until the risk of hypoglycaemia is over. Additional feeds may be needed if the blood glucose falls. The blood glucose level should be checked before feeds every 2 hours in the first 12 hours, and thereafter every 8 hours until the end of the 2nd day. If the blood glucose value falls below 2.5 mmol/L (45 mg/dL), the treatment detailed below should be followed.

As these babies have plenty of stored liver glycogen, an intramuscular injection of glucagon 100 µg/kg body weight may raise the blood glucose level within 10 minutes if needed, but an additional feed should be given also – to prevent a further fall – about 30 minutes later. The hyperinsulinism usually resolves within 48 hours and it is unusual for hypoglycaemia to persist after the second day of life.

Hypoglycaemia

Glucose is the infant's major source of immediate energy and is necessary for all metabolic activity and growth. Most organs can cope with short periods of glucose deprivation, and some organs, e.g. muscles, utilise alternative energy sources such as lactate or fat for short periods. However, glucose is essential for the baby's brain, and without it, even for short periods, brain function may be affected or brain growth and development impaired. This may result in immediate central nervous system effects such as fits, hypotonia, lethargy or depressed consciousness; in the longer term, it may permanently impair brain function, leading to learning difficulties, cerebral palsy or epilepsy (Hawdon 1999, Cornblath & Schwartz 1999).

The blood glucose level is maintained within normal limits by the combination of regular intake of lactose and other simple sugars in the diet and the rapid utilisation of the glucose, to which all carbohydrates are converted before absorption into the blood. Any glucose beyond the baby's immediate needs is stored as glycogen in the liver or muscles, under the influence of insulin and other hormones. At times when circulating glucose is falling to low levels, this stored glycogen is rapidly reconverted to glucose to maintain normal blood glucose values. The hormones mainly responsible for this are adrenaline (epinephrine), growth hormone and cortisol. Under most normal circumstances, these mechanisms prevent a fall of the blood level to dangerous values, but occasionally the system fails and the blood glucose falls below normal. It is, therefore, of great importance to be aware of the situations in which this may occur, the clinical features of hypoglycaemia, and the methods of preventing and treating it.

Hypoglycaemia is common in infants in the first 48 hours of life. In normal babies, the blood glucose falls from the normal maternal levels before birth to levels around 3 mmol/L (55 mg/dL) in the first 2 days, rising again towards more normal levels after the third day, so long as the baby is receiving an adequate calorie intake. Although no baby is immune from the problem, certain groups of babies are more at risk of developing low blood glucose levels than others. There are two groups of such infants:

1. Infants with hyperinsulinism and plentiful stores of glycogen:
   —infants of diabetic mothers
   —babies of mothers with gestational diabetes.
2. Infants whose glycogen stores are limited or depleted:
   —babies with intrauterine growth retardation
   —preterm infants who are unable to feed adequately
   —infants with serious infections
   —babies deprived of enteral feeds (e.g. when the breast milk supply is inadequate)
   —hypothermic infants
   —certain babies with rare metabolic disorders.

In all such infants, regular measurement of capillary blood glucose should be carried out for the first 2 days of life and treatment given if the blood glucose falls significantly. Though it is difficult to define what constitutes an abnormal blood glucose level, any value below 2.5 mmol/L (45 mg/dL) should be regarded as significant hypoglycaemia whether the infant has symptoms or not. If clinical signs appear at all, they will consist of jitteriness, apnoea, lethargy, sleepiness, altered conscious level, cyanosis or fits. In many cases the signs are extremely subtle or may even be absent, but such asymptomatic hypoglycaemia is not benign and it should be taken just as seriously. As there are no symptoms, it can only be identified by testing the blood. Even if there are no symptoms, low blood glucose levels may cause brain damage, and the risk is greater if the baby has suffered asphyxia, is infected, or the hypoglycaemia is prolonged. Since there may be no clinical indication that the infant has a low blood glucose, it is necessary to consider the possibility and measure the blood level whenever any infant is in one of the risk groups or is behaving in any unusual way.

Prevention and treatment

Prevention of hypoglycaemia should be the aim in all babies. In higher-risk infants, a feed should be given within an hour of birth, by nasogastric tube if necessary, or an intravenous infusion of 10% dextrose should be established if the risk is assessed to be particularly high or gastric feeding is inappropriate. Giving the first feed to the normal infant within the first 4 hours and leaving no more than 4 hours between feeds will usually maintain a normal blood glucose level.

Exceptions to this include babies under an additional physiological stress such as hypothermia or infection and those suffering from significant intrauterine malnutrition. If despite these measures the blood glucose falls below 2.5 mmol/L (45 mg/dL), urgent action is needed to restore it to normal and maintain it there until its cause is resolved. An action plan is given in Table 4.3.

The risks from symptomatic hypoglycaemia are high, and vigorous intervention is required urgently. For asymptomatic babies, a more gentle approach is justified unless the measures fail to raise the blood glucose value rapidly. From the table it can be seen that if a baby has a fit or other symptoms clearly related to a low blood glucose value, an intravenous bolus of 10 mL/kg of 10% dextrose must be given urgently. This should be followed by a dextrose infusion at a rate of 60–90 mL/kg/day, or more if this does not raise the glucose level sufficiently. As the blood glucose level becomes more stable, the infusion rate should be slowed and feeds increased until a value in excess of 2.5 mmol/L (45 mg/dL) can be maintained by feeds alone.

By contrast, if a baby develops asymptomatic hypoglycaemia, she should be given an immediate feed of 15–20 mL/kg of breast or formula milk and the blood glucose measured again in an hour. If the level has risen above 2.5 mmol/L (40 mg/dL), a further check should be made before the next feed; if it does not, the infant must be assumed to be suffering from persistent hypoglycaemia and be given an intravenous infusion of 10% dextrose as for symptomatic babies. Glucagon and steroids are not usually effective in raising the blood glucose level in cases where glycogen stores are depleted but may be very useful in the infants of diabetic mothers.

Table 4.3 Management of neonatal hypoglycaemia

Outcome

It is usually possible to maintain the blood glucose at normal values by the means outlined above, and in most cases the hypoglycaemia resolves within 48 hours. Persistence of the condition despite these measures can rarely result from idiopathic hypertrophy of the insulin-producing cells in the pancreas, a condition known as nesidioblastosis, in which the severity and duration of the hypoglycaemia may have serious effects on brain development (Rahman & Kuhule 1999, Cresto et al 1998). Surgery may be required if the condition does not resolve.

After successful treatment of neonatal hypoglycaemia, all babies should be followed up to assess their development, considering the potential impact on their brain function.

The heavy for dates infant

Babies with a birth weight over the 90th percentile are termed *heavy for dates*. Most are simply well-grown infants of larger mothers or the consequence of poor control of maternal diabetes during the pregnancy. Some, however, have features rather like the offspring of diabetic mothers and behave in the same way, developing hypoglycaemia in the first day or two of life. This should be treated similarly. These babies should be allowed to breast feed on demand unless the development of hypoglycaemia calls for additional feeding. Formula-fed infants should be offered the full amount for their weight but they will frequently take less than this. Commonly, their weight gain over the first few months is less than expected and they fall towards their genetic centile on the growth chart, a feature which may occasionally be difficult to distinguish from failure to thrive caused by genuine underfeeding. Other rare causes of heavy for dates infants are Beckwith's syndrome and transposition of the great arteries.

Twins and higher-order births

Twinning happens about once every 80 births in the UK, though its incidence has increased recently as a result of the use of fertility treatments and ovulation-stimulating drugs. It can result either from the splitting of a single fertilised ovum in early pregnancy (monozygotic twins) or from the simultaneous fertilisation of two separate ova (dizygotic twins). There are considerable extra risks for the infants of any multiple pregnancy. Over half of all twins are of low birth weight. Premature labour is common, and each infant is subject to the complications of prematurity, the risks being greater if the twins were a result of assisted conception (Zuppa et al 2001). Breech position for one twin is frequent and may add to the risk of asphyxia. As a result of these risks, the perinatal mortality for twins, particularly the second-born baby, is significantly greater than that in singletons (Hacking et al 2001), but appears not to be significantly greater in the short term than for higher-order births (Suri et al 2001). The incidence of congenital malformations is approximately double that in singleton births, and birth trauma is more common, particularly to the second twin. One member of the pair commonly has a poorer share of available nutrition in utero as a result of placental insufficiency, is born with all the signs of fetal malnutrition (Plate 3), and is therefore at greater risk of asphyxia during labour (p. 33). As a result of this, there is a higher incidence of cerebral palsy in twins than in singleton births, though, in contrast to the mortality statistics, it occurs equally in the first and second baby.

Occasionally there is a connection between the circulations of the two twins in the placenta. This can result in cross-transfusion of blood between the two fetuses, giving rise to a high haemoglobin level and polyhydramnios in one baby and anaemia and growth retardation with a diminished liquor volume in the other. In severe cases, repeated aspiration of excess amniotic fluid may prolong the pregnancy and thus reduce the risks from premature delivery. After birth, the polycythaemic twin runs into more difficulty from the increased blood volume and consequent cardiac strain than the anaemic one. If the polycythaemic twin has a packed cell volume of over 70%, a dilution exchange transfusion using 20 mL/kg body weight of plasma is often advisable to reduce the blood viscosity and improve blood flow (p. 184). The anaemic twin may occasionally need a top-up blood transfusion if she becomes symptomatic from the physiological fall of haemoglobin which occurs in all infants over the first few weeks of life (p. 184) (Cincotta et al 2000, Seng & Rajadurai 2000).

Feeding of twins

There is no reason why both twins should not be breast fed so long as the mother is producing enough milk to maintain adequate growth of the babies. The mother may wish to feed one from one breast and then the second baby on the other side, or feed both of them at the same time (Fig. 4.6). Sometimes there may not be enough milk for both infants, and supplements of formula milk must then be given. The babies may be given the breast and a formula feed alternately or a part breast and part cup feed on each occasion. So long as the infants are contented and growing, the method of coping with the feeding is not crucial. The principles of good breast feeding are, however, more important, since inevitably there is unlikely to be much excess milk when two infants are partaking.

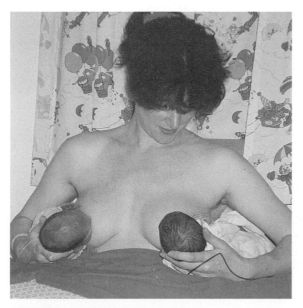

Figure 4.6 Tandem feeding of twins.

If the infants are preterm, either or both may have any of the usual perinatal complications and they may recover at different rates. Cerebral palsy occurs much more frequently in twins than in singleton babies and may only affect one of the pair.

Caring for twins

On the whole, it is probably better to keep the twins together until they are both ready to be discharged, since it is inevitably more difficult to visit the twin who remains in hospital. However, since one of the pair may need additional treatment for a congenital abnormality, this is not always possible and it can cause the parents to have a difference of approach to the two infants. It can also be particularly difficult for the parents if one of the twins dies, since they will then have to cope simultaneously with the joy of having the surviving infant and the grief over the one who has died. Each set of parents will handle this difficult situation differently and it requires a particular sensitivity on the part of the professionals involved to recognise and help the parents with these dual emotions. Many parents find help and assistance from joining a local twins club and in the UK there is a national organisation which can also give advice.

Triplets and more

The problems encountered in these higher-order births are similar to those of twins, although the greater the number of babies, the more likely they are to be preterm and the more immature they will be. There is, of course, a higher risk of one or more of the infants dying and the family may be faced with a multiple bereavement, perhaps with one or more of the surviving infants having a risk of permanent handicap. For example, the risk of cerebral palsy in triplet survivors is about 7%. In many instances, such pregnancies are the result of in-vitro fertilisation and thus are conceived after a period of infertility, which adds to the confused emotions such families suffer. Fortunately, improved techniques have reduced the risk of such large numbers of fetuses growing and this problem may diminish as further experience is gained.

REFERENCES

Agrawal R K, Lui K, Gupta J M 2000 Neonatal hypoglycaemia in infants of diabetic mothers. Journal of Paediatrics and Child Health 36(4):354–356

Ahluwalia I B, Merrit R, Beck L F et al 2000 Multiple lifestyle and psychosocial risks and delivery of small for gestational age infants. Obstetrics and Gynecology 97(5):649–656

Barker D J 2001 A new model for the origins of chronic disease. Medical Health Care Philosophy 4(1):31–35

Bonellie S R 2001 Effect of maternal age, smoking and deprivation on birthweight. Paediatric and Perinatal Epidemiology 15(1):19–26

Cincotta R B, Gray P H, Phythian G et al 2000 Long term outcome of twin-twin transfusion syndrome. Archives of Disease in Childhood Fetal and Neonatal Edition 83(3):F171–F176

Cornblath M, Schwartz R 1999 Outcome of neonatal hypoglycaemia: complete data are needed. British Medical Journal 318:194–195

Cresto J C, Abdenur J P, Bergada I et al 1998 Long term follow up of persistent hyperinsulinaemic hypoglycaemia of infancy. Archives of Disease in Childhood 79(5):440–444

Eriksson J, Forsen T, Tuomilehto J et al 2000 Fetal and childhood growth and hypertension in adult life. Hypertension 36(5):790–794

Grosso L M, Rosenberg K D, Belanger K et al 2001 Maternal caffeine intake and intrauterine growth retardation. Epidemiology 12(4):447–455

Hacking D, Watkins A, Fraser S et al 2001 Respiratory distress syndrome and birth order in premature twins. Archives of Disease in Childhood Fetal and Neonatal Edition 84(2):F117–F121

Hawdon J M 1999 Hypoglycaemia and the neonatal brain. European Journal of Pediatrics 158(Suppl 1):S9–S12

Jensen D M, Sorensen B, Feilberg-Jorgensen N et al 2000 Maternal and perinatal outcomes in 143 Danish women with gestational diabetes mellitus and 143 controls with a similar risk profile. Diabetic Medicine 17(4):281–286

Office of National Statistics 1999 DH3 No 32. HMSO, London

Rahman A R, Kuhule U 1999 Management and short term outcome of persistent hyperinsulinaemic hypoglycaemia of infancy (nesidioblastosis). Singapore Medical Journal 40(3):151–156

Seng Y C, Rajadurai V S 2000 Twin-twin transfusion syndrome: a five year review. Archives of Disease in Childhood Fetal and Neonatal Edition 83(3):F168–F170

Suri K, Bhandari V, Lerer T et al 2001 Morbidity and mortality of preterm twins and higher order births. Journal of Perinatology 21(5):293–299

Walkinshaw S A 2000 Very tight versus tight control for diabetes in pregnancy. Cochrane Database of Systematic Reviews (2):CD000226

Zuppa A A, Maragliano G, Scapillati M E et al 2001 Neonatal outcome of spontaneous and assisted twin pregnancies. European Journal of Obstetrics Gynaecology and Reproductive Biology 95(1):68–72

Chapter 5

Clinical assessment of the newborn baby

CHAPTER CONTENTS

Introduction 59
Inspection at birth 60
   Signs which may indicate a sick baby 60
   Selection of babies for admission to
   the neonatal unit 60
   Routine nursing observations 61
General examination of the baby 61
   Observation of the baby as a whole 61
Systematic examination of the baby 61
   The skin 61
   Head and neck 63
   Chest 67
   The heart and circulation 67
   Abdomen 68
   Genitalia 69
   Spine 69
   Limbs 70
   Dislocation of joints 70
Neurological assessment 71
   Normal behaviour and response
   to environment 72
   Wakefulness and sleep 72
   Sucking 72
   Crying 72
   Formal neurological assessment 72
   Interpreting the neurological examination 75
Testing the baby's hearing 75
Laboratory screening tests 76
Biochemistry of the neonate 77

INTRODUCTION

Since most babies are healthy, have no congenital malformations and behave normally, it may be thought that routine medical examination is an unimportant chore. However, this is far from true (Box 5.1). An accurate record of the health of the baby at birth is vital as a baseline for the regular child health and development checks which will occur throughout childhood. It should be recorded in the baby's Child Health and Development Record which the parents will keep at home (Dunn 2001). The ongoing routine baby health checks and immunisations will all be recorded in this document.

Routine examination at 24–48 hours of age identifies most babies who need further observation, investigation or treatment, though some serious malformations of the heart and renal tracts cannot be identified at this stage. It can also alert medical and nursing staff to areas of concern about the relationship between the mother and her infant.

Box 5.1 Purposes of the routine examination of newborn babies

- To check the growth, health and behaviour of the baby
- To confirm the infant's maturity
- To identify any effects of birth on the baby
- To detect congenital malformations
- To recognise the ill baby and institute treatment
- To inform the parents of any problems the baby may have or reassure them that the baby is healthy
- To provide the initial information for the child's ongoing health record

---

For the examination to be effective, it must be carried out by an adequately trained practitioner with full knowledge of the mother's medical history, especially those factors that can adversely affect fetal development (p. 203) (Lee et al 2001). There may be a family history of a genetic disorder and prenatal diagnosis may have been performed (p. 21). The mother herself may have had a complication of the pregnancy or a medical condition which could cause a malformation, alter fetal growth or affect the health of the newborn baby (p. 27).

The mother's age, the family structure and the support available from others will be noted from the social history, and further discussion with the parents at this point may reveal previously undisclosed facts which could affect the health or care of the baby.

The examination also gives the opportunity to explore any concerns the parents may have and to discuss the routine immunisation schedule, about which an increasing number of parents have questions. Maternal doubts, concerns and uncertainties are common at this stage and it is a unique opportunity to answer genuine questions and identify those areas of concern which will need further discussion (Wolke, Dave et al 2002).

INSPECTION AT BIRTH

A brief examination of the baby should be carried out immediately after delivery to confirm the sex and identify any visible abnormalities such as spina bifida, cleft lip, cleft palate or talipes, and to identify conditions requiring urgent attention such as anal atresia which may not be immediately obvious. It is important to provide a sympathetic initial explanation to the parents about any major defect noted at this time. If the baby is vigorous, alert and well, he should be given to the mother and fuller examination should be left until 24–48 hours of age. If it is clear that the baby is unwell or needs more urgent attention, this should be explained to the parents; however, so long as the infant is well enough, it is more important for the parents to see, touch and hear their child at this time than to carry out nursing or medical tasks.

Signs which may indicate a sick infant

Following the birth, there may be an indication that the baby is not completely healthy. Signs that may indicate a serious underlying condition include:

- a delay in the onset of breathing
- grunting respiration
- tachypnoea
- cyanosis
- hypotonia
- hypothermia
- pallor.

They should all be taken seriously and their cause diagnosed if necessary by investigation in the neonatal unit.

Selection of babies for admission to the neonatal unit

In general, newborn babies should be allowed to stay with their mothers unless some action needs to be taken for which facilities are available only in the neonatal unit. Babies at high risk of developing serious illness or needing highly trained nursing should be cared for in a special unit, but ideally services should provide as much care as possible on the postnatal wards. For example, most babies requiring phototherapy for jaundice or observation for hypoglycaemia and some needing tube feeding can be nursed at their mother's side and those with uncomplicated congenital malformations should not be removed.

There is no justification for admission for observation alone, since even temporary separation can interfere with the growth of the normal parent–child relationship and the development of good parenting. It may also reduce the chance of successful breast feeding and give the parents the incorrect impression that their baby will continue to be frail or vulnerable after discharge from the unit. Although the exact criteria for admission will vary from one unit to another, babies with the following conditions are at sufficient risk to justify separation from their mothers:

1. Immediately:
   —under 1800 g birth weight

—less than 34 weeks of gestation
—respiratory symptoms such as grunting, tachypnoea or costal recession
—severe rhesus haemolytic disease.

2. As symptoms appear:
—symptoms from a congenital abnormality
—convulsions
—persistent vomiting or abdominal distension
—hypoglycaemia which does not respond to oral or nasogastric feeding
—any ill baby (pp. 60 and 167).

For some infants, such as those who are dying, an individual decision about where and how to care for the baby will need to be made, remembering to take account of and respect the parents' wishes (p. 244).

Routine nursing observations

During the first few hours, it is necessary to note that the baby passes urine and meconium, to observe the heart rate and the infant's breathing and to check the rectal temperature to exclude hypothermia.

GENERAL EXAMINATION OF THE BABY

The first formal examination of the baby should always be carried out in the presence of the mother and she should undress and dress the baby so that her confidence in handling the infant and how she relates to him can be assessed. It also gives an opportunity to discuss with the mother any concerns she may have about the baby. The examination must be performed by an experienced doctor or midwife with knowledge of the normal infant and with an understanding of the range of normal findings and able to distinguish those which are benign from those with medical significance. At or after the examination, reassurance should be given about features related to the birth – such as superficial bruising, including forceps marks on the face (Plate 4), a caput succedaneum, moulding of the head or suction cap marks (Plate 5) – which will resolve leaving no lasting

effect on the baby, and about any minor anomalies which will not affect the baby's health.

Observation of the baby as a whole

The growth and state of nutrition of the baby can be assessed both by observation and by plotting the weight, length and head circumference on standard growth charts suitable for the ethnic group from which the baby comes. Most well-grown babies will have a moderate covering of fat, but this is greatly increased in poorly controlled maternal diabetes mellitus (p. 52). By contrast, the baby who has suffered from late intrauterine malnutrition will be noticeably thin, though often head growth is spared and the head circumference centile may be greater than the weight centile (p. 50). More prolonged fetal growth retardation can result in a small but apparently healthy baby with reduction of all parameters of growth, the degree of which may only be seen when the figures are plotted on the growth chart (p. 48).

SYSTEMATIC EXAMINATION OF THE BABY
The skin
Colour

Usually, in mature infants from white ethnic groups, the skin is pale over the body but in the first 24–48 hours the hands and feet may be slightly cyanosed. Thereafter its colour varies markedly from pale during sleep to deep red while crying vigorously. Central cyanosis, jaundice or unusual pallor should always be regarded as abnormal and investigated. In darker-skinned infants, such features may be seen only on the mucous membranes, particularly in the mouth. Darker racial colouring, particularly in babies of mixed race, may not be obvious at birth, but the scrotum is often noticeably pigmented.

Superficial skin peeling

In the first week, the superficial skin of the hands and feet often peels. It is most common in post-term babies or those who have suffered intrauterine malnutrition (p. 50). It requires no treatment and gives no indication of the future condition of the baby's skin.

Milia

The whitish pinhead-sized spots, often seen on or around the nose, are known as milia. They are tiny sebaceous retention cysts which last for only a few weeks and resolve without treatment.

Subcutaneous fat necrosis

This is a localised area of induration, usually on the back but sometimes over the face or thighs. The skin over the area has a blotchy reddened appearance and seems to be attached to hardened fat below it. Sometimes it may result from trauma – for example, following forceps delivery – but often there is no recognisable cause. It has no serious significance and gradually resolves spontaneously within the first year

Traumatic cyanosis

This is a term used to describe the appearance of cyanosis confined to the face and head resulting from masses of tiny petechial haemorrhages in the skin. It occurs after there has been congestion of the head, and is often due to partially obstructed delivery or a tight umbilical cord around the neck. It is usually harmless and resolves within a few days.

Urticaria neonatorum (Plate 6)

Urticaria neonatorum, or erythema toxicum, is very common in the first few weeks of life. It occurs mainly on the trunk and consists of rapidly varying irregular blotchy red patches or yellowish pinhead spots resembling pustules surrounded by a round flare of erythema. The spots are sterile and contain eosinophil cells. The baby is apparently unaffected by the spots and, although alarming in appearance, the rash is harmless. Its cause is uncertain and it disappears usually within a few days.

Occasionally, transient skin flushing of one half of the infant occurs with a clear demarcation down the midline separating it from the normal half. Known as the harlequin change, this odd phenomenon has no serious significance and rapidly resolves.

Birthmarks

'Mongolian blue spots' (Plate 7)   One or more well-defined irregular patches of bluish-black discoloration of the skin over the lower back occurs in up to 70% of darker-skinned babies and up to 10% of ethnic white infants (Cordova 1981). These dermal melanocytic naevi, known as Mongolian blue spots, can be mistaken for bruising but do not change in the neonatal period. They eventually fade during childhood.

Pigmented naevi   Pigmented naevi are rare but can be very large and multiple and may be hairy (Plate 8). Their presence can be very shocking to the parents and have a long-lasting psychological impact (Koot et al 2000). They are formed from abnormal dermal melanocytes and eventually become malignant in up to 30% of cases (Ammed et al 2001). Excision and skin grafting during childhood is often recommended, but it may not eliminate the risk of malignant change. Pigmented moles do not occur at birth, nor are marks such as café-au-lait spots or depigmented patches present until later in infancy. Thus, the diagnoses of neurofibromatosis and tuberous sclerosis, both of which are inherited conditions, cannot be reliably excluded by neonatal examination.

Haemangiomas   Haemangiomas are formed by abnormal proliferation of blood vessels in the skin which produce a patch of dicoloration. Some are transient and benign while others can have more serious significance. Especially when such lesions affect the face, parents will need much support and reassurance (p. 241).

'Stork marks', 'pressure marks' or 'salmon patches'   These are names traditionally given to the reddish-purple superficial capillary haemangiomas seen in about one-third of normal babies. They occur over the midline of the lower forehead just above the nose, on the nape of the neck, and sometimes on the upper eyelids.

The facial marks always fade within the first year but those on the neck may remain for life.

Port-wine stains   The port-wine naevus is a flat and dark reddish-purple capillary haemangioma. The overlying skin may be coarse and thickened. Occasionally such lesions are associated with a similar intracranial haemangioma on the same side. This can be familial and is known as the Sturge–Weber syndrome. It can cause developmental delay and epilepsy. Laser therapy can reduce the colour to some extent, but this is not usually advised in infancy, and careful cosmetic covering is often the best solution.

Strawberry marks   Since the 'strawberry mark' (Plate 9) is rarely present at birth, it cannot strictly be called a birthmark; it develops in the first week or two as a small bright red spot which enlarges to a variable extent during the first 3–6 months, forming a raised vivid red mottled capillary haemangioma, occasionally with an underlying subcutaneous cavernous haemangioma extending beyond its margins. After this it gradually regresses by flattening and becoming paler and most become barely visible by the age of 8 years. In preterm infants these naevi are more commonly multiple. Because they resolve so completely, the best treatment is to leave them strictly alone. But if, for example, the enlarging lesion will obstruct the baby's eyes, early excision or laser therapy is justified to ensure the normal development of his sight.

As such blemishes and disfigurements are distressing to parents, it is very important for nursing staff to give the family increased support, especially if the lesions are on the baby's face. They should try to build up parental confidence by encouraging them to see how beautiful their baby is, despite the birthmarks (p. 242).

Head and neck

The skull and head

The bones of the skull, being relatively soft and connected only by fibrous tissue, alter in shape readily in response to external pressure. The mode of presentation can often be deduced from the moulding that has taken place, the vertex being prominent in cephalic delivery but rather flattened after a breech birth. These changes are more marked in infants of primipara than multipara and are sometimes accompanied by overriding of the cranial bones. The *caput succedaneum* is the oedematous thickening of the scalp in the presenting area, which is more obvious after prolonged labour and disappears within 2 days.

The *anterior fontanelle* is a diamond-shaped depression at the point where the frontal and parietal bones converge, and may measure anything from 0.5 cm to 5 cm across. Normally it is slightly concave and may visibly pulsate, whereas if there is abnormally raised intracranial pressure, it becomes first tense, then convex. The sagittal suture passes from the posterior angle towards the occiput, and the coronal sutures continue from the lateral angles towards the ears. Their position is identifiable, but there is not usually a palpable gap between the bones. A persistent metopic suture (felt as a gap running forward from the anterior fontanelle and dividing the frontal bone) is common. If the sutures are palpably separated, hydrocephalus should be excluded by ultrasound examination of the ventricles (p. 232) or regular plotting of the head circumference.

A softening of the skull bones along the margins of the sutures is known as craniotabes. The bones indent easily but spring back to their normal shape. It is a common normal finding; however, when it is more generalised, it may be a sign of one of the rare disorders of bone calcification like osteogenesis imperfecta or early rickets. In the rare condition of cleidocranial dysostosis, the fontanelle may be 10 cm in diameter and the sutures 2 cm wide from a dysplasia of the membrane bone of which the skull is formed. The clavicles are also impalpable and their absence can be confirmed on a chest X-ray.

Cephalhaematoma   This localised subperiosteal collection of blood is a common occurrence and often follows a normal delivery with no apparent trauma. It develops over the first few days as a soft fluctuant swelling, usually over one of the parietal bones of the skull. It is strictly confined to the area of the bone concerned and within a few days a hard rim can be felt at its edge, giving a false impression that there is a hole in the skull. It is gradually absorbed and becomes firmer and smaller until it disappears entirely by the age of 3 months. Very occasionally the whole swelling becomes calcified and forms a hard, bony protuberance which takes over a year to absorb. No treatment is required and on no account should aspiration be attempted. In a small proportion of cases, a fracture of the underlying skull can be found on X-ray.

Plagiocephaly   After moulding of the skull has disappeared, only minor asymmetry of the cranial vault usually remains, but it is not uncommon to see asymmetry of the chin and mandible so that the alveolar margin is not quite parallel to that of the maxilla. This appears to be the effect of the baby's posture in utero. It usually resolves but may occasionally persist as malocclusion into later childhood.

There is an unexplained tendency for some infants to prefer lying with their head slightly rotated towards one side more than the other, and this may lead to postural deformity descriptively termed 'parallelogram skull' or plagiocephaly, with flattening of one side of the occiput and the opposite frontal region and face (Fig. 5.1). It becomes more noticeable towards the end of the first month and increases to a maximum towards the ninth month, after which symmetry returns over the next 2 years. Treatment is usually not needed, though some units use head turning, helmets or band therapy to accelerate recovery (Ellenbogen et al 2000). It is important to distinguish it from unilateral craniosynostosis – the much rarer asymmetry resulting from premature fusion of one of the coronal sutures in the first few weeks with consequent lack of growth on that side. In this condition, the whole of the side of the vault appears to be shorter from back to front than the other side, and the fused sutures can be seen on an X-ray. Early surgical treatment may be necessary to prevent further deformity.

The face

The appearance of most babies reflects the characteristics of both the family and racial group from which they come. Some infants, however, have a group of facial features which are obviously unusual, the best-known example being the child with Down syndrome. There are many such dysmorphic syndromes and each baby should be investigated (p. 209) since some are genetically determined and associated with developmental delay. Examples of such features are shown in Box 5.2.

Hair

The fine facial and body hair known as *lanugo* (Plate 10), which is a feature of preterm infants and is more common in dark-skinned infants

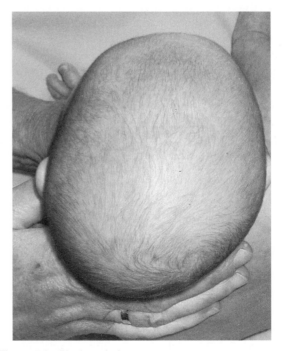

Figure 5.1 Plagiocephaly.

Box 5.2 Examples of facial dysmorphic features

- Epicanthic folds
- Upturned nose
- Downturned mouth
- Small, simple or low-set ears
- Prominent eyebrows
- Upslanted eyes
- Long philtrum

at term, is gradually lost during the first month along with some scalp hair. In ethnic white babies, the hair colour at birth may not reflect its eventual shade.

Nose

The nose varies in width and depth of the nasal bridge and it frequently forms epicanthic folds over the inner borders of the eyes, giving the false impression that the baby has a squint. Most babies can only breathe through the nose, and if breathing seems difficult, obstruction of the nasal passages from choanal atresia should be excluded by passing a fine polythene tube through the nose into the pharynx (p. 219).

Ears

The upper margin of the ears should be at the same level as the eyes and complex in form. Occasionally, accessory auricles, in the form of small pedunculated skin tags, may be seen in front of the ears. These can be dealt with by tying them off at the base (Fig. 5.2).

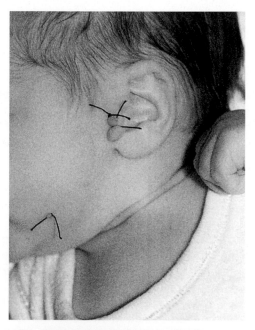

Figure 5.2 Preauricular skin tags showing ties.

Eyes

Vision The term infant can see from the first day of life and it is possible to demonstrate that the eyes follow a moving object or turn towards the light. Fixation of the gaze is at first slow and patience is required to show that it is present at all. Gradually it improves, and the baby obviously fixes and follows with the eyes at about 6 weeks of age. It is worth noting that a human face is often followed some time before a brightly coloured object or a light.

Eye movements Eye movements are at first poorly coordinated and the eyes may sometimes move independently, producing a squint. However, it is only a persistent squint which requires urgent referral for surgical correction to prevent permanent loss of binocular vision since the majority resolve spontaneously. The pupils react to light from birth. Tears are rarely seen during crying in the newborn baby.

Visual inspection of the eyes Formal examination of the eyes can be difficult and little useful information can be obtained if they are forced open. Holding the baby upright often results in spontaneous opening of the eyes. Their size and position and the angle of the palpebral fissures should be noted. The iris should form a complete circle around a black pupil.

Neonatal eye abnormalities are listed in Table 5.1. Crescentic subconjunctival haemorrhages are often seen on the sclerae around the margins of the iris, particularly after a difficult

Table 5.1 Visible abnormalities on neonatal eye examination

Abnormality	Common causes
Haemorrhages and abrasions	Birth/trauma or forceps damage
Crusting or discharge	Infection (p. 166)
Squint or nystagmus	Eye muscle imbalance
Microphthalmia	Isolated congenital abnormality
Macrophthalmia	Congenital glaucoma (p. 233)
Hypertelorism	Congenital dysmorphic syndrome (p. 209)
Colobomata of the iris	Congenital malformation or syndrome
White or grey pupil	Cataract or retinoblastoma
Retinopathy	Congenital infection (p. 176) Genetic retinopathy

vaginal delivery, but they are benign and resolve within 2–3 weeks. More rarely, orbital haemorrhage may result in proptosis of the eye, but spontaneous reabsorption of the haemorrhage almost always occurs without any residual damage. Forceps injury to the cornea may very occasionally produce permanent corneal opacities, and haemorrhage into the anterior chamber may cause a secondary glaucoma.

Sticky and crusted eyes commonly occur in normal infants, but pus indicates an infection which needs urgent attention (p. 166). The following eye abnormalities may eventually result in impaired vision and should be referred to an ophthalmologist to assess the cause and the impact on the baby's vision.

Shining a torch from 2 ft (0.61 m) straight into the eyes should give a point of light reflected in the same position in both pupils. If it is not, the baby may have a squint. A fixed squint or nystagmus is always abnormal. A grey or white pupil, or loss of a red reflex on shining the light into the eye may indicate that cataracts are present (p. 233). Congenital glaucoma (p. 233) causes the eyes to be unusually large.

Ophthalmoscopy Examination of the optic fundi should be carried out when other congenital abnormalities are found, to identify associated eye defects. The normal neonatal fundus is pale with a greyish tinge and is relatively streaky, especially at the periphery, but the appearance of the disc and vessels is similar to that in the older child. Congenital infections (p. 176) often cause a retinopathy. Examination is much easier if each pupil is dilated with cyclopentolate hydrochloride.

The mouth

The mouth is normally held closed and should open symmetrically. If it is drawn to one side during crying, this may indicate a facial palsy. A small receding jaw may cause feeding difficulties. To exclude a cleft, the palate is best examined while the infant is crying (Plate 11) since it is often difficult to depress the tongue sufficiently with a spatula. Small white retention cysts on the palate, known as Ebstein's pearls, are common

normal findings which require no treatment. Rarely, a submucosal mucus retention cyst under the tongue, called a ranula, may be seen. An epulis is a firm fibrous swelling protruding from the gum margin, which may interfere with feeding and require surgical excision.

Tongue tie is uncommon and is only significant if the frenulum is so short it causes limitation of movement sufficient to interfere with sucking or later speech development. Where a thickened frenulum grooves the tongue tip and obviously limits protrusion or upward movement, it may require surgical division.

Macroglossia A large protruding tongue can be a feature of congenital hypothyroidism (p. 212), but is more likely to be an isolated normal feature. It may form part of Beckwith's syndrome (p. 56). Tongue darting is common in Down syndrome but occurs in some healthy infants also.

Rounded thickened areas on the middle part of the upper lip are known as sucking blisters. They are not true blisters as they contain no fluid, and resolve without treatment.

Teeth The eruption of one or more lower incisor teeth before or soon after birth occurs about once in 2000 births. They are usually loose and do not interfere with feeding, so, unless they are obviously about to become detached, they may safely be left alone.

The neck

The neck is commonly rather short at this time but it should be fully mobile. Webbing of the neck posteriorly and an excess of skin at the nape of the neck commonly accompany some chromosome disorders such as Turner's syndrome (p. 209). In other cases, an X-ray may identify anomalies of the cervical vertebrae. The clavicles should be palpated to identify fractures which may occur during difficult deliveries.

Sternomastoid tumour Some babies prefer to hold the head to one side and in most cases it simply results from an unusual intrauterine posture. Occasionally it results from a diffuse or localised firm rounded swelling in the middle third of the sternomastoid muscle, known as a sternomastoid tumour. These develop some days or weeks after birth and may follow a difficult delivery involving traction to the head. This swelling may be due to interference with the circulation in the muscle. The lump resolves after about 2–4 months, but it may be accompanied by a degree of torticollis which seldom lasts beyond the first birthday. Physiotherapy is often used in treatment, with stretching of the involved muscle, but its efficacy is uncertain. Surgical correction may be required if the shortening of the muscle causes head tilt beyond the first year.

Other cervical swellings such as *dermoid cysts* and *thyroglossal cysts* are uncommon but show as midline swellings, whereas *branchial cysts* or sinuses appear just in front of the upper third of the sternomastoid muscle.

Chest

The ribs slope downwards less in the newborn than in later childhood and thus the chest is relatively deeper from back to front and narrower from side to side. They are soft and are easily indrawn during respiration, particularly if it is laboured or the lungs are stiff. The normal infant breathes more with the diaphragm than with the thorax, which can appear to be rather distended and barrelled.

The healthy sleeping baby breathes at about 20 breaths per minute, but apnoeic pauses of up to 12 seconds due to immaturity of the respiratory centre are common. The carbon dioxide builds up during the apnoeic phase and stimulates the respiratory centre to trigger breathing again. Provided these pauses are not associated with bradycardia or cyanosis, they are harmless and will cease spontaneously within a few weeks.

On auscultation the breath sounds are bronchovesicular, being similar in pitch and duration during both inspiration and expiration. Watching the baby's breathing pattern identifies most abnormalities and conditions affecting the lungs. Tachypnoea, grunting on expiration, or indrawing of the sternum, intercostal spaces or ribs on inspiration are common indicators of many lung diseases. An X-ray is often needed to clarify the underlying cause (p. 42) as little useful additional information is gained from other conventional

techniques of lung examination in these circumstances. Fine râles (crackles) may occasionally be present if a part of the lung is consolidated. Localised dullness on percussion is sometimes present when there is complete collapse of one lobe, or hyperresonance with a major pneumothorax, but even then this investigation can be misleading. Detection of mediastinal shift by an alteration in the site of the maximal heart sounds is often more useful diagnostically.

Breasts

At term in both sexes, a firm nodule of breast tissue 6–8 mm in diameter can be felt under the nipple, which may become engorged and even produce a little colostrum after the third day of life, due to changes in hormonal balance after birth. It usually resolves within a few weeks but may occasionally last a few months. No treatment is needed for the engorgement, and expression of the breasts should be avoided as it predisposes to the development of infective mastitis which requires antibiotic treatment (p. 165).

The heart and circulation

The heart lies relatively transversely and if the apex can be detected (which is difficult by palpation) it is in the midclavicular line in the left fourth intercostal space. There is often an easily palpable parasternal cardiac pulsation at this stage, due to the dominance of the right ventricle during intrauterine life.

The heart rate should be counted using a stethoscope over the heart. It is extremely variable, especially over the first 2 days. The usual resting rate at birth is about 180 beats per minute, but subsequently between 80 and 120 beats per minute is normal. It may rise with stress and activity up to 200 beats per minute.

Sustained rates below 80 beats per minute or above 200 beats per minute are uncommon. Persistent bradycardia may indicate congenital heart block, and high rates a supraventricular tachycardia. Both require investigation and treatment (p. 221). By contrast, occasional benign premature beats causing an irregularity of heart rhythm occur in 1% of normal babies and rarely cause problems.

Auscultation should be carried out while the baby is quiet. The first and second heart sounds are of about equal intensity at both the apex and the base of the heart. Transient soft systolic heart murmurs can be heard in about 50% of all infants at some time in the first week. They are thought to arise from variations in the dynamics of the circulation, or an incompletely closed ductus arteriosus. A persistent cardiac murmur is a common indication of a congenital cardiac malformation, though in many septal defects the murmur cannot be heard until the second week or later (p. 225). *The pulse* is best felt either at the elbow from the brachial artery or in the groin from the femoral artery and both should be palpated. Impalpable femoral pulses suggest the diagnosis of coarctation of the aorta; they are always difficult to feel in the first few days of life, but with practice can usually be detected if the baby is lying quietly on a firm base with the hips gently flexed and abducted.

Abdomen

In well-grown infants the abdomen is often prominent, especially after a feed, but an unusual degree of gaseous distension could suggest intestinal obstruction. The umbilicus should be inspected for unusual features. The groins should be examined for herniae, which appear as soft swellings in the groin, angled down towards the scrotum or labia. On abdominal palpation, the liver edge is normally palpable 1 cm below the costal margin, and normal kidneys can frequently be felt between the fingers of the two hands palpating simultaneously deep in the lateral aspects of the upper abdomen and in the loin. Enlarged kidneys are even more readily palpable. The tip of the spleen is also commonly felt beneath the left costal margin by gentle superficial palpation. The rectus muscles are often separated in the midline of the upper abdomen at this time, allowing some bulging of the abdominal structures between them. A full bladder is often palpable, but if it persists after micturition, urethral valves should be suspected. The identification of other abdominal

masses always indicates a serious pathology, such as a tumour, which requires immediate investigation, usually by ultrasound scanning.

Rupture of the liver or spleen with intra-abdominal haemorrhage is a rare complication of a difficult delivery, but should not be forgotten when there is increasing pallor, restlessness and tachypnoea. There may be superficial bruising, but other signs are not often present.

Umbilicus

The umbilical cord normally contains two arteries and one vein, which are readily visible on the cut end of the cord. A single umbilical artery is associated with an increased incidence of other congenital malformations (p. 203) (Rinehart et al 2000, Pierce et al 2001). The cord dries and sloughs off between the sixth and tenth days, the time being influenced to some extent by the method of care. Some moistness of the stump remains for a day or two, and although this does not mean that there is sepsis, the area is a ready culture medium for bacteria, particularly the staphylococcus. Excessive granulation tissue sometimes accumulates and delays the healing of the stump, which then discharges and forms a small granuloma. Treatment with one or two applications of a silver nitrate stick usually effects a cure within a week, but it is important to distinguish it from the much rarer umbilical polyp. This remnant of the mesenteric duct consists of intestinal mucosa and has a bright-red smooth-shining surface. A persistent urachus may present a similar appearance and may discharge urine. Both require surgical exploration but are fully correctable.

The cord stump may be covered by abdominal skin for 1–3 cm from the abdominal wall. This cutis navel differs from an umbilical hernia in feeling solid on palpation. No treatment is required, as it becomes flatter with time.

An umbilical hernia developing in the first month of life is very common (especially in preterm infants) and it generally requires no treatment. Spontaneous cure by the age of 2 years is the rule. However, a supraumbilical hernia, which protrudes from a palpable defect just above the umbilicus, will require surgical correction since it never closes spontaneously.

Anus

The anus should be checked to confirm that it is correctly situated and that meconium passes through it. It can be anteriorly placed and rarely even opens into the vagina. Though it is not often necessary, a very gentle rectal examination should be performed if the anus is thought to be stenosed.

Genitalia

The scrotum in the male and the labia minora in the female are relatively large in the newborn, an appearance which is exaggerated in the preterm infant or, temporarily, by transient oedema in a breech baby.

Male infants

The penis varies in size and shape but the foreskin should form a complete covering to the glans. No attempt should be made to retract it, as it adheres to the glans in infancy, gradually separating, until 90% are retractable by the age of 3 years. There are no medical indications for circumcision in the neonatal period. The shaft of the penis should be straight and this can be seen most clearly if the baby has an erection. In hypospadias, the glans penis is partly uncovered and the urethral meatus opens on the underside of the penis at some point below the tip (p. 228). It is useful to confirm that the baby has a good urinary stream, to exclude urinary obstruction, which is often shown by either dribbling micturition or an unusually powerful fine stream of urine. Often the mother will be able to give a good description of it.

The scrotum varies in size and should contain both testes in the full-term infant. If they are not in the scrotum, it is important to note whether the testes are ectopic, in the inguinal canal or absent (Plate 12A). The testes normally descend from the abdomen at the eighth month of fetal life, and by 36 weeks lie at the neck of the scrotum. In 98% of boys at term, they lie in the scrotum or can easily be manipulated there on examination. The majority of those which are not down descend within the first month but those which do not are true undescended testes (Hamza et al 2001). Occasionally, testes which appear normal at one time may become apparently undescended later (Lamah et al 2001). The degree of descent helps to determine the gestational age of preterm infants (p. 109). The testes are often surrounded by soft transilluminable fluid swellings known as congenital hydroceles (Plate 12B). These rarely need treatment and most resolve within the first few months of life.

Bruising of the external genitalia is not uncommon after breech delivery. Occasionally there is a large haematoma which causes temporary difficulty with passing urine, but this always subsides spontaneously within a few days.

Female infants

In the term infant, the labia majora completely cover the labia minora but they can be easily separated revealing a mucoid hymen covering the vaginal opening. Occasionally, some endometrial bleeding occurs from the hormonal changes after birth, reaching its maximum between the third and fifth days. This generally ceases without intervention during the second week.

Ambiguous genitalia

Ambiguous genitalia, which are neither clearly male nor clearly female, are always an indicator of a serious underlying abnormality such as congenital adrenal hyperplasia or testosterone insensitivity and need urgent investigation (p. 228). They are also very worrying for the parents, who naturally wish to know the sex of their child; nevertheless, it is vital to avoid guessing the sex of the baby.

Spine

The spine should be inspected for evidence of a scoliosis or kyphosis, either of which may indicate malformation of the vertebrae. A post-anal dimple at the base of the spine occurs in about 1% of babies and is usually of no significance so long as the base is clearly seen to be skin covered and there is no discharge from it. A hairy patch or haemangioma over the lower lumbar region may indicate an underlying spina bifida occulta, which should be investigated radiologically later in the first year.

Limbs

The arms and hands should be checked for normal shape and posture, for deformities or limitation of movement of the joints and to confirm normal symmetrical movements. Accessory digits may be found often at the base of the little fingers, and missing digits may be noticed. Unless the baby has Down syndrome, there is no significance in the isolated finding of single transverse palmar creases.

The legs retain the flexed fetal posture for some days after birth and often they cannot be extended completely at the knee. The feet should be examined for talipes, though in many cases this is purely a postural deformity resulting from the cramped intrauterine environment and will resolve without intervention (Fig. 5.3). If the foot cannot be easily placed in a normal position without force, talipes is confirmed and treatment will usually be needed (p. 235). Overriding toes and syndactyly (fusion of two toes) are common benign features which are often familial. They need no more treatment than reassurance to the

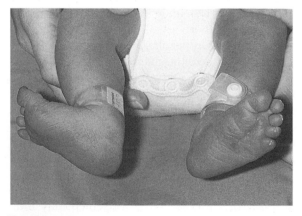

Figure 5.3 Postural right talipes calcaneovalgus.

parents. The limbs may be disproportionately short in achondroplasia and other rarer bone dysplasias.

Fractures of the long bones

The bones most often broken during delivery are the clavicle, humerus and femur. Such fractures occur most commonly after a breech birth in large babies or those where shoulder dystocia has complicated the delivery. The fractured clavicle, if not noticed at delivery, is often missed for it causes little swelling and practically no interference with arm movements. Fractures of the other bones are usually recognised by the sound or feel of the break at the time, and later confirmed by the immobility of the limb, with perhaps bruising or swelling at the site of the fracture. Occasionally, crepitus is the only sign.

When a fracture is suspected, ultrasound examination is often better than X-rays for diagnosis in the early stages. Analgesia should be considered, though babies often appear to have little pain even after major fractures. Remarkably, healing of fractures occurs, with complete remodelling of the bone to a normal contour in spite of severe displacement, and accurate reduction of the fracture is not often necessary. Immobilisation need not be complete, and strapping the arm to the chest is all that is required for fractures of the humerus. For the femur, bandaging the leg to a light lateral splint extending upwards beyond the pelvis is sometimes advocated, but healing almost always results in normal ultimate alignment even if no immobilisation is used. The parents will need advice about how to handle the baby and what analgesia to give him.

Dislocation of joints

Congenital dislocation of the knee results in an alarming reversed angulation of the leg at the knee. Unstable knees can be held in place with a splint until the damaged ligaments heal. A fixed dislocation can be gently manipulated and splinted in place by the physiotherapist until its correct alignment is achieved. Usually, normal function is restored. Occasionally, other joints such as the elbow can be dislocated during delivery, but physiotherapy and crêpe bandaging usually restores the joint to normal.

Hips

The importance of identifying the dislocated or unstable hip within the first 48 hours of life cannot be overstated. No system so far devised is perfect, but every maternity department must have a programme to screen all babies by clinical examination (Dunn 1992) or ultrasound imaging techniques (p. 233). Whichever system is used, it is vital for all those involved in assessing babies to become proficient in the clinical examination techniques. It is probably the most difficult part of the neonatal examination and reliable only in experienced hands. For the examination to be successful, the baby must be relaxed, and this can usually be achieved by allowing the baby to suck on an empty sterile feeding teat and by ensuring that the examiner's hands are warm. It should be performed very gently and, if it is carried out properly, it should cause the baby minimal discomfort. Forceful abduction of the hips can damage the hip joint or the head of the femur and must be avoided. Shortening of the leg or asymmetrical skin creases on the posterior thighs are sometimes present when there is established dislocation of one hip.

The infant is examined lying on his back with his hips and knees flexed to a right angle. The examiner should first note any inequality of length of the thighs, then proceed to Ortolani's test (Fig. 5.4). The legs and thighs are grasped between the thumb and first finger while the middle finger is placed over the greater trochanter of the femur at the hip. Both hips are then gently abducted as far as they will comfortably go. If a hip is unstable or dislocated, it may relocate in the acetabulum with a palpable 'clunk' during the manoeuvre under the gentle pressure exerted on the trochanter from behind. Ligamentous 'clicks' are normal findings and can be ignored. In Barlow's test, an attempt is made to push the head of the femur backwards out of the joint with a similar 'clunk' as the abducted hip is slowly adducted.

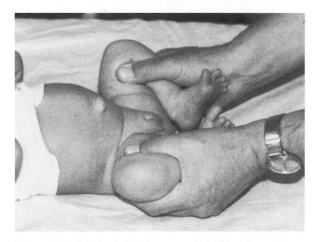

Figure 5.4 Ortolani's test for congenital dislocation of the hip.

The range of abduction is then tested. If the baby is relaxed, it should be possible gently to abduct each hip through 80–90°, i.e. to move the thigh to a position with its outer side almost flat on the table. A definite restriction of this movement usually indicates established congenital dislocation, though if it is bilateral it may be caused by adductor muscle spasm (spasticity). The management of the unstable hip is discussed on page 234.

NEUROLOGICAL ASSESSMENT

A great deal of information about the neurological state of the baby can be deduced from simple observation and a discussion with the mother about the baby's behaviour. The ability of infants to latch on and suck at the breast, how much they cry, how well they sleep and how readily they wake all suggest how their brain is functioning. The maturity of the baby affects his response to the environment and handling, and progressive maturation of such activities is used in the assessment of gestational age (p. 108). Considerable experience of the newborn is needed to evaluate the normality of the baby's movements and reactions to stimuli. They change with development and gestational age, so what is normal at, say, 34 weeks of gestation may be quite abnormal at term, hence their value in assessing maturity (p. 109).

Normal behaviour and response to environment

No two healthy newborn babies behave in exactly the same way, even when they are identical twins, but there is a broad pattern which can be regarded as normal and from which only minor deviations occur. At first it is a relatively simple pattern of sleep, wakefulness and semi-purposeful movements with some reflexes, such as sucking and swallowing, which enable the baby to survive. From the moment of birth, however, infants are able to respond to their carers and the environment in their own individual way and begin the process of learning which will enable them to progress in their development.

Wakefulness and sleep

At times during the day, the baby lies awake and quiet; at others, he is active and crying. For between 16 and 20 hours each day the baby will be asleep, though the depth and duration of sleep vary considerably from one infant to another. Some arouse easily and are wakeful even though well fed, while others wake only to be fed and changed. In most cases the early sleep pattern has no predictive value in assessing later characteristics.

Sucking

The normal term infant can suck and swallow almost immediately after birth. The touch of the nipple on the baby's face initiates rooting, latching on to the nipple and the coordinated movements of lip, tongue, palate and pharynx required to feed successfully (see Fig. 5.6). Failure to suck when the stomach is empty always means something is amiss and is an important sign of brain stem damage.

Crying

Crying is the baby's main means of communicating his needs in the first weeks of life. He cries vigorously and spasmodically without tears and often without any obvious reason. At birth, crying is a response to the dramatic sensations of light, sound, cold and gravity, experienced for the first time. Thereafter it generally means hunger, thirst or pain, but also may indicate a need for protection or comfort. Most mothers will rapidly learn to recognise their own baby's need from the types of cry he makes, though such factors as negative experiences around the time of birth or maternal depression after it may diminish the mother's sensitvity to her infant's needs and perpetuate the crying. Various other discomforts can initiate it – for instance, contact with a cold hand, sudden movement or a bright light. Infants appear to be more sensitive to visceral pain (e.g. distension with wind) than to somatic pain, though there is clear evidence to suggest that they feel significant pain from invasive procedures such as heel pricks and venepuncture (p. 144).

Formal neurological assessment

The formal neurological examination of term infants must be interpreted in the light of not only their gestational age but also their degree of arousal, and is best carried out after a feed with the infant in a state of quiet wakefulness. The muscle tone of infants is best assessed by confirming that they flex their head on arm traction from the supine position and briefly hold their head up to the horizontal on ventrosuspension (see below). Noticeable floppiness or hypertonia is abnormal and should be investigated further (p. 158). They should respond to handling without distress and be alert and suck well. They should gaze at the examiner's face, at least briefly.

Normal posture, movements and general responses

When lying on the back at rest, the legs of the normal infant are semi-flexed and the head turns to one side (Fig. 5.5A). If the arms and legs are extended, they should recoil readily, and the elbow should not cross the midline when the arm is 'wrapped' around the neck.

When prone, the legs are even more flexed and tend to be drawn up under the abdomen

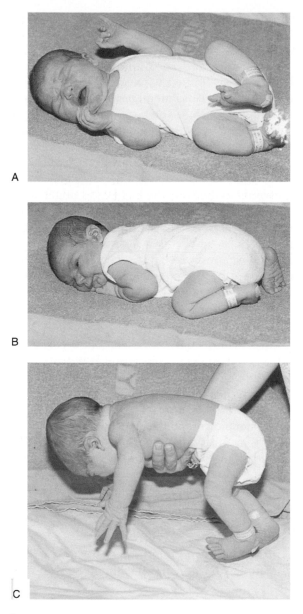

A

B

C

Figure 5.5 Normal posture of the newborn infant when placed (A) supine; (B) prone; (C) in ventrosuspension.

back of the hand is stroked. The thumb is often tucked in under the fingers.

Spontaneous movements of all four limbs occur when the baby is awake, usually alternating flexion and extension, which can appear to be semi-purposeful.

Jittering movements of the limbs often accompany a general increase in the deep reflexes and may occasionally be caused by hypoglycaemia or hypocalcaemia. They are very common and, in the absence of other signs of a neurological disorder, are of no serious significance. If jitteriness is accompanied by hypertonia and irritability, it may be a symptom of hypoxic-ischaemic encephalopathy or withdrawal from illicit drugs, even if this is not known from the maternal history (p. 18).

Specific responses

Certain stimuli produce consistent response patterns. Some of those that are well known, like the Moro response, are elicited regularly during routine examination of the newborn in the belief that the neurological integrity of the baby has thereby been tested. Since they depend only upon spinal reflexes, they give little information relevant to the future developmental progress of the infant, which is dependent more on the integrity of the cortex of the brain. However, persistence of these primitive reflexes beyond their normal time may indicate an emerging cerebral palsy. Some of the responses depend on the state of alertness at the time and the baby's gestational age.

The feeding responses are present from birth and are most easily elicited when the baby is hungry. The rooting reflex (Fig. 5.6) is the deviation of the opened mouth and turning of the head towards a touch on the cheek. Stimulation of the upper lip causes opening of the mouth, pouting of the lips, and tongue movements. Latching on, sucking and swallowing are reflex responses and the whole coordinated pattern is developed by 32 weeks of gestation, though it only becomes strong enough for adequate feeding around 36 weeks. Failure of this complex mechanism in a hungry term infant may indicate severe neurological damage at a midbrain level.

(Fig. 5.5B). The arms are held flexed to the chest. If the infant is held up by a hand under the chest (ventrosuspension), the posture is semi-flexed and the head is momentarily extended in line with the trunk (Fig. 5.5C).

The fingers are often fully flexed at rest but open spontaneously when feeding or when the

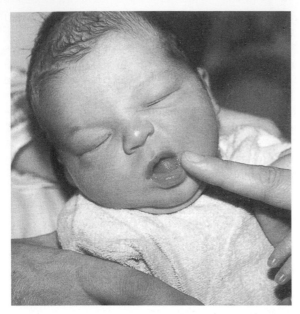

Figure 5.6 Rooting reflex.

Primitive reflexes

Grasp responses The palmar and plantar grasp responses are spinal reflexes. The 'grasp', with flexion of the fingers and adduction of the thumb when the palm is touched, is developed as early as 12 weeks' gestation and is very strong in the term infant; similarly, the toes flex in response to stimulation of the sole.

Traction response The traction response, the flexion of the elbows in response to pulling the baby by the hands towards the sitting position, reflects the development of flexor tone at around 37 weeks.

Asymmetric tonic neck reflex The asymmetric tonic neck reflex is seen most prominently during the phases of development when the extensor tone is dominant, from 30 to 36 weeks of gestation and again some 4–6 weeks after term. If the head is turned to one side, the arm and leg on that side extend while the others remain flexed. Although this is a normal response, requiring only an intact medulla and spinal cord, if it is very obvious and obligatory in a baby at term, it is an indication of abnormally increased extensor tone. This can be due to many different forms of neurological disturbance, including metabolic disorders like hypocalcaemia, increased intracranial pressure, cerebral birth injury or asphyxial brain damage (p. 151).

The Moro reflex The Moro reflex, though easy to obtain, has limited value except as a means of demonstrating a unilateral nerve lesion such as an Erb's palsy (p. 159). The body is supported in the supine position by one hand while the other hand supports the head. The head is suddenly allowed to drop back a little way by lowering the hand while the baby is relaxed. The arms are thrown outwards to the side, the hands and fingers open and the legs extend. During the manoeuvre, the baby will look startled and may cry, but within moments he returns to a normal flexed posture. The reflex may be absent in severe asphyxial brain damage or heavy sedation. The flexion component is absent in many preterm infants.

Progression responses

Crossed extension reflex The crossed extension reflex is obtained by stimulation of the sole of one foot, which causes withdrawal of that leg and flexion of the other leg, followed by strong extension and adduction.

The stepping response The stepping response (Fig. 5.7) has a similar mechanism: when the baby is held in the standing position with the sole of one foot on a firm surface, the leg extends and the opposite leg makes a stepping movement, which can be continued on alternate feet. The trunk and head tend to straighten at the same time. Present by 34 weeks, this reflex is not always easy to elicit until near term and it indicates only the presence of mature extension and flexion mechanisms.

Cranial nerves

The cranial nerve responses are not all easy to obtain, but, with patience, a considerable amount of information can be gained.

Vision (II) Healthy term infants will turn their head towards a bright light, and will often fix their gaze on the observer's eyes and follow through a few degrees. Initially, the baby can see clearly only to about 30 cm, but this increases rapidly over the next few weeks. The pupils contract to light from 30 weeks of gestation.

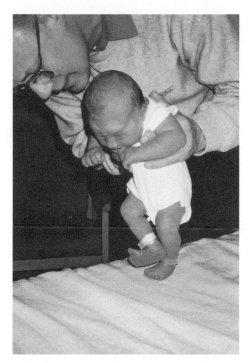

Figure 5.7 Stepping reflex.

Eye movements (III, IV, VI) When the head is turned to one side, the eyes tend not to move with it ('doll's-eye phenomenon'). If the baby is held erect facing the observer, who then rotates himself, the eyes move in the direction of the movement, but at times the gaze may be briefly fixed. This is known as *optico-kinetic nystagmus* and shows that the baby has adequate vision, and can be used to demonstrate which ocular movements are abnormal if the baby has a squint.

Glabella tap (V, VII) A tap just above the bridge of the nose causes the baby to blink. This reflex appears at 32 to 34 weeks of gestation.

Bulbar reflexes (IX, X, XII) These include the gag reflex, sucking and swallowing.

Interpreting the neurological examination

Predicting the future development of a child from neurological examination around the time of birth is very difficult. The neonatal reflexes do not depend on higher (cortical) brain function and therefore may be normal in the presence of quite serious cerebral damage. It is more often through a knowledge of predisposing factors and observing an altered pattern of behaviour that the baby who will have lasting cerebral damage can be identified. The risk factors include low birth weight, abnormal delivery, asphyxia, congenital abnormalities such as hydrocephalus, and infants with dysmorphic syndromes (p. 209).

The following features may be associated with significant cerebral injury and indicate that the baby should be evaluated more fully:

- persistent failure to latch on to the breast or suck
- irritability, staring or persistently clenched fists
- a high-pitched cry
- persistent head retraction
- hypotonia or hypertonia
- lack of spontaneous activity or asymmetry of movements
- convulsions.

Any baby showing such signs should be investigated for underlying causes (p. 152) in a neonatal unit.

Neurological assessment at this early stage of life cannot always detect those babies who are at risk of developing a handicap later. Some who appear quite normal in the neonatal period will be brain damaged, whereas many with clear signs of cerebral dysfunction, such as cerebral irritability (p. 151), in the first days of life, will have no permanent sequelae. It is important that in counselling the parents unnecessary anxieties should not be generated by attributing too much significance to minor variations in neurological signs or behaviour. Moreover, there is some evidence that early developmental treatment directed by a skilled paediatric physiotherapist and implemented at home can improve the eventual outcome for their child (p. 155). This subject is also discussed in Chapter 10.

TESTING THE BABY'S HEARING

The inner ear can be damaged by trauma or asphyxia at birth, infection by the rubella virus in

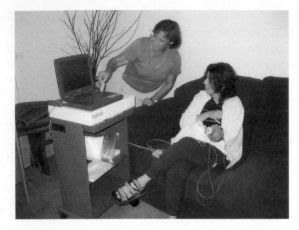

Figure 5.8 Otoacoustic response testing for congenital sensorineural deafness.

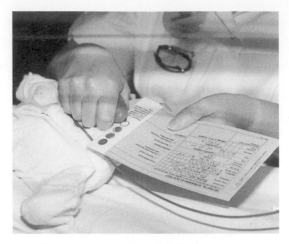

Figure 5.9 Heelprick capillary blood collection for hypothyroidism and phenylketonuria screening.

pregnancy or by aminoglycoside antibiotics such as gentamicin (p. 175). There also appears to be an increased incidence in some ethnic minority groups in the UK. Hearing can now be tested with reasonable accuracy in the newborn period using otoacoustic responses (Fig. 5.8) or by performing auditory brain-stem-evoked response tests (Owen et al 2001). In some geographical areas, all babies are screened for severe hearing loss using these techniques. Overall, around one baby per 1000 has congenital sensorineural deafness identified in this way. Severe deafness from birth is followed in many cases by very poor speech development: the early provision of hearing aids and speech training may improve the acquisition of speech. It is recommended that babies in the following categories should be considered for neonatal hearing testing:

- a family history of sensorineural deafness
- moderate or severe hypoxic-ischaemic encephalopathy
- identification of parenchymal brain damage on ultrasound scans
- following treatment with aminoglycoside antibiotics
- evidence of intrauterine infections
- preterm infants
- chromosomal anomalies
- congenital malformations of the head and neck, including cleft lip and palate

- parental consanguinity
- neonatal hyperbilirubinaemia
- following meningitis.

LABORATORY SCREENING TESTS

In addition to the clinical examination of the baby, certain potentially treatable inherited metabolic disorders can be identified in the neonatal period, before they produce any harm in the baby, by employing specific laboratory tests on a small sample of blood obtained from a heelprick and collected onto a filter paper (Fig. 5.9). As there is no family history in most cases, they are applied to the whole population or, in some disorders, to all the ethnic group susceptible to the condition. It is possible to detect many disorders, but so far only a few tests have been shown to be sufficiently accurate, economical and beneficial to the infant to justify their introduction as a universal routine screening procedure. The reasons for carrying out such screening procedures are:

- to detect the disorder at an early enough stage to introduce effective treatment to prevent the disease from affecting the baby's development
- to enable genetic counselling to be given to the parents at an early stage, with the possibility of prenatal diagnosis in subsequent pregnancies

- to reduce the morbidity of the condition by early detection – for instance, in cystic fibrosis or sickle cell disease.

The conditions for which such tests are used include:

- phenylketonuria (p. 211)
- primary hypothyroidism (p. 212)
- cystic fibrosis (p. 210)
- Thalassaemia (p. 188)
- Sickle cell disease (p. 188)

These conditions are described in detail later in this book.

Many other genetic conditions are amenable to neonatal screening programmes and may be included in the future when treatments such as gene therapy become more effective in improving their prognosis.

BIOCHEMISTRY OF THE NEONATE

The blood biochemistry for those constituents commonly estimated in the newborn period is summarised in Table 5.2. The concentration of many of these alters with almost every hour after birth and varies widely from one baby to another, but the quoted figures may be regarded as the normal range of values for term infants at 1–2 weeks of age.

Table 5.2 Blood chemistry values at 1–2 weeks of age in healthy term infants (from Clayton Round 1984, with permission.)

Constituent	Range
Sodium	130–145 mmol/L
Potassium	3.6–5.8 mmol/L
Calcium	1.90–2.85 mmol/L
Magnesium	0.59–1.05 mmol/L
Chloride	92–109 mmol/L
Phosphate	1.8–3.2 mmol/L
Urea	1.0–5.0 mmol/L
Creatinine	62–106 µg/L
Glucose (fasting)	3.2–4.9 mmol/L
Other units	
Blood gases:	
pH	7.33–7.47
$PaCO_2$	4.4–6.0 kPa
PaO_2	6.0–9.0 kPa
base deficit	− 5 mmol/L
Total protein	43–76 g/dL
albumin	28–49 g/dL
Immunoglobulins:	
IgG	4.8–13 g/L
IgA	15.6–124 mg/L

REFERENCES

Ammed H, Pindiga U H, Onuora C U et al 2001 Giant congenital pigmented naevus with unusual presentation and early malignant transformaton in a Nigerian infant. Nigerian Postgraduate Medical Journal 8(1):26–31

Clayton B, Round J 1984 Chemical pathology and the sick child. Blackwell, London

Cordova A 1981 The Mongolian blue spot: a study of ethnic differences and a literature review. Clinical Pediatrics (Philadelphia) 20(11):714–719

Dunn PM 1992 Diagnosing congenital dislocation of the hip. British Medical Journal 10:305

Dunn PM 2001 Examination of the newborn infant in the UK: a personal viewpoint. Journal of Neonatal Nursing 7:55–57

Ellenbogen R G, Gruss J S, Cunningham M L 2000 Update on craniofacial surgery: the differential diagnosis of lambdoid synostosis/posterior plagiocephaly. Clinical Neurosurgery 47:303–318

Hamza A F, Elrahim M, Elnagar B et al 2001 Testicular descent: when to interfere. European Journal of Paediatric Surgery 11(3):173–176

Koot H M, de Waard-van der Spek F, Peer C D et al 2000 Psychosocial sequelae in 29 children with giant congenital melanocytic naevi. Clinical and Experimental Dermatology 25(8):589–593

Lamah M, McCaughey E S, Finlay F O et al 2001 The ascending testis: is late orchidopexy due to failure of screening or late ascent? Paediatric Surgery International 17(5):421–423

Lee T W, Skelton R E, Skene C 2001 Routine neonatal examination: effectiveness of trainee paediatrician compared with advanced neonatal nurse practitioner. Archives of Disease in Childhood Fetal and Neonatal Edition 85(2):F100–F104

Owen M, Webb M, Evans K 2001 Community based universal neonatal hearing screening by health visitors using otoacoustic emissions. Archives of Disease in Childhood Fetal and Neonatal Edition 84(3):F157–F162

Pierce B T, Dance V D, Wagner R K et al 2001 Perinatal outcome following fetal single umbilical artery diagnosis. Journal of Maternal and Fetal Medicine 10(1):59–63

Rinehart B K, Terrone D A, Taylor C W et al 2000 Single umbilical artery is associated with an increased incidence of structural and chromosomal anomalies and growth restriction. American Journal of Perinatology 17(5):229–232

Wolke D, Dave S, Hayes J et al 2002 Routine examination of the newborn and maternal satisfaction: a randomized controlled trial. Archives of Disease in Childhood Fetal and Neonatal Edition 86 (3): F155–F160

FURTHER READING

De Vries L 1992 Routine neurological examination of the newborn. Current Paediatrics 2:183–185

Ladewig P, London M, Old S 1998 Maternal newborn nursing care, 4th edn. Longman, New York

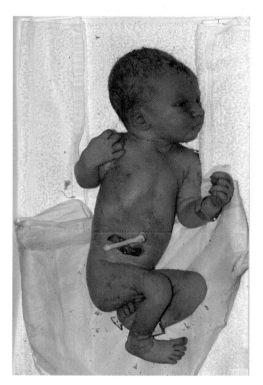

Plate 1 Term light for dates infant.

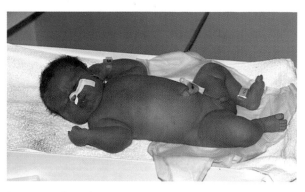

Plate 2 Infant of a diabetic mother, showing macrosomia and polycythaemia.

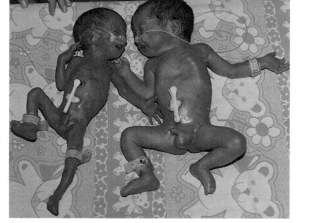

Plate 3 Disproportionate growth in twins. The smaller shows all the signs of intrauterine malnutrition.

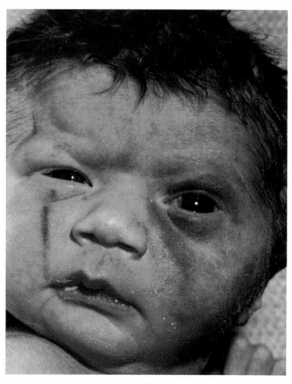

Plate 4 Facial bruising from forceps delivery.

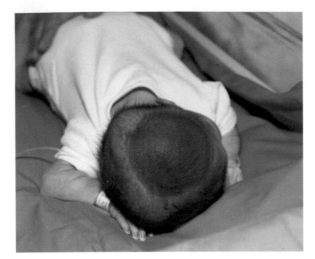

Plate 5   Suction cap bruising of the scalp.

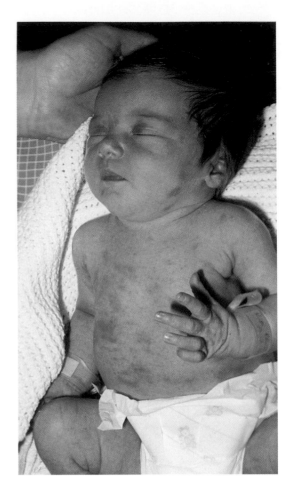

Plate 6   Urticaria neonatorum.

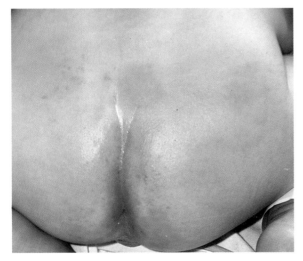

Plate 7   'Mongolian' blue spot.

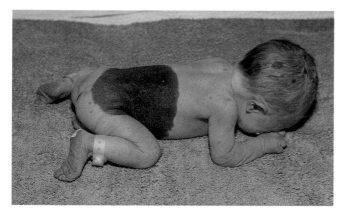

Plate 8   Giant pigmented naevus with satellite smaller lesions.

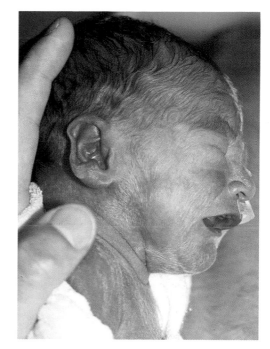

Plate 10   Lanugo.

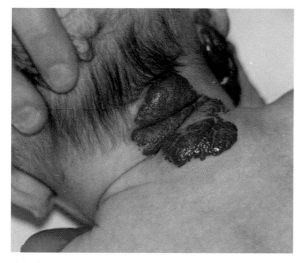

Plate 9   Strawberry marks.

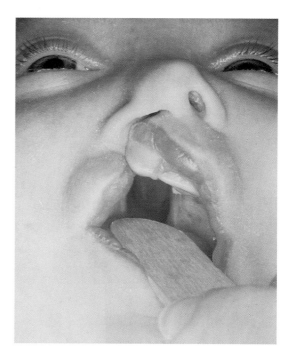

Plate 11   Cleft lip and palate.

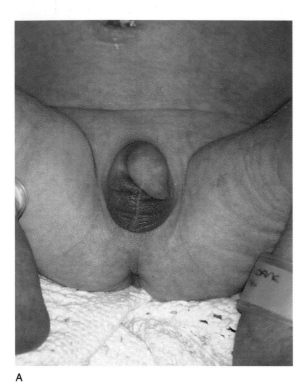

A

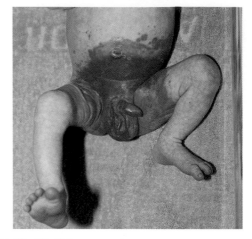

Plate 13 Monilial nappy rash.

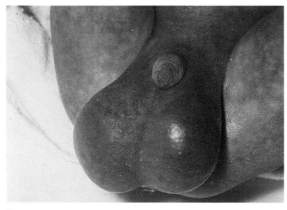

B

Plate 12 A: Bilateral undescended testes. B: Bilateral hydroceles.

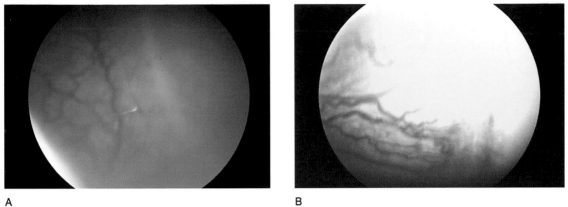

A   B

Plate 14   Fundal photographs in retinopathy of prematurity. A: Mild disease – an avascular (pale) peripheral retina with a visible ridge. B: Active progressive disease showing engorgement of the posterior pole vessels. (By kind permission of Mr David Clark.)

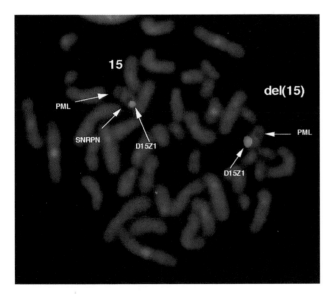

Plate 15   Fluorescent in-situ hybridisation (FISH) demonstrates the deleted gene SNRPN in Prader–Willi syndrome. The red signal from a probe for the SNRPN gene is present on the normal chromosome (15) and absent from the deleted chromosome (del(15)). (By kind permission of Ms Christine Joyce.)

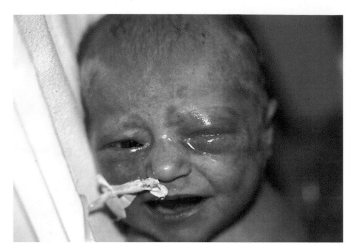

Plate 16 Chlamydial conjunctivitis.

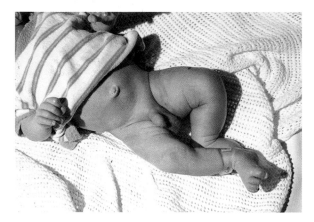

Plate 17 Large haematoma in the left thigh caused by femoral venepuncture in a baby with haemophilia.

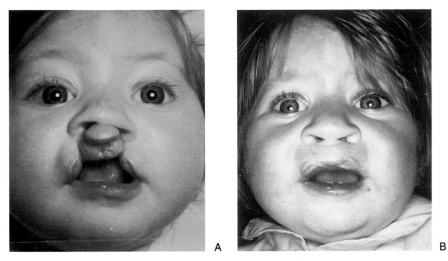

Plate 18 A: Bilateral cleft lip. B: After surgery at 3 months of age.
(By kind permission of Mr R McDowall.)

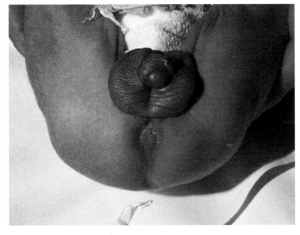

Plate 19 Anal atresia (note also the bifid scrotum).

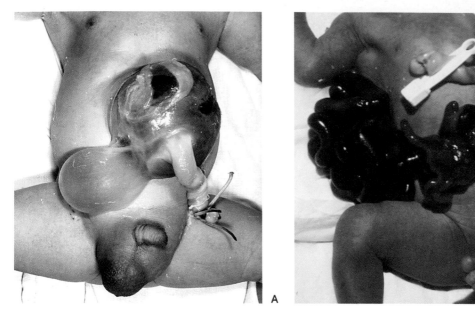

Plate 20 A: Exomphalos. B: Gastroschisis.

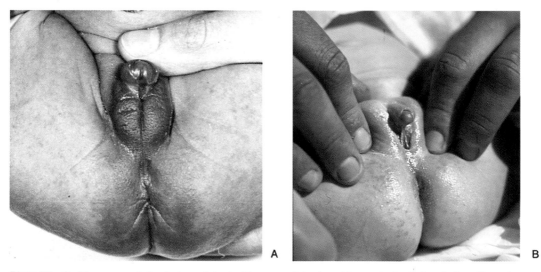

Plate 21 Ambiguous genitalia. A: In an infant with congenital adrenal hyperplasia. B: In a baby with androgen-insensitivity syndrome.

Chapter 6
Essential care of the newborn baby

CHAPTER CONTENTS

Introduction   79
Procedure at a normal birth   79
Maintenance of body temperature   80
    The role of the skin   80
    Temperature regulation   80
    Clothing the baby   81
    Hypothermia   82
Caring for the healthy newborn infant   83
    Fostering the bonding and attachment process   83
    Factors which affect parenting ability   84
Minimising the risk of infection   85
Alimentary tract function – stools   86
Renal function – urine   86
Care of the skin and umbilicus   87
    Cleansing the infant   87
    Nappy rash   87
    The umbilical cord   88
Sleeping posture and prevention of cot death   88
Weighing the baby   89

INTRODUCTION

The care of the baby at birth should ensure a safe transition from the intrauterine environment to the point where the parents can safely take care of their infant without professional help. Even with careful preparation, the parents will often feel a mixture of anxiety and anticipatory wonder during the birth, and unnecessary actions by the midwife, obstetrician or paediatrician can adversely affect the development of the relationship between the parents and their infant and should be avoided. Planning for the birth is a vital part of antenatal care, and, increasingly, the parents' wishes about the place and mode of delivery and the care of the infant after birth are incorporated into a plan pre-agreed with the midwife. This is particularly necessary in a multicultural society where religious or cultural customs related to birth may be important to the family (Gatrad & Sheik 2001). Yet, although about two-thirds of deliveries progress in a natural manner and the baby is born without medical intervention, it is not always possible to identify in advance the baby who may suffer harm, and all caregivers must watch for potential hazards and act when necessary.

PROCEDURE AT A NORMAL BIRTH

In the normal course of events, the baby is delivered after only a minor degree of oxygen deprivation – caused by interruption of blood flow through the placenta at each uterine contraction – and breathing starts spontaneously within a few seconds. The only immediate actions required are to ensure that the airway is clear, so that debris and fluid from the mouth and nose are not inhaled into the lungs with the baby's first breaths, and to dry the baby with a warm towel to prevent heat loss (p. 80).

As soon as the head is delivered, therefore, the nose and mouth are gently wiped clear of mucus and debris. Vigorous nasal suction with a catheter can damage the mucosa and cause the heart rate to fall from vagal stimulation and is not often necessary. Vernix and blood should be wiped away from the eyes. As long as the vessels of the umbilical cord are pulsating, some blood continues to flow into the baby through this structure thus supplementing the infant's blood volume. This provides the baby with additional red cells, which maintain a higher haemoglobin level and extra iron stores. Even if the baby is delivered up onto the mother's abdomen, the cord may be left unclamped until cord pulsation stops, unless asphyxia or the risk of hypothermia necessitates immediate resuscitative measures. Two cord clamps should then be applied 5 and 6 cm from the umbilicus, and the cord divided between them.

Fluid material from the fetal lungs will often accumulate in the baby's mouth and pharynx and this should be removed by a soft suction catheter attached to a mechanical sucker regulated to a pressure of no more than 100 cmH$_2$O. Higher pressures may damage the mucous membranes. Mouth-operated mucus extractors should not be used unless no alternative exists and should have a filter fitted to protect the operator from aspirated material. When there is a risk that blood or mucus is infected, they should not be used.

MAINTENANCE OF BODY TEMPERATURE
The role of the skin

The skin is one of the largest organs in the body and has several functions which are vital for protection and maintenance of homeostasis. It is the most important structure in the maintenance of body temperature. By varying the state of the arteriolar circulation, the skin can enable the baby to lose or retain heat as needed. Sweating, which increases heat loss by evaporation of water from the skin surface, is also well developed in

the newborn infant, though it is only in rare situations (e.g. acute heart failure) that it is visible. Smaller babies are more likely to become cold than are larger ones, because the former have a relatively larger surface area of skin in relation to weight, and the ambient temperature should be adjusted to take account of this.

Larger babies in incubators and normal babies in hot climates can equally become overheated easily because their relatively smaller surface area-to-weight ratio limits their ability to lose heat. The subject of maintenance of body temperature is discussed more fully on page 115.

Temperature regulation

The newborn baby's temperature regulation is less efficient than that of the older child and there is a risk both of excessive cooling leading to hypothermia and of overheating.

Before birth, the baby has grown in a wet environment at a constant temperature of 37°C, his temperature being regulated by minimising metabolic activity and by disposal of heat through the mother's body. At birth, he usually encounters dry air and a dramatically lower environmental temperature. Immediately, he starts to lose heat rapidly by:

- evaporation from his wet skin
- radiation to his surroundings
- convection to the air
- conduction to his coverings.

These losses are usually counteracted physiologically by four main heat-conserving mechanisms:

- constriction of the skin arterioles, which reduces blood flow and therefore diminishes heat losses
- enhanced heat production by increased muscular activity (though the newborn's capacity to produce heat by shivering is very limited)
- the liberation of heat chemically from a form of fat peculiar to the newborn baby, known as brown fat
- accelerated metabolism of circulating glucose.

Because babies have a large surface in proportion to their weight and volume, they can lose heat very rapidly, especially if their birth weight is low (p. 115), and hypothermia will quickly follow if heat production fails to keep up with losses. The increased metabolic activity required can rapidly exhaust the circulating glucose and render the baby hypoglycaemic (p. 54). It also requires additional oxygen, which may not be available if the baby has a lung disorder (p. 41).

Prevention of hypothermia immediately after birth by employing good care practices is therefore essential. Delivery should be in a room with a temperature of at least 20°C which is draught-free. The baby must be dried carefully with a warm towel immediately after birth. Placing the infant skin-to-skin on the mother's abdomen and covering the baby in warm blankets can also help to reduce immediate losses of heat. Should resuscitation be needed (p. 36), it must be performed under a radiant heat source and with great attention to keeping the infant warm, since the usual heat production mechanisms may not be operating effectively in an asphyxiated baby. For transfer to a neonatal unit, heat loss can be reduced by wrapping the baby in a metal foil sheet or, for longer journeys, warm blankets and placement in a warmed transport incubator (p. 115; Fig. 6.1).

The baby is exposed to the same risks later on during nappy changes, while being bathed, during clinical or radiological examination or an operation, or if he is simply nursed in a cold room.

However, the greatest risk is immediately after birth, when the adjustment required is dramatic and has to be achieved in such a short time.

By contrast, large well-nourished infants have little difficulty coping with the temperature adjustments at birth but in the subsequent days can become overheated in hot climates, in incubators or if they are overwrapped. Avoidance of hyperthermia is just as important, as it has been implicated in some cases of sudden infant death syndrome (cot deaths) (p. 88).

Despite this, in most circumstances the healthy well-grown term baby has a remarkably stable temperature at 37°C and significant variations from this figure require an explanation. Either high or low temperature may indicate an infection, and appropriate examination and investigations should be carried out (p. 168). If no evidence of infection is found, the probable explanation is that the baby has either too much or too little clothing for the surrounding room temperature.

Clothing the baby

Although most parents clothe their babies with an appropriate number and type of garments instinctively, a more formal assessment can be made by calculating the tog values, which gives a numerical figure to the insulating quality of the clothes. The higher the value, the greater the heat

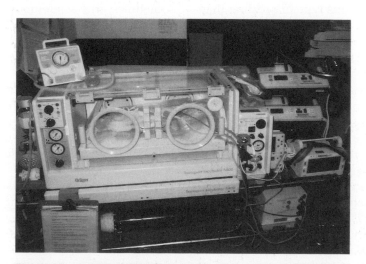

Figure 6.1 Modern transport incubators provide full supportive care for even the most preterm infant.

Table 6.1 Tog values of baby clothing and bedding

Item	Tog value
Vest	0.2
Babygro	1.0
Jumper	2.0
Cardigan	2.0
Trousers	2.0
Disposable nappy	2.0
Sleeping suit	4.0
Sheet	0.2
Old blanket	1.5
New blanket	2.0
Quilts	Variable, but about 9

retained. Table 6.1 gives the tog values of commonly used baby wear and bedclothing. For most infants a value of 6–10 tog will keep them safe from hypothermia and hyperthermia in an ambient temperature of 16–20°C, though it must be remembered that in cold weather the room temperature of an unheated room may fall considerably during the night. In practice this means that at night an average well-nourished baby should have a vest, nappy, babygro, cardigan and two blankets (tog value 8.2–9.2); if the cardigan is replaced by a sleeping suit, only one blanket is needed (tog value 8.7–9.2). A very slim baby may need more and a fatter baby fewer clothes to keep warm. If the temperature falls significantly or the infant feels cold, additional coverings should be used. Blankets are preferred since it is easier to adjust the tog value of this type of bedding than it is when a duvet is used. On the other hand, swaddling the infant with blankets and covering the head increases the risk of overheating by preventing the baby from adjusting his own temperature through increasing heat loss from the head.

If a steady room temperature cannot be maintained, it is usually possible to ensure a stable body temperature during the night by clothing the infant for the cooler, rather than the warmer, expected room temperature. It must be remembered, however, that cold clothes will initially take heat from the baby, so it is preferable to put on warmed garments if the room is cool. Heating the cot itself is not necessary apart from the initial warming before the baby is placed there. For a well-fed thriving infant, there is probably more risk of

hyperthermia from overwrapping than hypothermia from too little clothing. Midwives and health visitors now check on these features routinely.

During the first week, regular temperature recording, either by a rectal thermometer or from the axilla, ensures that a harmful drop in temperature, which can be one indication of neonatal infection, is not missed. Thermometers that read as low as 30°C are an essential part of the midwife's equipment.

Hypothermia

Neonatal cold injury has become less common in the last few years. There is a recognisable clinical picture associated with hypothermia, which may remain undetected for several days unless the condition is kept in mind. Although sepsis, underfeeding and intracranial bleeding may all be associated causes, the principal factor is usually inadequate heating or clothing in the home in winter. The baby makes good initial progress but in the first week or two of life begins to show apathy, refuses some feeds and fails to gain weight. The cry becomes feeble and whimpering. At this time, if felt, the skin is cold to touch, though surprisingly enough the baby may not look ill and there is often a misleading redness of the face and extremities. The rectal temperature is found to be below 34°C (94°F), sometimes in the region of 30–32°C (85–90°F). Hard oedema or, sometimes, true sclerema (p. 121) develops and, if untreated, death ensues. Pulmonary haemorrhage is the usual terminal complication.

The treatment involves rewarming the body gradually, maintaining the infant's nutrition by giving tube feeds of milk with additional glucose to counteract the associated risk of hypoglycaemia (p. 54), using a glucose intravenous infusion with hydrocortisone in severe cases, and treating any identified infection by giving an appropriate antibiotic.

The warming process must be slow, taking several hours to return the infant to normal body temperature. If it is done quickly, the increased metabolic activity of the body will outstrip the available glucose and make the infant more hypoglycaemic and increase the risks of long-term cerebral complications such as learning difficulties or epilepsy. It is best done by keeping the infant lightly dressed in an incubator with the surrounding temperature just a few degrees above his body temperature, and increasing the heat setting as the body temperature rises. The metabolic processes of the body will produce heat by metabolising the administered glucose. Changes in the blood glucose should be closely monitored to ensure that enough is being given to maintain a normal blood level at all times.

CARING FOR THE HEALTHY NEWBORN INFANT

After birth, the baby should be allowed to stay with the mother at her bedside so that she can get to know him, have the opportunity to enjoy his company and learn to love and care for him. She will also learn the way he behaves, how he expresses his feelings, and the significance of the sounds and cries he makes, since no two babies are the same. It also offers the mother the opportunity to express her feeling for the baby as and when she wishes and to learn how often the infant wants a feed or other attention. Only rarely is there a clinical reason for separating the mother and her healthy baby, though occasionally a court order which requires such may be in place where, for example, a previous child has been abused. However, because it is often a new and unfamiliar experience for the mother, it is essential for there to be qualified nursing support on hand when needed.

The baby's needs in the first few days of life are to be kept warm and comfortable, to be fed and cleaned, clothed and protected, but above all to be loved, cared for, cherished and enjoyed. Both physical and emotional care are vital for the infant's future health and development and from the start these should take precedence over any other routine procedures required by professional carers.

Good parenting involves providing the baby with his physical needs, ensuring a consistent caring relationship which avoids confusion, and understanding the baby's wants and responding promptly, appropriately and sensitively to them.

It is not always an easy task and both parents may need much encouragement and support before they become confident in caring for their infant. Many parents will have experienced how to provide good care for a baby within their own families, though poor practices may be learned if their own childhood was emotionally deprived. It is, therefore, wise to allow most parents to develop their own ways of caring for and responding to their baby, based upon their own experience and cultural practices and influenced by the information gained from the midwife or antenatal classes during the pregnancy. By encouraging the good features, the parents' confidence in nurturing their baby can be effectively increased. The risk of 'spoiling' the infant by responding promptly to his needs is small, and both mother and baby will become more content if these needs are met appropriately. It should only be necessary to recommend to a mother that she changes the way she handles her baby if it is clear that her ways are detrimental to the baby's well-being.

The medical and nursing care of healthy babies consists of teaching the parents the necessary skills to enable them to prevent avoidable illness, to provide proper nutrition, to encourage appropriate developmental stimulation of the infant and to ensure that the parents' love for the child can evolve and grow. So long as this is happening satisfactorily, little intervention is needed, though it is important to respond appropriately to the parents' requests for help or advice and to provide encouragement when new parents lack confidence in caring for their new baby.

Fostering the bonding and attachment process

The development of love between parents and their baby originates long before birth. For some mothers it starts at the moment pregnancy is confirmed, for others at the time of quickening at about 16–20 weeks. In yet other cases it is not until the baby is seen that the real feeling for him develops. Attachment to the infant gradually develops over the early months of life, and the ease with which it grows can be greatly

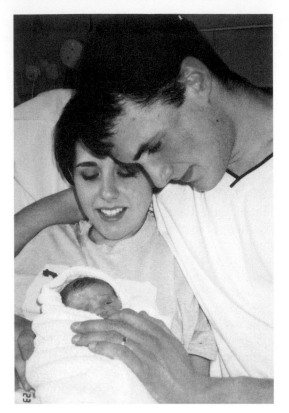

Figure 6.2   A time to admire and wonder at the new baby.

If the baby has a visible abnormality, is sick or of low birth weight, this procedure may have to be modified or curtailed. The general principles, however, apply even more strongly and meeting the emotional needs of the parents and family without physical risk to the baby is a matter for careful judgement in each individual case.

The midwife or doctor may usefully carry out the brief preliminary examination of the baby in the view of the mother, before rewrapping the infant in warm blankets and placing him in the cot. In maternity units, identification bracelets or security devices should be put on and the infant given 1 mg of vitamin K intramuscularly or orally, with parental consent, to prevent haemorrhagic disease of the newborn (p. 186) before the baby leaves the delivery room.

Factors which affect parenting ability

The psychological well-being of the mother before and after birth can have a profound effect on the care she can provide for the baby. Where her confidence is diminished by unhelpful or negative remarks from professional caregivers or unsupportive family members, inadequate mothering can follow. The baby needs good eye contact with the parents, gentle affectionate handling, to hear the sound of the parents' voices and to be given the opportunity to see and hear what is going on in the surroundings while he is awake. If the parents are not able to provide this stimulation, the baby's developmental progress may be hindered. Social factors, too, may adversely affect the infant's progress. Poor maternal educational attainment, young maternal age, lone parenthood, the reduction in family income which often accompanies the arrival of a baby, unemployment, social isolation and psychiatric disease (Stocky & Lynch 2000) may also take their toll. When several of these factors are present, there may be an increased risk of the infant failing to thrive or suffering delayed psychosocial development.

Not all mothers have a straightforward puerperium, some having had a medical complication of the pregnancy or an abnormal delivery, while others may develop the 'blues' or true puerperal depression or psychosis. These can seriously

influenced by the events during pregnancy, delivery, and the first few hours and days of the infant's life. Although safety of the infant must be paramount at all times, it is important to recognise and respond to the emotional needs of the parents and infant throughout this period. Observational studies suggest that physical contact between mother and baby encourages the attachment between them, and research shows that putting the baby to the breast immediately after birth improves the chances of successful breast feeding.

This time offers the parents their first opportunity to look at, feel, hear and wonder at their new infant (Fig. 6.2). A brief initial examination by the midwife can reassure the parents that there is no visible abnormality. It should not be necessary to hurry this phase of care, and after the infant is wrapped up warmly again, it should be possible for the baby to stay close to the mother for as long as she wishes.

impair the mother's ability to care for her infant and it is vital for the infant that such conditions are recognised by the midwife or health visitor and the mother referred for treatment or given additional support (Zuckermann & Beardslee 1987, Kuller et al 1996). It is often at this time that a supportive father can make a most important contribution to the care of the baby and mother. Sometimes it is only through noting that the baby is failing to thrive, is less responsive than expected or is unsettled or miserable that the maternal condition is identified, or other adverse social factors come to light. Further enquiry into this situation, with appropriate counselling and advice from the health visitor, could reduce the risk of child abuse or neglect.

MINIMISING THE RISK OF INFECTION

Before birth the baby has been largely protected from bacterial and viral infection, but during and after birth he is exposed to many organisms which may cause minor, or even major, infection. As the baby has limited protection against infection (p. 163), prevention of unnecessary exposure to pathogens is very important (Modi & Carr 2000). During the process of a vaginal birth, the infant encounters the bacterial flora of the mother's birth canal and perineum, with which the baby becomes colonised harmlessly during the first few days of life. Unless the mother has an active infection with a pathogenic organism, she is unlikely to be the source of serious infection for the baby, since the infant has received her antibodies through the placenta (p. 163). The infant's main sources of infection in hospital are members of the hospital staff, clothing, feeding utensils and, occasionally, other infants. In maternity hospitals where the babies may be cared for in large nurseries, ensuring that there is sufficient space between cots reduces the risk of cross-infection from other infants. The main practical precautions to prevent infection after birth are as follows:

1. Where possible, the mother should give the baby all the necessary care. Handling of the baby by health professionals should be limited to essential care – e.g. bathing, changing nappies, feeding.

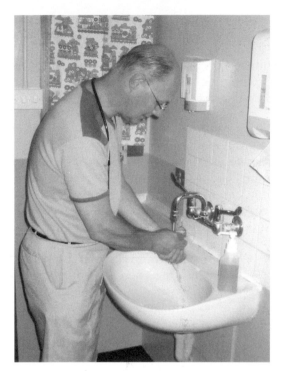

Figure 6.3   Hand washing is the most effective method of preventing cross-infection.

2. Hand washing is the single most effective measure against cross-infection of infants in hospital (Fig. 6.3). Mothers should wash their hands with ordinary soap before handling their infant. All other caregivers must wash their hands thoroughly with an antiseptic soap or apply a suitable antiseptic lotion before dealing with each baby, including children who are visiting.

3. The umbilical cord stump should be kept clean with boiled water or alcohol-based wipes, though some units prefer to use an antibiotic application at birth or an antiseptic powder at each nappy change (p. 88).

4. Good facilities are essential for preparation of sterile feeds. Where bottles and teats must be reused (e.g. special teats for an infant with a cleft palate), they should be used only by the same infant and sterilised carefully (p. 102).

5. Nappies and excreta should be carefully disposed of in sealable identifiable bags.

6. Cot blankets and infant clothing must be effectively sterilised in laundering. Cotton blankets are easiest to keep bacteriologically clean.

7. Special attention is paid to minor infections in those who come into contact with the babies; for example, a nurse, midwife or doctor with a bacterial skin infection, throat infection or mild gastroenteritis should be excluded temporarily.

8. Wherever possible, any infected infant or one carrying a pathogenic organism must be isolated from the others, preferably being cared for by the mother in a single isolation ward. If circumstances make this impossible, extra pre-cautions against cross-infection (barrier nursing techniques with plastic aprons) should be used whenever the baby is handled. Disposal of infected material, particularly faeces, must be carried out with great care.

9. Any infant admitted from outside the hospital should be regarded as a potential source of infection and isolated initially. If bacterial cultures show no pathogens, isolation is no longer required.

10. Healthy visitors, including young siblings of the new baby, are rarely a source of infection, though parents should be encouraged to report minor illnesses in family members to the hospital staff so that advice can be given to deter those with significant infections from visiting.

The use of face-masks and the routine wearing of gowns by hospital staff or the parents does not protect the infants from infection.

ALIMENTARY TRACT FUNCTION – STOOLS

Meconium is a viscid semi-fluid substance which consists mainly of mucus with an accumulation of swallowed amniotic fluid, desquamated epithelial cells and bilirubin which gives it the characteristic blackish-green colour. The first stool is normally passed within the first 24 hours but, exceptionally, it may be delayed for up to 3 days in normal infants. A firm plug of meconium may obstruct the anus and cause abdominal distension, which is relieved after gentle stretching of the anal sphincter by rectal examination.

If feeding is taking place normally, 'changing stools' of a light greenish-brown colour replace the meconium on about the third or fourth day.

Thereafter, there is a gradual change to the mustard-coloured stools of the breast-fed, or the paler yellow stools of the formula-fed infant. There is great individual variation in the number and consistency of the stools, which bears little relation to the rate of the infant's weight gain. A vigorous gastrocolic reflex may cause the breast-fed baby to pass one or two stools at each feed, but occasional infants pass only one large soft stool as infrequently as once every 2 or 3 days. Much more regularity is found in formula-fed babies, and variations in the number and consistency of stools in this group are more likely to reflect an alimentary disorder.

RENAL FUNCTION – URINE

Urine secretion takes place in the latter half of pregnancy and much of the amniotic fluid is fetal urine. The baby may also micturate during delivery, when it may go unnoticed. Normally, infants pass urine first at any time up to 48 hours, or even exceptionally as late as the third day, though most infants will do so within 12 hours. Serious causes for delay are rare in the absence of other clinical signs such as enlargement of the bladder. The nature of the urinary stream should be observed since dribbling micturition is the most useful sign of urethral valves in a boy or ectopic ureters in a girl.

The amount and frequency of urine passed gradually increases with the quantity of feed taken during the first week and the bladder may empty up to 20 times a day during the second week. The volume is immensely variable and depends on the fluid intake. Breast-fed infants average 20 mL on the 1st day, rising to 200 mL on the 10th day.

Urate crystals may colour the urine at this age, leaving a brick-red stain on the nappy which can be mistaken for blood. Albumin is not normally present in more than slight traces but false-positive tests due to urates can sometimes be misleading.

The normal term infant has a glomerular filtration rate of about 40 mL/min per 1.73 m^2, or about a third of adult values, and it only slowly increases over the first year of life. The kidneys can neither rapidly excrete a water load nor concentrate the urine to conserve fluid well in the first month, although the tubules are capable of responding normally to antidiuretic hormone. The term infant can conserve sodium but the premature baby's kidney often leaks sodium even when the serum level is low. Consequently, it is important that the term baby is not given feeds with too high a sodium concentration which could render him or her hypernatraemic and damage the developing brain. All reputable formula milks contain adjusted mineral levels to reduce this risk.

CARE OF THE SKIN AND UMBILICUS
Cleansing the infant

Any faecal soiling should be wiped gently from the skin as soon as possible after it occurs, particularly in the nappy area to prevent nappy rash, using cotton wool and water only. Most modern paper-based disposable nappies soak up urine and prevent the skin from remaining in contact with it. However, the nappy must be changed and the skin washed about 4-hourly as the urea in the urine can be broken down by faecal organisms to form ammonia which may cause nappy rash.

The first full bath should be given only when feeding is well established and the baby's temperature is stable, since before this time there is a risk of the baby becoming cold. For the term infant, this need not be until the end of the first week of life, though if careful attention is paid to prevention of heat loss, much earlier bathing is permissible (Varda & Behnke 2000). For the preterm infant, bathing can be delayed for several weeks. The use of a moisturising baby soap will prevent the skin from becoming dry and uncomfortable, especially in babies who are post-term or growth retarded. The infant should be gently patted dry and wrapped in a warm towel to prevent heat loss. After the first week or so, bathing becomes largely a social event which should be pleasurable for both mother and baby.

Nappy rash

Rashes in the nappy area at this early period of infancy are most commonly around the anus and are often attributable to irritation of the skin by faeces rather than urine. This perianal excoriation often accompanies a change from breast to artificial feeding. Babies withdrawing from maternal drug misuse are at an increased risk of developing sore buttocks due to the constant loose stools they excrete (Ladewig et al 1998). There is also an increased tendency for babies undergoing phototherapy to develop nappy rash from the associated loose stools (p. 197). It is important for nurses and midwives to ensure they teach good nappy care to parents. Nappy rash can usually be prevented, but if it does occur it can be treated successfully by exposure of the affected area to the air in warm surroundings or by the use of a silicone barrier cream to protect it from additional moisture when the nappy is reapplied.

Monilial dermatitis

Monilial dermatitis (thrush) in the perineum is also common, especially in infants who have received antibiotics, and may occur even in the absence of visible thrush in the mouth. It typically affects the moist areas and flexures as a localised shiny redness with superficial desquamation of skin (Plate 13). Such a rash here is most unlikely to have any other cause and treatment with local application of nystatin cream, together with oral nystatin suspension (p. 167), is usually successful. A number of other antifungal preparations are available as alternatives. Sometimes, a sensitisation reaction of the skin to the *Monilia* requires a short period of local steroid application as additional treatment.

Ammoniacal dermatitis

Ammoniacal dermatitis is commoner after the first month and consists of erythema, peeling, or ulcerating eruptions over the projecting parts of the nappy area, sparing the flexures. Treatment is by reducing the duration of contact of the skin with urine by frequent washing with a moisturising soap, drying and putting on a dry nappy. Secondary monilial infection is common and should be treated with topical nystatin cream. The use of highly absorbent paper-based disposable nappies significantly reduces the frequency of this condition, but if towelling nappies are being used, they must be washed thoroughly and used with a water-repelling nappy liner to keep the skin as dry as possible.

The umbilical cord

Soon after the initial clamping with forceps, a sterile disposable clamp is placed on the cord 1–2 cm from the umbilical skin. The possibility of a single umbilical artery and its associated congenital malformations (p. 203) should be rechecked at this time. The cord is then cut about 1 cm beyond the clamp, which is left on until the stump is dry, usually around 2 or 3 days. Separation usually occurs between 7 and 10 days of life. The stump is occasionally moist when the cord separates and it can become colonised by potentially pathogenic bacteria. Cord care practices vary (Graham & Hundley 2000) and relatively little research has compared the methods of prevention of umbilical infection. Some units allow the stump to dry naturally with no interference, some wiping with water only, others using isopropyl alcohol swabs and application of 0.3% hexachlorophane powder with each nappy change, while others recommend an antibiotic spray at birth with no other active intervention. Current evidence suggests that simply keeping the cord clean is as effective as applying antimicrobial agents (Zupan & Garner 2000). Whichever method is chosen, it is important to inspect the cord daily and note any periumbilical erythema or discharge so that an infection can be treated before it becomes generalised.

SLEEPING POSTURE AND PREVENTION OF COT DEATH

Research in several developed countries has confirmed a connection between sudden infant death syndrome (SIDS; cot death) and placing babies face down to sleep (Ponsonby et al 1995). In Britain, the overall incidence of the condition halved after it was recommended that all infants should be placed on their backs to sleep and this reduction has been maintained. Although the

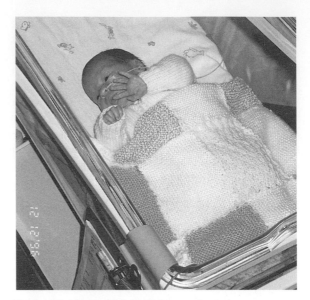

Figure 6.4 'Back to sleep and feet to foot'.

exact reasons for this are not clear, it is known that hyperthermia from overheating, which has been found in some cot-death victims, is more likely in the prone position, particularly if the infant has a virus infection. All infants should be placed on their back to sleep (Fig. 6.4) unless there is a clear medical reason to do otherwise, such as gastro-oesophageal reflux. In the absence of reflux, there is no evidence of a serious risk of inhalation in the supine position. Putting babies on their side to sleep also carries an increased risk and should be avoided (Fleming et al 1996).

The risk is substantially increased if the baby sleeps with the parents in a sofa or chair, and bed sharing increases the risk if the parents smoke (Beal & Byard 2000), have drunk alcohol, have taken drugs or are of large size (Carroll-Pankhurst & Mortimer 2001). Although bed sharing is not in itself a risk factor, parents in these higher risk groups should be advised against the practice (Blair et al 1999, Nelson et al 2001).

Other factors which recent research has shown to be related to cot death include overheating the infant, antenatal and postnatal exposure of the baby to tobacco smoke, low birth weight, poor socioeconomic circumstances and maternal substance abuse. Preterm infants are 8 to 10 times

---

Box 6.1 Risk factors for and prevention of sudden infant death syndrome

Risk factors
- Cigarette smoking:
  —before birth
  —in the baby's room
  —if the baby sleeps with the parents
- Parental drug misuse
- Bed sharing if the parents:
  —have drunk alcohol
  —have taken drugs
  —are smokers
  —are of large size
- Sleeping with a baby on a sofa or easy chair
- Overheating the baby
- Poor socioeconomic circumstances
- Preterm babies
- Male babies

Positive preventive measures
- Place the baby to sleep:
  —feet to foot in the cot
  —on his or her back (Fig. 6.4)
- Tuck in blankets
- Avoid loose bedding and duvets
- Keep the baby in the parents' bedroom at night for the first 6 months of life
- Seek medical advice promptly if the baby is feverish

---

more likely to die from SIDS than term babies (Fleming et al 1996,) and male babies are at greater risk than females.

Actions which can be recommended to parents include the measures listed in Box 6.1, though there is no complete guarantee that they will prevent sudden unexpected death. Nursing and medical staff should ensure that all parents are aware of the latest government-recommended guidelines. The Confidential Enquiry into Stillbirths and Deaths in Infancy (CESDI) report found that in 60% of SIDS cases the parents were not following the official guidelines, either because the information had not been made available to them or because they were ignoring it.

WEIGHING THE BABY

The baby must be weighed accurately within a few hours of birth and thereafter on alternate days. Weighing should always be carried out immediately before a feed and at the same time of day on each occasion so that the weights are comparable. All babies will lose a little weight in the first 4 days, but if this exceeds 10% of birth weight an explanation should be sought. So long as the weight begins to rise from the fourth day, alternate daily measurements can be reduced to weekly weighing after 10 days of age, by which time most infants should have regained their birth weight. Rates of weight gain thereafter vary considerably, and apparently unusual gain must be interpreted carefully (p. 46). Where intrauterine growth has been poor because of placental insufficiency, weight gain may accelerate through the chart until the baby reaches his genetic centile. Overgrown babies may show lag down growth (p. 56).

REFERENCES

Beal S M, Byard R W 2000 Sudden infant death syndrome in South Australia 1968–97. Is bed sharing safe for infants? Journal of Paediatrics and Child Health 36(6):552–554

Blair P S, Fleming P J et al 1999 Babies sleeping with parents: case control study of factors influencing the risk of sudden infant death syndrome. British Medical Journal 319(7223):1457–1461

Carroll-Pankhurst C, Mortimer E A 2001 Sudden infant death syndrome, bedsharing, parental weight and age at death. Pediatrics 107(3):530–536

Fleming P J, Blair P S, Bacon C et al 1996 Environment of infants during sleep and risk of the sudden infant death syndrome: results of 1993–5 case-control study for confidential inquiry into stillbirths and deaths in infancy. British Medical Journal 313(7051):191–195

Gatrad A R, Sheikh A 2001 Muslim birth customs. Archives of Disease in Childhood Fetal and Neonatal Edition 84:F6–F8

Graham W, Hundley V A 2000 Cord care practice in Scotland. Midwifery 16(3):237–245

Kuller J A, Katz V L, McMahon M J et al 1996 Pharmacological treatment of psychiatric disease in pregnancy and lactation: fetal and neonatal effects. Obstetrics and Gynecology 87(5):789–794

Ladewig P, London M, Olds S 1998 The newborn at risk. In: Maternal newborn nursing care, 4th edn. Addison Wesley, Longman, New York, Ch 25:617–671

Modi N, Carr R 2000 Promising strategems for reducing the burden of neonatal sepsis. Archives of Disease in Childhood Fetal and Neonatal Edition 83:F150–F153

Nelson E A, Taylor B J, Jenik A et al 2001 International child care practices study: infant sleeping environment. Early Human Development 62(1):43–55

Ponsonby A-L, Dwyer T, Kasl S V et al 1995 Correlates of prone infant sleeping position by period of birth. Archives of Disease in Childhood 72:204–208

Stocky A, Lynch J 2000 Acute psychiatric disturbance in pregnancy and the puerperium. Baillières Best Practice Research in Clinical Obstetrics and Gynaecology 14(1):73–87

Varda K E, Behnke R S 2000 The effect of timing of initial bath on newborn's temperature. Journal of Obstetrics and Gynaecology Nursing 29(1):27–32

Zuckermann B S, Beardslee W R 1987 Maternal depression: a concern for paediatricians. Pediatrics 79(1):110–117

Zupan J, Garner P 2000 Topical umbilical cord care at birth. Cochrane Database of Systematic Reviews (2): CD001057

Chapter 7
Feeding the baby

CHAPTER CONTENTS

Introduction   91
Physiology of feeding   91
   Digestion and absorption   92
Principles of neonatal nutrition   92
Breast or bottle?   93
   Why should breast feeding be encouraged?   93
   Reasons for not breast feeding and common
   problems   95
   Antenatal education for infant feeding   97
   Maternal nutrition   97
   Feeding in the immediate postnatal period   97
   Physiology of milk secretion   98
   Making breast feeding more effective   98
   Care of the breasts   99
   Breast engorgement and mastitis   99
   Cup feeding   100
Feeding difficulties   100
   Underfeeding   100
   Overfeeding   100
   Problems related to sucking   100
Artificial feeding by the bottle   101
   Alternatives to breast feeding   101
   Cow's milk formulae   101
   Preparing the feeds   102
   Giving the feeds   103
   The amount and frequency of feeds   104
   Cow's milk intolerance   104
Common problems related to feeding   104
   Wind, posseting and vomiting   104
   Distension of the abdomen   105
   Unusual bowel actions and stools   105

INTRODUCTION

It is important to recognise that feeding not only is a process designed to provide nutrition for the baby but also it contributes to the protection of the infant from infection and fosters and develops the relationship between the baby and the parents. In the case of breast feeding, it also assists in the mother's recovery from the pregnant state. A great deal could be written about infant feeding, but only those features which are important in the newborn period will be described, including ways of making feeding more effective and alleviating some of the common difficulties.

PHYSIOLOGY OF FEEDING

Whether the baby is breast or bottle fed, the milk is obtained by a wavelike movement of the tongue compressing the nipple from front to back while the areola is held in a firm grip by the lips. When the milk hits the palate, it induces swallowing, which is completed before the next suck occurs (Fig. 7.1). The coordination to 'latch-on' and obtain the feed in this way develops near term, and most infants over 35 weeks of gestation are able to suck adequately to obtain enough milk to grow. The normal infant swallows a variable quantity of air during feeds, most of which is expelled afterwards, sometimes with a little milk. Vomiting of a more persistent nature should be regarded as abnormal and a cause sought (p. 105).

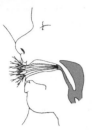

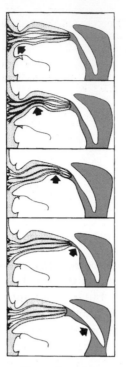

Figure 7.1   Diagram showing the rolling action of the tongue during breast feeding. The nipple is compressed between the tongue and the anterior part of the palate from which a wave of compression (arrowed) progresses backwards towards the pharynx, thus expelling the milk and initiating swallowing. (From *Successful breastfeeding*, with permission of the Royal College of Midwives.)

Digestion and absorption

There is relatively good development of secretory and absorbing surfaces in the infant gut from well before term. This results in efficient absorption of food, but the gut may become distended with wind because of a lack of supportive tissues in the bowel wall. Digestive enzymes are fully active at term except for pancreatic amylase, so that digestion of starch is theoretically not possible.

PRINCIPLES OF NEONATAL NUTRITION

At birth a baby has stores of brown fat and glycogen, which are metabolised to produce heat, which in turn maintains body temperature. The principal nutritional importance of the feeds given within the first few hours of life is to maintain a safe blood glucose level, whereas after the first few days the provision of sufficient calories, proteins and minerals for growth and increasing activity becomes more important. From the end of the first week, the rate of growth and weight gain of the infant is faster than at any other time and the average term baby gains between 180 and 210 g each week, slowly reducing to around 110 g per week at 6 months of age. To achieve this gain, at least 1.5 g/kg per day of protein are required with sufficient calories from carbohydrate to utilise it, and approximately one-third of the total calorie intake is expended on growth. An inadequate supply of energy will, therefore, decrease weight gain, though brain growth is usually spared until intake is grossly deficient. Human milk contains appropriate amounts of all the necessary nutrients, minerals and vitamins, including fats, which provide about half the baby's energy needs, and the essential fatty acids, such as arachidonic and linoleic acids, which are needed for optimal brain development. These fatty acids are also present in all reputable baby milk formulae as currently recommended by international bodies such as the World Health Organisation, though evidence of cognitive benefit is hard to find (Auestad et al 2001). Certain long-chain polyunsaturated fatty acids also are important for optimal brain growth, particularly in the preterm infant, and they are now included in many baby milk formulae.

The amount of feed required varies from one baby to another depending on the rate of metabolism, how active the baby is and on the need to produce heat to keep warm. In addition, a baby whose intrauterine growth was reduced may need to make 'catch-up growth' which requires additional nutrients. These differences cannot be accurately calculated, but, fortunately, except when the baby is ill or preterm, he usually obtains the amount he needs by showing when he is hungry or satisfied. The feed must meet all the metabolic needs of the baby without exceeding the capacity of the body to handle specific components. The kidneys have a limited ability to dispose of the urea produced by protein metabolism, and an excessive intake may result in the baby becoming uraemic. Too much lactose in the gut can cause diarrhoea. Excess vitamin D produces hypercalcaemia.

Table 7.1 Selected daily nutritional requirements of a newborn baby at 1 week of age

Calories	120–140 kcal/kg
Protein	1.5–4.0 g/kg
Carbohydrate	8–15 g/kg
Sodium	2.5 mmol/kg
Calcium	0.5–1.0 mmol/kg
Phosphate	2–3 mmol/kg
Vitamin A	5000 IU
Vitamin D	400 IU

Average daily requirements of some important nutrients in the neonatal period are shown in Table 7.1.

BREAST OR BOTTLE?

When asked the question, those concerned with the care of the newborn generally express no doubt that breast feeding is the method of choice. Yet, although it is the cheapest and most convenient way of feeding and it has been promoted vigorously by health professionals and others, only around 63% of mothers in Britain start breast feeding, and fewer than 50% successfully breast feed beyond 2 weeks and fewer than 25% by 4 months. The UK has among the lowest breast-feeding rates in Europe.

The factors affecting the parents' decision whether to breast or bottle feed have more to do with social and cultural attitudes, whether the mother encountered problems breast feeding previous babies, support from the family and whether the mother needs to work after the birth, rather than with professional recommendations (National Breastfeeding Working Group 1995). Mothers from skilled or professional backgrounds and those from Asian backgrounds are more likely to start breast feeding than are teenage mothers (Botting et al 1998, Lawson 1998) and unskilled mothers, especially if the latter already have several children, have no partner, finished full-time education before the age of 16 or smoked during pregnancy. One study showed how the media do not promote a positive image of breast feeding: on analysing the content of television programmes, bottle feeding appeared to be the infant feeding of choice (Henderson et al 2000). There is now good evidence that locally based initiatives can increase

Box 7.1 Initiatives which have improved breast-feeding rates

- Breast-feeding training for medical staff
- Introducing cup feeding for babies not able to go to the breast
- Information booklets for the mother
- Breast-feeding counsellors on postnatal wards
- Introducing the baby-friendly initiative
- Encouraging fathers to accept breast feeding
- Producing guidelines for postnatal wards
- Providing rooms for breast feeding
- Promoting study days on breast feeding
- Helplines accessible by mothers
- Encouraging mothers to attend breast-feeding support groups

the rates of breast feeding if midwives and medical staff are committed to them (Box 7.1). Mothers who are undecided know that bottle-fed babies thrive and may feel tempted to bottle feed because they can see how much the baby has taken; they also know that someone else will be able to take over if they are unable to give an occasional feed themselves, particularly at night, and these factors may sway the mind of those uncertain about which method of feeding to choose. To assist in the promotion of breast feeding, the United Nations International Children's Fund (UNICEF) has suggested a number of factors which may be introduced into a hospital to make it more 'baby-friendly' and to encourage more mothers to start and continue to breast feed their babies (Box 7.2). In those hospitals which succeed in putting all the points into action, rates of breast feeding can rise by 10% (UNICEF website). In 1999, the British Government recommended increasing breast-feeding rates through health professionals providing accurate factual information about it to both school-age boys and girls to try to persuade more young mothers to breast feed their babies.

Why should breast feeding be encouraged?

The nutritional advantages of human milk are numerous (Box 7.3). It has a varying composition which alters over the days and weeks to provide for the changing needs of the growing baby.

Box 7.2   UNICEF-designated 'baby-friendly' initiative: ten steps to successful breast feeding

Every facility providing maternity services and care for newborn babies should:

1. Have a written breast-feeding policy which is routinely communicated to all health staff
2. Train all health staff in skills to implement this policy
3. Inform all pregnant women about the benefits and management of breast feeding
4. Help mothers initiate breast feeding within half an hour of birth
5. Show mothers how to breast feed, and how to maintain lactation even if they are separated from their infant
6. Give newborn infants no food or drink other than breast milk, unless medically indicated
7. Practice rooming-in 24 hours a day
8. Encourage breast feeding on demand
9. Give no artificial teats or pacifiers (dummies) to breast-feeding infants
10. Foster the establishment of breast-feeding support groups and refer mothers to them on discharge from the hospital

---

Box 7.3   The benefits of breast feeding

- Provides optimum nutrition for growth and development
- Content of the milk adapts to baby's changing needs
- Protects the baby against some infections
- Promotes a good relationship between mother and baby
- Associated with better acquisition of cognitive skills
- Reduces risk of later childhood eczema and diabetes
- Assists the mother to lose weight
- Reduces the risk of some breast and ovarian cancers in the mother

---

Initially the energy content of the milk provides around 115 kcal/kg/day, falling to 100 kcal/kg/day after about 3 months. The proteins, initially consisting predominantly of lactalbumin with little casein, are readily digested and absorbed. The relative amounts change, and as breast feeding continues, the proportion of casein increases. Breast milk contains the correct amounts and ratios of certain lipids including long-chain polyunsaturated fatty acids, which are thought to be essential for optimal development of the brain and retina. Other individual components of breast milk, including iron, are in a form well suited to the healthy full-term baby's requirements such that deficiency states rarely emerge. The low concentration of sodium prevents the development of hypernatraemia, which can cause brain damage. Neonatal convulsions from hypocalcaemia and hypomagnesaemia are prevented by the low phosphate content of breast milk (p. 157).

Colostrum and breast milk contain numerous factors, including secretory IgA, lysozymes, lactoferrin and white cells, which have a considerable protective effect against gastroenteritis and infections of the middle ear, respiratory tract and urinary tract (Wang & Wu 1996), which is particularly important in babies in developing countries. The high lactose content, by producing a relatively acid pH in the large intestine, favours the growth of lactobacilli and inhibits that of potentially harmful *Escherchia coli*, and the oligosaccharides, which form about 15% of the carbohydrate in mature breast milk also inhibit bacterial growth. The stools are inoffensive and constipation is rarely a problem. Other factors such as hormones, growth factors and certain enzymes are also present, though their precise function is as yet unknown.

Breast feeding exclusively from the start reduces substantially the risk of introducing the allergens of cow's milk protein, which, if taken in the first few weeks of life, can be a contributory cause of later atopic disease such as eczema. The incidence of childhood asthma is also reduced, especially in those from atopic families (Gdalevich et al 2001). Thus, it is especially important to encourage breast feeding in cases where there is a strong family history of allergic disease. In preterm infants, breast feeding is associated with better neurodevelopmental outcome and it reduces the risk of necrotising enterocolitis (p. 140). There also appears to be some measurable cognitive benefit in healthy term infants (Angelsen et al 2001). The incidence of insulin-dependent diabetes mellitus in later childhood is lower if the infant has been breast fed.

Breast feeding also has psychosocial advantages. Not only is the milk readily available whenever the baby requires it, but also the mother is likely to lose any excess weight gain more readily. It also assists in the return of the uterus to the non-pregnant state. However, perhaps the main

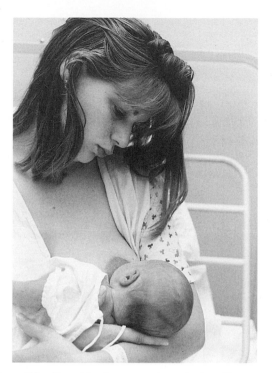

Figure 7.2 Breast feeding strengthens the bond between mother and baby.

value of breast feeding lies in the act itself, for when it goes well, there is often an emotional satisfaction to the mother, which is reflected in the reactions of the baby, and this can strengthen the strong attachment between the two (Fig. 7.2). Although bottle feeding by no means precludes this, the closer contact of breast feeding often provides an easier way of fostering the normal stable relationship.

The disadvantages are few. Haemorrhagic disease of the newborn due to vitamin K deficiency occurs mainly in breast-fed babies, but can be prevented by giving a supplement of the vitamin at birth (p. 188). Extra vitamin D may be required to prevent the possible onset of rickets after 6 months of age and it is probably wise to supplement those infants from dark-skinned ethnic groups and those living in cities in temperate lands. In a small proportion of infants, physiological jaundice is prolonged by breast feeding, but the condition is usually benign and seldom requires treatment other than reassurance (p. 197). On rare occasions, allergy may be enhanced by exposing the baby

to an allergen in the milk. For example, recent evidence has shown that peanut allergens are secreted in breast milk (Vadas et al 2001). Around 80% of children who suffer an allergic reaction to peanuts do so on their first exposure and must have been sensitised before their initial contact, possibly from breast feeding. Breast-feeding mothers who have allergic disease should avoid nuts from their diet during lactation.

Reasons for not breast feeding and common problems

The size of the breast has no bearing on its potential for producing milk, though structural abnormalities such as non-protractile nipples may make breast feeding more difficult. Cosmetic breast surgery is usually compatible with successful breast feeding unless the nipple has been repositioned. Maternal ill-health or some defect in the infant may account for a few failures. Some mothers have clear social reasons for choosing artificial feeding – for instance, the return to a job. A few give up because they find breast feeding distasteful. For some mothers it is painful, particularly in the first few weeks, but changes in positioning of the baby on the breast often alleviate the problem. The majority of mothers who discontinue breast feeding do so because they are faced with a discontented baby in the third or fourth week, resulting from an apparently – but possibly only temporary – inadequate supply of milk. If the mother feels that her baby is being starved, she may be ready to accept a suggestion that a change to the bottle would be wise. There are several possible causes for this reduction of milk secretion and, although prolonged engorgement of the breasts during the first week predisposes to it, improving the feeding technique or allowing more frequent suckling often improves the supply (p. 99). The worry of managing the home as well as the new baby also contributes. Some research suggests that excessive weight gain in pregnancy – over 30 lb (13 kg) – may impair the ability to breast feed. This is partly due to physical difficulties related to the size of the mother's breasts, making it difficult for the baby to latch on. In addition, the excess fat acts as a source of circulating progesterone, which delays the onset of lactation.

There are a few conditions which render breast feeding inappropriate or unwise. Milk secretion adds a considerable load to the metabolic activity, thus any severe chronic maternal illness may be a contraindication. Examples of such include cardiac disease, chronic nephritis with hypertension, and chronic respiratory infection. However, most acute infective maternal illnesses require only brief separation from the infant, during which time breast-milk production is maintained by expression.

Many drugs taken by the mother are secreted in the milk but, fortunately, the concentration is often small and may not affect the baby adversely. It is advisable, however, to avoid breast feeding when the mother has to be on full-dosage treatment with any of the drugs listed in Table 7.2. This list is not exhaustive, and for further information the current edition of the British National Formulary (BNF), Internet resources or telephone information services should be consulted (Spencer et al 2001). In addition, commonly taken drugs such as alcohol, nicotine, caffeine and marijuana all enter breast milk, hence it is wise for breast-feeding mothers to limit their intake of such substances (Liston 1998). Some of the by-products of cigarette smoking, e.g. cotinine, are found in breast milk and may increase the risk of respiratory problems in the infant (Stepans & Wilkerson 1993).

Although it is not an absolute contraindication, current recommendations suggest that mothers who are infected with the human immuno-deficiency virus (HIV) or have acquired immuno-deficiency syndrome (AIDS) should not breast feed, to reduce further the small risk of infecting the infant through the milk (p. 179). Hepatitis B carriers with the e antigen in the blood can also transmit the infection to the infant through their milk and should not breast feed. Hepatitis C virus can be excreted in breast milk but the estimated vertical infection rate is around 7% (Gibb et al 2000) and at present the view is that the benefits of breast feeding outweigh the possible risks (Hadzic 2001). Occasionally, cytomegalovirus and Epstein-Barr virus are excreted in the breast milk of acutely infected mothers and this may infect

Table 7.2 Maternal drugs and breast feeding. The baby should not breast feed if the mother is taking the following drugs:

Non-steroidal anti-inflammatory drugs	Indometacin
	Phenylbutazone
Anticoagulants	Phenindione
	Dicoumarol
Anticonvulsants	Carbamazepine
	Primidone
Antithyroid drugs	Carbimazole
	Thiouracil
Antibiotics	Chloramphenicol
	Metronidazole
	Novobiocin
	Tetracyclines
	Trimethoprim
Cortisone	
Cytotoxic agents	Cyclophosphamide
Ergotamine	
Hypotensive agents	Propranolol
	Reserpine
Lithium	
Radioactive isotopes	Radioiodine
Sedatives	Chloral hydrate
	Diazepam
	Phenothiazines
Tolbutamide	
Vitamins	A & D in high dose
Drugs of addiction	Heroin
	Methadone
	Cannabis

the baby (Golding 1997). Small amounts of illegal drugs such as heroin and cocaine are secreted into breast milk and can affect the infant, but each situation should be assessed individually, as often the benefits to the infant of breast feeding will be greater than the risk.

Preterm birth or severe neonatal disease and some congenital abnormalities (e.g. cleft lip and palate) may render breast feeding impossible initially, though a mother who is very keen to breast feed can keep her milk flowing by either hand expression or the use of a breast pump until the baby is able to feed from her, and the milk given to the baby by another means. Social contraindications can only be judged individually, but it must be recognised that there are mothers who feel such an antipathy to the idea of breast feeding that forcing the issue may only do harm. Finally, inadequate breast-milk secretion may be a good reason for a change to artificial feeds, especially where an attempt at improving the feeding technique

(p. 99) fails to increase the infant's weight gain after a reasonable trial period.

Antenatal education for infant feeding

During pregnancy, infant feeding should be discussed with the parents in Education for Parenthood classes and in the antenatal clinic, and excellent visual aids are now available to assist in this task. It is important that the advantages and disadvantages of breast and formula feeding are explained in these forums, so that the mother and her partner can make an informed decision about how to feed the infant, since leaflets alone have been shown not to be successful. It should be explained to the parents that the first few weeks of caring for the new infant will be exacting and that some mothers do not find breast feeding easy and emotionally fulfilling initially (Hatfield 2000). Breast feeding should not be romanticised but be portrayed in a realistic fashion, since if it fails to live up to expectations, mothers will feel it was not successful.

Many mothers give up breast feeding early because they fear that the baby is not thriving on it (p. 46), and the attitude of mind in which discussion of feeding is approached both by the mother and by the midwife has an important influence on its success. If the young mother realises that breast feeding is not always straightforward but learns that those who look after her understand these difficulties and can give continuing consistent guidance and practical help, she is the more likely to want to carry it through.

Maternal nutrition

The extra intake of food in pregnancy, which is necessary for the developing fetus, should continue during lactation. The fatty-acid pattern of the milk and its content of many vitamins and minerals are adversely affected if the maternal diet is deficient. In addition to her own normal diet, the mother should take an extra 15 g of protein per day and additional carbohydrate, calcium, vitamins and water. These needs can be supplied by consuming at least one pint of milk a day together with a good mixed diet containing meat, fish or cheese, and fresh fruit and vegetables. Extra vitamin A, C and D and folic acid (p. 230) should be added, and the mother should be encouraged to take fluids liberally.

Feeding in the immediate postnatal period

It is now common practice to put the baby to the breast within a few minutes of birth. There is good evidence that this both influences the success and duration of breast feeding and provides an early opportunity for the relationship between the mother and infant to develop. There is only a small nutritional content in the colostrum obtained, but even a few moments of suckling will provide the infant with a valuable amount of the substances which give some protection against infection (p. 163). Even if the baby does not suckle immediately after birth, feeding should begin at some time within the first 4 hours and for a healthy term infant the first feed should be at the breast. In some cultures there is an erroneous belief that the colostrum is not good for the infant, which may be a barrier to effective breast feeding. The first feed should be supervised by a midwife skilled in the techniques of breast feeding to ensure that mother and baby both learn good methods from the beginning.

For successful breast feeding, the mother should be comfortable and the baby physically well supported. Either lying or sitting, she should support the baby's back and buttocks in the crook of her arm, allowing the nipple to touch the cheek, thus stimulating the rooting reflex (p. 73). Correct attachment may be achieved by keeping the infant's lower jaw as low on the areola as possible so that the maximum amount of the nipple is taken into the mouth (Fig. 7.3). It may also be assisted by holding the breast underneath or behind the areola to aid protrusion of the nipple, but the mother should not push the nipple towards the baby.

Correct positioning of the infant at the breast will help to prevent nipple damage and ensure that breast feeding is maintained (Short 1994). Subsequently, the infant should be allowed to determine the frequency of feeds and, so long as

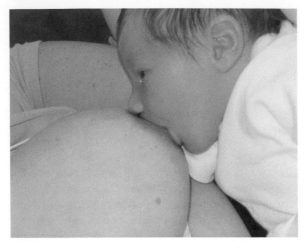

Figure 7.3 Correct positioning of the baby on the nipple prevents sore nipples and maximises the effectiveness of breast feeding.

a correct feeding technique is used, the suckling time should not be limited. One additional benefit of unrestricted suckling is that more bilirubin is excreted in the increased number of stools passed, which may reduce the severity of jaundice in the infant.

Physiology of milk secretion

Successful breast feeding depends upon the secretion of two maternal pituitary hormones. Prolactin from the anterior pituitary gland acts upon the glandular tissue of the breast to promote milk production, and oxytocin from the posterior pituitary gland stimulates the ejection of milk from the breast during feeding. Oxytocin is released in response to the sucking of the baby at the breast, but secretion may be inhibited by stress, anxiety and other emotional factors. Breast feeding should, therefore, take place in a relaxed atmosphere and the mother should be positively encouraged throughout feeding. This should promote adequate oxytocin secretion during suckling, a phenomenon known as the let-down reflex. This enables the milk in the alveoli of the breasts to be pushed forward through the duct system to the place where the mechanical rolling action of the baby's tongue can remove the milk from the breast.

Breast milk is not a uniform secretion. It varies in constitution from beginning to end of each feed and over time to adapt to the infant's changing needs. Colostrum, which is secreted initially, is small in quantity and low in nutritional value. This is in part why healthy babies lose weight initially, as they utilise the excess water the body contains at birth to counteract the small initial milk volume. Within 2 to 3 days, the milk comes in and the volume available rises rapidly. From this point on, the milk taken at the beginning of a feed is high in protein, lactose and water content; although the volume decreases as the breast empties, more fat, which has a higher calorie content, is secreted. Provided the baby is satisfied and gaining weight, it is appropriate for him or her to feed at only one breast at each feed – this is certainly preferable to a short time on both breasts, which may deny the baby the important hind milk.

Over two-thirds of the volume of a feed is taken in the first 3 minutes, but the hind milk is only available after this. Enabling the baby to feed long enough to take the hind milk is advised, since breast engorgement is less likely to occur if at least one breast is emptied at each feed. Individual babies also differ in the volume they take at each feed. Some may demand feeding every hour or two for several feeds and then sleep for a longer interval, and the duration of the feed may vary from only 5 minutes to over 20. Responding to this irregular pattern can be tiring, but unrestricted feeding increases the likelihood of successful breast feeding and reduces nipple trauma. After a week or two, the baby usually settles into a more regular pattern of six to eight feeds each day. Feeding the baby on a timed schedule does not allow the mother to respond to her infant's needs and should be discouraged. Even at this age babies will learn to be confident whether their crying will be answered sensitively, and responding swiftly to their needs will not get them into bad habits.

Making breast feeding more effective

It is imperative that those who give professional advice to a mother about breast feeding should

---

Box 7.4 Effective breast feeding

Breast feeding can be made more effective by:

- Consistent advice from professionals
- Advice based upon sound knowledge
- Personal support for the mother
- Unrestricted breast feeding on demand
- Correct positioning of the baby at the breast
- Correct fixing on the nipple
- Fully emptying at least one breast at each feed
- Avoidance of formula-feed supplementation
- Avoiding routine supplements of water
- Supplementation by cup feeding

---

avoid laying down dogmatic rules and regulations. Rather, they should have an adequate understanding of the principles underlying successful breast feeding so that they can provide personalised support and give consistent advice based on sound knowledge (Box 7.4). Little discourages a mother from breast feeding more than being given simplistic, hurried and conflicting advice rather than listening to her concerns and responding sensitively to them.

Supplementary and complementary feeds of formula milk are not necessary for healthy full-term infants and they may hasten the abandonment of breast feeding. Only rarely is even additional water really needed except during phototherapy for jaundice, when additional fluid losses occur from the exposed skin as a result of the heat from the lamp (p. 196). Supplementary feeds may interfere with lactation and have the ability to change the bacterial flora of the gut and potentially encourage the growth of pathogenic bacteria.

Care of the breasts

The breasts, if heavy, may need support during the process of a feed and therefore a nursing brassière which supports the breast while the cup is open should be encouraged. Otherwise, a nursing brassière which opens at the front, giving adequate support without pressing on the nipple, should be worn. Breast pads may be used within the brassière to absorb leakage of milk and protect clothing, but they should be changed frequently to prevent the nipple from being constantly wet.

Nipples and breasts should be washed daily as advised in the antenatal period. The use of soap and alcohol have been shown to increase nipple soreness and should be avoided. There are many protective creams and sprays available commercially, but there is little firm evidence to show that their continued use prevents nipple damage or promotes healing if damage occurs.

Breast engorgement and mastitis

The breasts are subject to two types of engorgement, 'vascular' and 'milk', although there may be an overlap between them. Vascular engorgement occurs 2–4 days after delivery and is due to the increased blood flow to the breasts which normally occurs at this time. Milk engorgement occurs as a result of the increased milk production accompanied by only limited removal of the milk by the baby. If this continues, overdistension of the alveoli will lead to eventual suppression of milk production and may even cause rupture of the alveoli and the symptoms of non-infective mastitis. It results in a painful lump covered by a red flush together with fever and reduction of secretion, but may often be dramatically cured within a few hours by emptying the breast from which no pus, but only milk, flows. If this is not done, however, staphylococcal infection may supervene and a true breast abscess develop. Treatment consists of early and repeated emptying of the breast, but if after 48 hours there is no improvement, an antibiotic may be necessary.

Milk engorgement rarely occurs if the mother is encouraged to feed her baby on demand day and night and the baby is properly fixed and removing the hind milk adequately. It may occur when the baby becomes ill and is separated from the mother. In these circumstances, the mother should continue to remove milk for the baby's use, either manually or through the use of a breast pump. Infective mastitis may also result from organisms infecting a break in the skin, especially if the mother is in a debilitated condition due to anaemia or malnutrition. It is treated with antibiotics but is not an indication to discontinue breast feeding.

Cracked nipples may follow engorgement or prolonged vigorous sucking at a stage when secretion is not established. Non-protractile nipples (p. 95) are the more likely to become cracked because they are not drawn properly into the baby's mouth and may be subject to more trauma. The use of a latex nipple shield is often successful in promoting healing but it may be unacceptable to the mother and reduce the milk flow. Other treatments include resting the affected breast with expression of the milk or repositioning the infant at the breast for the feeds. In either case, breast feeding can usually be maintained and the use of bottle feeding in this phase should be avoided if at all possible since the technique of feeding from a bottle is quite different from that required to take milk from the breast.

Cup feeding

This technique is an alternative to both bottle and tube feeding in breast-fed infants, particularly in some preterm infants, if supplementary feeds are required or when breast feeding must be interrupted.

The baby should be wrapped securely and a bib placed under his chin. He should be awake and alert if possible and held upright on the mother's lap with her hands supporting the baby's back and neck. The cup should be half full and the rim gently placed against the baby's upper lip, leaving the lower lip and jaw to move freely. It is then tipped until the milk just touches the upper lip, but is not poured into the mouth (Fig. 8.5, p. 116). The baby is allowed to suck the milk from the cup at his own pace until he is satisfied.

The advantages of this method are that it encourages good eye contact with the baby, avoids the confusion between the techniques of sucking at the nipple and a teat, and enables others to do it if the mother needs a rest. It also stimulates jaw movements and maximises the calorie intake.

FEEDING DIFFICULTIES
Underfeeding

Underfeeding is common and shows itself as excessive crying, poor weight gain, small stools and, sometimes, vomiting. By far the most common reason for this is that the feeding technique is not allowing the infant to take the feed adequately. Test feeding, even by weighing the infant before and after a feed with accurate electronic baby scales, has been shown to be an unreliable means of estimating the amount of feed the infant is taking and cannot be recommended. One important reason for this is the variation of volumes taken at different feeds at different times of the day. If underfeeding is suspected, the position of the infant at the breast should be modified as the first step, but if no increase in weight occurs with improving breast-feeding technique after 2–3 weeks, complementary feeds may be given from a cup after each breast feed, stopping when the infant appears satisfied.

Overfeeding

Some hold the view that overfeeding from the breast never occurs. It is certainly uncommon and is never a cause of really serious trouble. However, in the neonatal period, babies do sometimes become fretful, pass large frequent stools producing sore buttocks, and vomit small amounts after each feed, all of which cease when a small amount of milk is expressed from the breast before feeding is started. It should be remembered that about three-quarters of the feed is taken within the first 3 minutes of a breast feed and reducing the available milk may also reduce the speed with which it is taken yet stimulate the breast adequately to produce enough milk for the next feed.

Problems related to sucking

If the mother has received pethidine during labour, the baby may remain too sedated to suck adequately for a day or two, not only due to transplacental acquisition of the drug but also because it continues to be secreted into the breast milk for at least 2 days after birth (Weetman 2000).

An inability to suck may be caused by abnormalities in the infant such as cleft lip and cleft palate or underdevelopment of the lower jaw (micrognathia). Partial nasal obstruction can be a cause and is most commonly due to a temporary excessive secretion of mucus which may be reduced by applying one drop of 0.25% ephedrine in normal saline to each nostril before feeds for 2–3 days only. Obstruction of breathing from compression of the nose by the breast during feeding is avoided if the mother holds the breast away from the baby's face with her hand. In the absence of such a mechanical difficulty, more general causes must be sought, including the presence of infection somewhere (p. 168).

Sometimes, the unwillingness to suck may simply be due to tiredness from repeated fruitless attempts when the milk supply is inadequate or the baby too small to grasp the breast successfully. If alterations in feeding technique fail to improve matters, it is justifiable to feed the infant by either cup or bottle for a day or two, whilst maintaining breast milk production by expression, so that the baby may become strong enough to resume breast feeding.

Occasionally, breast feeding is not successful despite every attempt to support it or the mother may have other reasons for discontinuing it. In these circumstances, she may need considerable reassurance that she has not personally failed the baby and the benefits of changing to artificial feeding should be described.

ARTIFICIAL FEEDING BY THE BOTTLE

If the mother has decided not to breast feed her infant, or because it is medically recommended that she should not do so (p. 96), her lactation can, if necessary, be suppressed. Firm binding of the breasts using a firm brassière together with the use of a mild analgesic is often all that is required and little discomfort usually ensues. Prolactin-suppressing drugs are now regarded as inappropriate and unnecessary.

Alternatives to breast feeding

The majority of artificial baby feeds are based on cow's milk. Some specialised milks designed for people who wish their baby to have vegetarian feeds, either for religious or moral reasons, are available but they should only be used under the guidance of a dietitian. Certain medical conditions, such as cow's milk protein allergy, lactose intolerance, phenylketonuria and galactosaemia, require treatment with highly specialised dietetic products and the specific exclusion of cow's milk formula. These are not discussed further as they require careful medical and dietetic management and are beyond the scope of this book.

Cow's milk formulae

Most artificial infant feeds are derived from cow's milk, which in its natural state has numerous nutritional disadvantages compared with human milk (Table 7.3) and is not suitable for any baby until after the sixth month of life. The casein portion of the protein is relatively high, and there is less lactalbumin, which renders digestion somewhat more difficult; the high protein content produces more urea during its metabolism than the neonatal kidney can excrete effectively. The sugar (lactose) content is less, whereas the mineral salts (particularly sodium chloride and phosphate) are present in much greater concentration, with the consequent risk of hypernatraemia and neonatal hypocalcaemic tetany, respectively. This has led to the substantial modification of cow's milk by manufacturers so that it resembles more closely the composition of human milk and is suitable for babies in their first few months. Modifications required by such bodies as the European Community Council, the World Health Organisation and the Department of Health in Britain include changes in the amount, and in some cases the type, of proteins, fats, carbohydrates, minerals and vitamins (Table 7.3). More recent additions to some formulae include selenium, nucleotides, beta-carotene and even starch (as a thickener). It must be remembered, however, that even such greatly modified milk formulae have only a nutritional similarity to breast milk – they cannot provide the immunological advantages, the psychological benefits or the value to the mother of breast feeding.

In the modified formulae, total protein levels are reduced since the kidneys of the newborn

Table 7.3 Comparison of human and cow's milk, modified cow's milk formulae and preterm formulae

Component	Human milk	Cow's milk	EEC and WHO recommendations[a]	Preterm formulae	Preterm follow-on formula
Energy kcal	69	66	65–69	80	72
Protein g/100 mL	1.0	3.3	1.5–1.9[b]	2.0–2.2	1.85
Fat g/100 mL	4.2	3.7	2.5–3.8[c]	4.0–4.9	4.0[e]
Carbohydrate g/100 mL	7.4	4.8	6.9–8.60[d]	7.0–8.5	7.3
Vitamin A μg/100 mL	53–60	27	40–150	60–100	100
Vitamin D μg/100 mL	0.01	0.1	0.7–1.3	1.2–2.4	1.3
Sodium mg/100 mL	15	75	15–35	30–42	22
Calcium mg/100 mL	35	137	30–120	70–108	70
Phosphate mg/100 mL	15	91	15–60	35–54	35
Iron μg/100 mL	0.01	0.1	0.7–1.3	1.2–2.4	0.65

[a]All reputable commercial baby milk formulae in the UK conform to these international standards.
[b]In some milks, the curd:whey ratio is made similar to human milk.
[c]Some milks have only butterfat; most have added vegetable oil.
[d]Some milks have lactose and maltodextrin mixtures, others only lactose.
[e]Preterm formulae contain long-chain polyunsaturated fatty acids but their origins differ and they may vary in effectiveness.

infant are not able to handle large solute loads, and in some milks (often referred to as whey-based milks) the proportion of the more digestible lactalbumin is increased and casein decreased. In others (sometimes called casein-based milks), the total protein content is reduced, though the ratio of casein to lactalbumin is nearer that found in cow's milk. Because of the slightly increased renal solute load from these latter milks, it is usually recommended that they are introduced at around 6 weeks of age. Cow's milk fat is reduced in most milk formulae and some polyunsaturated vegetable oils are added. Lactose or maltodextrins (derived from hydrolysis of starch) are added to approximate to human milk and ensure adequate immediate energy for cerebral metabolism and growth. The phosphate concentration is reduced to decrease the risk of hypocalcaemia (p. 157) and the sodium level lowered to prevent hypernatraemia. Although most babies can maintain normal serum sodium levels on these low-salt milks, the preterm baby may lose excessive amounts because of immaturity of renal sodium handling mechanisms. Some specialised baby milks now contain live bifidobacteria which may help in certain babies suffering from infantile colic.

All the common baby milks suitable for home use are supplied in dried powder form to facilitate storage and transport without risk of deterioration. Manufacturers also supply these preparations sterilised and ready to give to the baby in disposable bottles to which disposable or resterilisable teats may be fitted. Although more expensive, they are eminently suitable for use in maternity units because of their safety without the need for costly milk-sterilising equipment and the trained staff to use it. The specialised milks designed for the preterm infant are described on page 117.

Preparing the feeds

During their stay in the maternity unit, all parents choosing to bottle feed should be instructed carefully on safe methods of preparing and storing artificial feeds. Great care is needed in preparing the feeds to ensure that the equipment and milk do not become contaminated by potentially pathogenic bacteria and that the milk is made up to the correct concentration as detailed on the container. Before handling any utensils or making up the feed, the hands must be washed thoroughly. The bottles, teats and other utensils can be sterilised by immersion in boiling water for 10 minutes or, more simply, by placing them in a solution of a commercial sterilising agent. There are many such preparations available, which are added to a specified quantity of water. They take several forms – tablets, crystals and solutions – which should be made up exactly according to the manufacturer's instructions. Most of these will sterilise the equipment within 30–60 minutes. Dishwashers and microwave ovens do not achieve adequate sterilisation of baby feeding equipment, but suitable specialised steamers are available including some for use in microwave ovens. Plastic liners in baby bottles cannot be adequately sterilised and should be used only once and then discarded.

The milks are reconstituted by adding scoops of powder to cooling boiled water in the feeding bottle, which is then sealed and shaken to ensure the milk is mixed. Usually, one levelled scoop is added to 30 mL (1 oz) of water, but the directions on the tin or packet must be followed exactly since the concentration of the feed will vary considerably if, for instance, the powder is packed into the scoop, heaped scoops are used, the water is added to the powder or the wrong number of scoops are added to the water. Such mistakes are commonly responsible for under- or overfeeding in the first few weeks of life. Provided the stored powder is quite dry, the milk itself is adequately sterilised by the use of boiling water in the reconstitution process, and a full day's requirement may be made up at one time. To ensure that bacterial contamination does not occur, the extra bottles must be stored in a refrigerator at or below 4°C and any left over after 24 hours should be discarded.

The water used for making up the feeds should be fresh and drawn from a rising main, boiled and allowed to cool. Reboiling water increases its mineral content and its use may result in unacceptably high levels in the reconstituted milk. Water from softening equipment has a high salt content and should not be used, since babies are not able to excrete salt adequately and they may become seriously hypernatraemic (p. 94). Both fixed and portable water filters can become contaminated with pathogenic bacteria, some of which produce toxins that are not destroyed by boiling, and water treated in this way is not recommended. Some bottled water has a low enough solute content to be safe, and it is suitable if it contains less than 35 mg/L of sodium, 20 mg/L of potassium and below 0.05 mg/L of both lead and nitrates. Carbonated water should not be used.

Giving the feeds

Warming of the bottled feed in a water bath has been common practice for many years, but it has been shown not to be essential and many people just prefer to bring it to room temperature if it has been in a refrigerator. Feeds should not be warmed in a microwave oven as they may continue to heat and produce a 'hot spot' in the milk. If the feed has been rewarmed, the temperature of the milk itself, not just the bottle, must be tested immediately prior to giving the feed, to ensure the milk is not too hot for the infant. Once a feed has been rewarmed, any milk remaining after the baby has completed the feed should be discarded, since it may have become contaminated by pathogenic bacteria during the feed.

It is important for both mother and baby that feeding times should be relaxed, unhurried and deliberate – a time during which they can get to know each other (p. 83). The baby is held comfortably either cradled in the mother's (or father's) arm, allowing no more than 15 inches (38 cm) between their faces so that the parent's face is within the infant's range of clear vision (p. 74) (Fig. 7.4), or sitting on her lap with her hand supporting the back and head. The baby's arms should be free and the infant in a flexed posture with the head supported. Before the bottle is offered to the infant, the rate of milk flow through the teat should be tested. With the bottle inverted, if the milk flows in a rapid succession of drops, the teat will be correct for most babies. Teats with different flow rates can now be obtained to suit the infant's requirements. If this is impractical, the teat hole size can be enlarged with a heated needle. The bottle should then be gently inserted into the mouth, ensuring that the teat passes above the tongue, and should be held at such an angle that the teat remains full of milk until the end of the feed to avoid air-swallowing. It is then held still to encourage the baby to work for the feed.

Sometimes a baby's lips have a weak grip on the teat which can be improved by gentle support

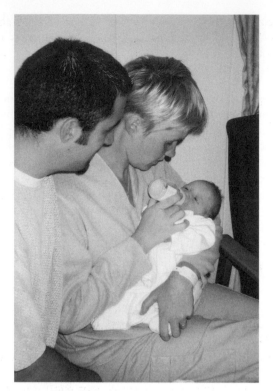

Figure 7.4 Correct position for artificial feeding of the newborn infant.

under the chin. If the milk flows too slowly, the teat hole size can be enlarged as described. An average time for a feed is 15–20 minutes and anything slower than this may mean that some modification of technique is required. The infant should be winded halfway through the feed, or more often if he is feeding rapidly.

The amount and frequency of feeds

As with breast feeding, individual babies differ greatly in the volume and frequency of feeds that they seem to need to satisfy their appetite and to ensure growth at a normal rate. The amount taken at one feed may also vary throughout the day. Feeding on demand is not quite so easy to carry out successfully from the bottle as it is from the breast, and some planning as to how much and how often is necessary for practical purposes.

An average term baby takes about 60 mL/kg body weight on the first day, divided into four or five feeds. This amount gradually increases to 150–180 mL/kg per 24 hours, divided into six or seven feeds, by the end of the first week, though the number of days taken to reach this varies considerably from baby to baby. This means offering 30–45 mL per feed to a newborn baby of an average birth weight, and by the end of the first week he will be taking about 75–90 mL at each feed.

Low birth weight babies require more food in relation to body weight to keep them thriving, particularly if they have suffered intrauterine growth retardation, and this is discussed in more detail in Chapter 4.

Not all formula milks suit every baby and constipation is a common problem. This can sometimes be remedied by giving extra drinks of water, but if this is not effective, medical advice should be sought.

Cow's milk intolerance

This problem can present as vomiting, diarrhoea or a skin rash, but it is not commonly seen within the first week or two of life. Some milks have been produced using soya protein instead of cow's milk protein to prevent exposure of potentially allergic babies to bovine antigens, though there is also a similar risk of the baby developing antibodies to the soya protein. The milks are not recommended for the newborn baby in the first month of life as their high aluminium and low calcium content make them unsuitable for routine use. They are, however, valuable for use under medical supervision in those babies who prove to have true cow's milk sensitivity.

COMMON PROBLEMS RELATED TO FEEDING
Wind, posseting and vomiting

The normal infant swallows a variable amount of air when feeding, which is normally easily expelled by sitting the infant upright or holding him over the shoulder after a feed. It is not usually necessary to pat the infant's back to achieve this, though some infants gain comfort from having the back gently rubbed. A teaspoonful or two of milk is often regurgitated within the first 10 minutes after a feed (posseting) and occasional larger vomits without serious cause are not uncommon in healthy infants in the first 2 weeks. If swallowed during the process of birth, amniotic fluid and mucus can irritate the stomach, and a simple stomach washout using a nasogastric tube and warmed normal saline will usually cure the problem.

Repeated small vomits, especially when they occur shortly after feeds, are often caused by gastro-oesophageal reflux, which is particularly common in preterm infants (p. 121). Rarely does this cause pain in the first weeks of life, but if the baby is failing to thrive from loss of calories in the vomit or has aspirated the milk into the lungs, treatment may be necessary. Food thickeners or antacids may help, but if they do not, ranitidine, a drug which suppresses acid production in the stomach, is often useful. Occasionally, reflux is associated with a hiatus hernia (p. 215). Feeding mismanagement is also a common cause. This can include underfeeding, mechanical problems with the breast such as engorgement, or an inappropriate hole size in the teat in bottle-fed infants.

Vomiting has many possible causes, most of which are simple and benign, and in general only *persistent vomiting* is likely to have a serious origin.

Vomited blood in the first day or two is almost always swallowed maternal blood and can be distinguished from the infant's blood by confirming that it contains no fetal haemoglobin.

If the vomit contains *bile* it must always be taken seriously and intestinal obstruction excluded with an erect plain abdominal X-ray. Obstruction can occur at many levels in the gut and all such infants require urgent attention from a specialist paediatric surgeon. Most lesions are readily amenable to corrective surgery within the first few days of life (p. 217). Bile-stained vomiting may also occur with a cerebral disorder such as intracranial bleeding (p. 150) or meningitis (p. 169).

Distension of the abdomen

Abdominal distension has many causes. If it is present at the time of birth it usually indicates enlargement of one or more of the intra-abdominal organs such as the kidneys, liver or spleen, the presence of ascites, or, rarely, an abdominal tumour. Sometimes the distension can compress the diaphragm and cause additional respiratory distress, and this requires urgent attention.

Distension developing over the first few days of life will most commonly result from gaseous distension of the gut caused by obstruction at some level, although the higher in the gut the obstruction occurs, the more likely it is to present with vomiting rather than distension.

Unusual bowel actions and stools

Green stools are not necessarily abnormal in breast-fed infants and the stool often turns greener after being passed. An infant taking more breast milk than usual may pass looser and more frequent motions which are often frothy due to the fermentation of excess lactose in the large gut. This need not be regarded as overfeeding unless there is an accompanying failure to gain weight. The stools of a breast-fed baby will often be affected by the dietary intake of the mother. For example, unusually spicy foods, some fruits and orange juice may increase stool frequency. Such effects result from some dietary components being secreted into the breast milk. Underfeeding commonly results in stools which are not hard but are characteristically small and dark coloured. Small streaks of blood are often present if the baby has to strain to pass a hard stool, e.g. when changing from breast to formula milk.

Failure to pass meconium within the first 24 hours is uncommon, and the longer the delay, the more likely it is to be associated with an abnormality. A plug of thick meconium in the rectum is the commonest cause and can be relieved by a small rectal washout or can be encouraged to pass by a gentle rectal examination.

The whole large bowel may be full of thick and sticky meconium which the baby is unable to pass in the condition known as meconium ileus; this is the mode of presentation for a minority of patients with cystic fibrosis (p. 210).

REFERENCES

Angelsen N K, Vik T, Jackobsen G et al 2001 Breast feeding and cognitive development at 1 and 5 years. Archives of Disease in Childhood 85(3):183–188

Auestad N, Halter R, Hall R T et al 2001 Growth and development in term infants fed long-chain polyunsaturated fatty acids: a double-masked, randomized, parallel, prospective, multivariate study. Pediatrics 108(2):372–381

Botting B, Rosato M, Wood R 1998 Teenage mothers and the health of their children. Population Trends 93:19–28

Gdalevich M, Mimouni D, Mimouni M 2001 Breast-feeding and the risk of bronchial asthma in childhood: a systematic review with meta-analysis of prospective studies. Journal of Pediatrics 139(2):261–266

Gibb D M, Goodall R L, Dunn D T 2000 Mother to child transmission of hepatitis C virus: evidence for preventable peripartum transmission. Lancet 356:904–907

Golding J 1997 Unnatural constituents of breast milk - medication, lifestyle, pollutants, viruses. Early Human Development 49(suppl.):S29–S43

Hadzic N 2001 Hepatitis C in pregnancy. Archives of Disease in Childhood Fetal and Neonatal Edition 84:F201–F204

Hatfield E 2000 It isn't working. Midirs Midwifery Digest 10(4):501

Henderson L, Kitzinger J, Green J 2000 Representing infant feeding: content analysis of British media portrayals of bottle feeding and breast feeding. British Medical Journal 321(7270):1196–1198

Hendrick V, Fukuchi A, Altshuler L et al 2001 Use of setraline, paroxetine and fluvoxamine by nursing women. British Journal of Psychiatry 179:163–166

Lawson M 1998 Recent trends in infant nutrition. Nutrition 14(10):755–757

Liston J 1998 Breastfeeding and the use of recreational drugs – alcohol, caffeine, nicotine and marijuana. Breastfeeding Review 6(2):27–30

National Breastfeeding Working Group 1995 Breastfeeding: good practice guidance to the NHS. DOH, London

Orlando S 1995 The immunological significance of breast milk. Journal of Obstetric and Gynaecological Neonatal Nursing 24:678–683

Short R 1994 What the breast does for the baby and what the baby does for the breast. Australian and New Zealand Journal of Obstetrics and Gynaecology 34:262–264

Spencer J P, Gonzalez L S, Barnhart D J 2001 Medications in the breastfeeding mother. American Family Physician 64(1):119–126

Stepans M B, Wilkerson N 1993 Physiologic effects of maternal smoking on breast feeding infants. Journal of American Academic Nurse Practice 5(3):105–113

Vadas P, Wai Y, Burks W et al 2001 Detection of peanut allergens in breast milk of lactating women. Journal of the American Medical Association 285(13):1746–1748

Wang Y, Wu S 1996 The effect of exclusive breast feeding on development and the incidence of infection in infants. Journal of Human Lactation 12:27–30

Weetman J 2000 Pethidine, difficult births and breastfeeding. The Practicing Midwife 3(10):18–19

USEFUL WEBSITES

UNICEF – www.unicef.org
World Health Organisation – www.who.org

Chapter 8
Preterm infants

CHAPTER CONTENTS

Prevalence of preterm and low birth weight babies 107
Causative factors of preterm birth 108
The assessment of gestational age 108
   General characteristics of the preterm infant 108
Effects of prematurity on the infant 110
   Skin 111
   Blood 111
   Heart and circulation 111
   Respiration 111
   Gastrointestinal tract function 112
   Renal function 112
   Poor resistance to infection 112
Management of the preterm infant 112
   Prevention 112
   Delivery and care in the delivery room 112
   Care of the preterm infant in the neonatal unit 113
   Feeding the preterm infant 116
   The important parental link 119
Common disorders of the preterm infant 120
   Respiratory problems 120
   Alimentary tract problems 121
   Jaundice 121
   Oedema 121
   Sclerema 121
   Anaemia 122
   Infections 122
   Other minor disorders related to preterm birth 122
   Routine immunisations in preterm infants 122
The outlook for surviving preterm babies 123

PREVALENCE OF PRETERM AND LOW BIRTH WEIGHT BABIES

Between 3% and 4% of babies are born before 37 weeks' gestation and these are called preterm infants. Almost all of them weigh less than 2500 g and are, therefore, low birth weight babies. They provide the great majority of work in neonatal units and it is in this group that 60% of all neonatal deaths occur. The incidence of preterm birth and low birth weight varies from one part of the country to another and according to ethnic group, and this contributes significantly to the difference in neonatal mortality rates in different places (p. 6).

Preterm infants may either have grown appropriately for their gestation or be light for dates and show the characteristics and problems of this group of babies in addition to their prematurity (p. 49).

Over the years, the gestational age at which an infant has been regarded as viable has been falling, and current technology and medical care can offer considerable hope to those down to 25 weeks. Even some babies at 23–24 weeks can now be saved by using the whole range of neonatal intensive care facilities presently available.

The lower the gestational age at birth, the greater the risk of neurological handicap in the survivors. Nevertheless, 90% or more of surviving infants born at 26–28 weeks' gestation, and higher proportions of more mature infants, will develop into healthy children.

CAUSATIVE FACTORS OF PRETERM BIRTH

Preterm delivery is about equally distributed between those that follow spontaneous early onset of labour and those in which the early labour is elective. Although the cause of most spontaneous preterm births is not identified, some predisposing factors are known. These have much in common with those that lead to low birth weight from impairment of intrauterine growth. They include:

- poor socioeconomic status
- pre-eclampsia
- infection
- smoking and alcoholism in pregnancy
- antepartum haemorrhage
- multiple pregnancy
- fetal developmental abnormalities
- primiparity
- short maternal stature
- maternal age below 18 years.

THE ASSESSMENT OF GESTATIONAL AGE

It is important to distinguish between the preterm and the light for dates mature infant as the care each requires is different. The more mature preterm infant at, say, 35 weeks, may be active, able to maintain her body temperature well, and feed from the breast from the beginning. By contrast, a 28-week infant will almost always require artificial ventilation to maintain adequate respiration, nasogastric or even parenteral feeding, and the full range of intensive care.

In about 80% of cases, the date of the mother's last menstrual period is the best guide to the length of gestation, giving an estimate to within a week either way, though the use of oral contraceptives can cause confusion. The size of the uterus and measurement of either the fetal crown–rump length or the biparietal diameter of the head using ultrasound in early pregnancy increases the accuracy of the assessment (p. 20).

After birth it is possible to estimate maturity with reasonable accuracy by examination of the baby, through assessment of the infant's neurological developmental stage and a set of physical characteristics which alter with increasing gestational age.

In one system of assessment, the progressive changes of just four physical features (skin texture, skin colour, breast size and ear firmness) is used to put the infants into one of four general categories, namely, very premature, premature, transitional and mature. Another method employs the progression of some neurological reflexes (pupil response to light, glabella tap, traction response and neck righting) to give similar general guidance about the degree of prematurity of the infant. For babies between 28 and 34 weeks of gestation, the progressive reduction in the number of surface blood vessels on the lens of the eye is probably the most accurate method of estimating maturity, but the technique requires considerable skill and experience with an ophthalmoscope.

In the more elaborate system devised by Dubowitz (Dubowitz 1969) and its modification by Ballard (Ballard et al 1991) (Fig. 8.1), a score is given to each of a series of neurological and physical features, the total score being converted on a rating scale to the baby's gestational age. These methods are more complicated than is needed for most routine care in neonatal units, where the purpose of the assessment is to confirm the accuracy of the antenatal assessment of maturity. They are, however, useful tools for teaching about the characteristics of preterm infants at different gestational ages.

General characteristics of the preterm infant

Figure 8.2 displays a chart for preterm infants, showing the range of dimensions of infants from 20 weeks to term. The weights of individual preterm babies at the same maturity vary widely and depend on the adequacy of fetal nutrition. Length is more closely related to maturity than is weight, but is not easy to measure accurately and is not by itself a reliable indicator of gestational age. The head circumference exceeds that of the chest, which tends to be relatively small and narrow. The length of the trunk in proportion to the limbs is greater than that of the term infant.

Figure 8.3 illustrates some of the clinical features of the preterm infant at birth. Fine hair on the face

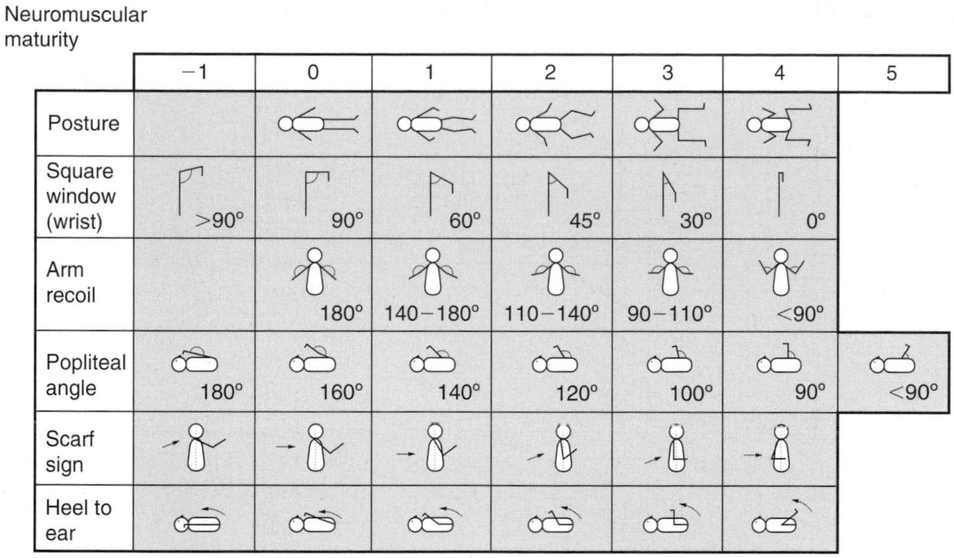

Neuromuscular
maturity

	−1	0	1	2	3	4	5
Posture							
Square window (wrist)	>90°	90°	60°	45°	30°	0°	
Arm recoil		180°	140–180°	110–140°	90–110°	<90°	
Popliteal angle	180°	160°	140°	120°	100°	90°	<90°
Scarf sign							
Heel to ear							

Physical
maturity

Maturity
rating

Skin	Sticky friable transparent	Gelatinous red, translucent	Smooth pink, visible veins	Superficial peeling &/or rash, few veins	Cracking pale areas rare veins	Parchment deep cracking no vessels	Leathery cracked wrinkled
Lanugo	none	sparse	abundant	thinning	bald areas	Mostly bald	
Plantar surface	heel-toe 40–50 mm:−1 <40 mm:−2	>50 mm no crease	faint red marks	anterior transverse crease only	creases ant. 2/3	creases over entire sole	
Breast	imperceptible	barely perceptible	flat areola no bud	stippled areola 1–2mm bud	raised areola 3–4mm bud	full areola 5–10mm bud	
Eye/ ear	lids fused loosely:−1 tightly:−2	lids open pinna flat stays folded	sl. curved pinna; soft; slow recoil	well-curved pinna; soft but ready recoil	formed & firm instant recoil	thick cartilage ear stiff	
Genitals (male)	scrotum flat, smooth	scrotum empty faint rugae	testes in upper canal rare rugae	testes descending few rugae	testes down good rugae	testes pendulous deep rugae	
Genitals (female)	clitoris prominent labia flat	prominent clitoris small labia minora	prominent clitoris enlarging minora	majora & minora equally prominent	majora large minora small	majora cover clitoris & minora	

Score	Weeks
−10	20
−5	22
0	24
5	26
10	28
15	30
20	32
25	34
30	36
35	38
40	40
45	42
50	44

Figure 8.1 Ballard's method of assessing gestational age in preterm infants. Each of the clinical and neurological features is assessed and scored. The gestational age is determined by comparing the total score with the maturity rating grid.

and trunk (lanugo) is more plentiful, especially if the baby is less than 30 weeks' gestation (p. 64). The nails are soft but not necessarily short. There is a rather shiny unwrinkled appearance to the skin, which is a darker pink colour than at term. The labia minora in the girl are protuberant and gaping, whilst in the boy the testes are usually incompletely descended. Below 34 weeks, the creases on the soles of the feet are almost absent except for a single one anteriorly. Ears are floppy and, lacking formed cartilage, tend to remain folded after the infant has lain on them. The palpable nodule of breast tissue at the nipple is absent before 34 weeks, 1 to 2 mm across from 34 to 36 weeks, about 4 mm from 36 to 38 weeks and about 8 mm at term. The skull is soft and easily indented around the fontanelles before 36 weeks, but becomes much harder towards term.

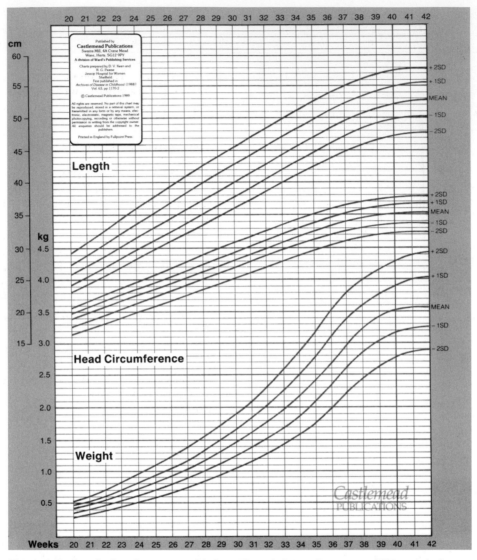

Figure 8.2 Growth chart for preterm girls from 20 weeks' gestation to term. (With permission from Casttemead Publications.)

EFFECTS OF IMMATURITY ON THE BABY

The major problems faced by preterm infants relate to the level of maturity of their organ systems, and the greater the immaturity, the more serious they are. Immaturity is shown most clearly by differences in the baby's physical activity and neurological responses. The shorter the gestation period, the less muscular activity is shown by the baby. In a preterm infant born before 34 weeks, the eyes remain closed for most of the time and the cry, if any, is weak. The movements of the body and limbs, when they occur, tend to be in little bursts of activity and are often jerky and frog-like. The posture of the preterm baby is generally extended, becoming more flexed towards term, and muscle tone is low but gradually increases as gestational age advances. It must be remembered that even these neurological responses are suppressed if the baby is sick.

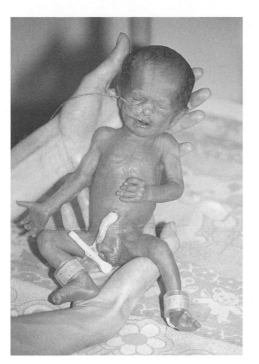

Figure 8.3   A preterm baby of 29 weeks' gestation.

Skin

The mature skin acts as a physical barrier which prevents both the loss of body fluid through surface evaporation and the absorption of toxic substances into the body. This function is not fully developed until the stratum corneum, the superficial layer of the epidermis, thickens and dries to form a barrier on the surface of the skin. This process, known as cornification, takes several days in the term infant but up to 2 weeks in the very preterm baby. Prevention of invasion of pathogenic bacteria by this physical barrier and the maintenance of an acidic pH by the skin secretions are also immature and are partly responsible for the increase in systemic infection in preterm infants (Rutter 2000).

Blood

Capillary walls are weak and this, combined with reduced clotting factors in the blood, leads to a greater tendency to bleed and bruise easily. Preterm infants, whether delivered vaginally or by caesarean section, are often born with bruising even after the most gentle handling. The cord blood haemoglobin is as high as in a term infant and there is no clear correlation between its level and maturity. The blood volume is around 80 mL/kg body weight, which limits the amount of blood that can safely be taken for testing.

Heart and circulation

After birth, the adaptations of the circulation occur more slowly and are less complete than in the term infant. The tone in the pulmonary arterioles is high, reduces more slowly and remains labile in preterm infants. Thus, the pulmonary blood pressure is high and varies widely. The systemic blood pressure is, by contrast, relatively low. The ductus arteriosus does not close firmly and is capable of opening again to allow shunting of blood between the pulmonary and systemic circulations. This instability may result in significant variation of the oxygen saturation in the peripheral circulation if an excessive elevation in the pulmonary blood pressure shunts desaturated blood across either the foramen ovale or the ductus arteriosus.

Respiration

The nasal airway is narrow and easily obstructed. The thoracic cage is soft, so that it is sucked in by a small rise in negative pressure during inspiration, and the respiratory passages are narrow, giving greater resistance to air flow (Fig. 9.2, p. 132). The infant breathes irregularly, using the diaphragm more than the chest. The cough reflex is poorly developed. Gaseous exchange is relatively inefficient in very immature babies because the alveoli are lined by thick cuboidal epithelium in contrast to the flattened thin cells in the mature lungs and are surrounded by a meagre supply of capillaries which only start to increase significantly after the 28th week. Production of pulmonary surfactant by the alveolar cells is also minimal, causing the alveoli to collapse progressively. The mechanisms that regulate depth and rate of breathing by stimulating the respiratory centre in the brain stem are not fully developed and the baby is thus liable to periods of apnoea, when she seems to 'forget' to breathe altogether (p. 67). The result is an unstable respiratory system.

Gastrointestinal tract function

The mechanism of sucking and swallowing is poorly developed in the smallest preterm babies, the mechanisms only becoming sufficiently coordinated for the infant to begin to feed from the breast at about 32–34 weeks and becoming fully effective around 36–37 weeks. The ability to digest food matures early, and only in babies of less than 25 weeks are digestive enzymes deficient. The lack of mucosal folds in the small bowel reduces the surface area for absorption of digested food. Sugar is well assimilated, while protein is less so and fat is least well tolerated. Immaturity of liver function is seen mainly as a reduced ability to conjugate bilirubin, which results in an increased incidence of jaundice in preterm infants (p. 195), though reduced liver glycogen stores limit the baby's production of glucose in respone to hypoglycaemia, and reduced bile secretion diminishes fat absorption from the gut. Immaturity of other liver enzyme systems may affect the rate of metabolism of many drugs and influence both the dose to be given and the frequency of administration.

Renal function

Although the kidneys are usually able to excrete urea and water adequately even in the very premature baby, they are unable to excrete large fluid loads and oedema may result. Metabolic acidosis can occur from excessive loss of bicarbonate from the renal tubules and an inability to secrete enough hydrogen ions into the urine. They are also less able to retain sodium than in the more mature baby and the sodium intake may need to be increased to overcome the resulting hyponatraemia. The immature kidneys may be unable to excrete some potentially toxic drugs, e.g. gentamicin, rapidly, so these should be given less frequently in preterm infants, to avoid accumulation in the blood (p. 249).

Poor resistance to infection

Transfer of maternal immunoglobulin (IgG) across the placenta starts slowly at about 28 weeks, the fetal blood levels only increasing rapidly after 34 weeks. The most immature infants therefore have limited passive immunity and their own ability to produce antibodies in response to infection is poorly developed, as are the cellular immune responses (p. 163).

MANAGEMENT OF THE PRETERM INFANT
Prevention

Bed rest is the mainstay of treatment for suspected preterm labour, with or without the use of a uterine muscle relaxing drug such as nifedipine or ritodrine (Vause & Johnston 2000). Once labour has started, provided that no complications develop which make immediate delivery necessary, it can sometimes be delayed for up to 48 hours by giving the same drugs intravenously or by giving a prostaglandin inhibitor. This delay grants time for the mother to be given a corticosteroid such as dexamethasone for 1–2 days, which reduces the risk of hyaline membrane disease in the baby by about 50%. In the UK, around 98% of maternity units give more than one course of steroids for repeated episodes of preterm labour (Brocklehurst et al 1999), though the benefits and potential risks are still being evaluated (Brocklehurst et al 2000).

Delivery and care in the delivery room

It should be possible in most cases to diagnose the onset of premature labour sufficiently early to arrange for delivery to take place where full paediatric back-up and a neonatal intensive care unit with appropriate facilities are at hand, thus avoiding the greater hazard of transfer after birth. The paediatric staff should be fully informed in advance of the history of the pregnancy and someone experienced in resuscitation of very immature infants must be present at delivery.

In preterm labour, it is wise to minimise narcotic analgesia and provide pain relief by either epidural or light nitrous oxide anaesthesia.

All equipment for resuscitation (including the extra-small endotracheal tubes of 2.5 and 3 mm width) and for maintenance of normal body temperature must be checked and made ready.

At birth, the baby must be handled very gently. She should be gently wiped dry to minimise evaporative heat loss, wrapped in a warm towel and placed under a correctly adjusted source of radiant heat. If possible, the umbilical cord is allowed to pulsate for at least 1 minute before clamping (p. 80).

A small number of preterm infants cry vigorously at delivery and in these cases additional respiratory support is unnecessary. If this does not happen, the baby should be promptly resuscitated with elective endotracheal intubation and ventilation. Preterm babies of less than 30 weeks' gestation should be electively resuscitated to provide maximal initial expansion of the alveoli and thus reduce the severity of the subsequent respiratory distress syndrome. Details of resuscitation procedures are as described on page 36. A single intramuscular injection of vitamin K 1.0 mg (Konakion) should be given once breathing is established, to improve blood coagulation by stimulating hepatic production of clotting factors.

Anxiety over the baby's physical welfare should not be allowed to obscure the emotional needs of the parents in their relationship with the infant at this time. Unless there is clearly a need for immediate intensive treatment elsewhere, it should be possible to allow the parents to hold their infant at least briefly before transfer to the neonatal unit. The infant should then be transferred in a transport incubator at 34–35°C (93–95°F) or in a specially warmed cot. Time must be set aside for a well-informed talk with the parents about the management of the baby and her outlook, and questions about the future answered as honestly and sensitively as possible.

If transfer to a distant intensive care unit is necessary, it is best to undertake the initial assessment and treatment in the hospital of birth and prepare for the journey when the infant's condition has been stabilised. In ideal circumstances,

an experienced team from the receiving neonatal intensive care unit should travel to the hospital of birth and provide the necessary treatment during the transfer. In some areas, ambulances have been equipped specially to undertake full intensive care during transfer of very sick preterm infants.

Care of the preterm infant in the neonatal unit

Preterm infants require care which is adapted to take account of the immaturity of their organ systems and homoeostatic mechanisms, but it must be remembered that they have similar human needs to babies born at term. They need sleep, feeding, to be kept clean, to feel secure, to be comfortable and to be subjected to as little stress as possible. Their sight, hearing, and senses of touch and smell are well developed. They can feel pain, both physical and emotional. They can respond to pleasant and unpleasant stimuli in appropriate ways. They can communicate their feelings. The ways in which preterm infants convey distress is through subtle changes of movement, alterations of body functions such as heart rate and blood pressure, or as periods of apnoea rather than crying. Inappropriate methods of care can delay the baby's progress, but providing a suitable environment and sensitive handling can promote a more normal pattern of physiological and emotional development.

Observation and recording of changes

During the first 24 hours, careful observation and frequent recording of the baby's core temperature, heart rate, the type and rate of respiration, skin colour and any abnormal movements is necessary, as it is in this time that most problems begin.

Environment

The ambient light in the neonatal unit should only be as bright as is needed to carry out normal care procedures and it is good practice to dim the light at night. Incubator covers can also reduce the intensity of light. The impact of sensory overload on the baby's physiology from excessive noise can be reduced by closing incubator doors gently, speaking quietly and by reducing the volume of equipment alarms and telephones. These measures have been shown to improve sleep and cardio-respiratory stability (Blackburn & Patterson 1991).

Emotional and developmental needs

Preterm infants tolerate disturbance poorly and they should be handled as little as their condition permits. They should be allowed adequate sleep and rest to conserve energy and to ensure the development of a proper sleep pattern. Placing the baby in a flexed posture, supported if necessary by towel rolls or padded flexible bars, not only is more comfortable for the infant but also promotes midline motor development which will prevent the tendency to develop an extended posture in the back arms and legs later. Gentle but positive handling of the infant and a technique known as containment will make the baby feel more secure and can settle a distressed infant. Containment involves placing the parent's hands firmly but gently on the baby to limit movement whilst talking to her. This method can also give parents confidence in handling the baby (Fig. 8.4). Stroking should be discouraged as some babies find it intolerable (Bond 1999). Some nursing and medical observations, investigations and interventions are essential, but it should be recognised that such procedures as venepuncture, heelpricks, chest physiotherapy and endotracheal suction are particularly uncomfortable for the baby and should be performed only when really necessary.

Care of the skin

The skin of the term infant provides an effective barrier against water loss through evaporation by rapidly developing a thick stratum corneum (p. 111). This process is much slower in the preterm infant and it may be 2 weeks before the permeability resembles that of a term infant. Insensible water loss through the skin and the risk of invasive infection or skin damage is greatly increased until it is fully cornified. Those who care for very preterm babies will recognise

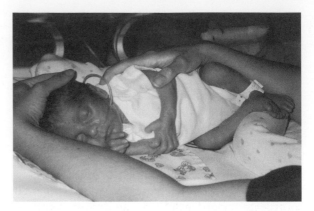

Figure 8.4 Containment reduces physiological stress in preterm infants.

how poorly adhesive monitoring pads stick to the infants' moist skin and how readily it can become sore. It is important for nurses and doctors to minimise skin damage and not to accept it as inevitable. Toxic substances applied to the skin may be absorbed rapidly, and adhesive tapes, monitoring pads and urine collecting bags can all traumatise the skin surface as they are removed. Damage to the skin can be minimised by using waterproof adhesive-free hydrocolloid dressings under adhesive tapes to secure, for example, intravenous cannulae, and splints or monitoring probes may be secured with self-adhesive latex-containing bandages. Practices vary considerably from one unit to another, but awareness of the impact of procedures on the immature skin should affect the way it is treated (Baker et al 1999, Darmstadt & Dinulos 2000).

The collection of urine into a cotton-wool ball placed at the urethtral opening and moistening of adhesive tapes with warm water before removal are other examples of how skin trauma can be limited.

Pressure marks occur readily if the position of the infant is not changed at least every 6 hours, and lying the baby on a sheepskin or soft mattress can also minimise skin damage and decrease neonatal head moulding.

The skin should normally only be cleaned if it is significantly soiled, using warm water and cotton wool. Only removal of excessive vernix is needed initially and full bathing is unnecessary

Table 8.1 Average incubator temperatures for babies nursed naked

Birth weight (kg)	Incubator temperature (°C)					
	37°	36°	35°	34°	33°	32°
Less than 1.0	1 d	2–14 d	14–21 d	over 21 d		
1.0–1.5			1–10 d	over 10 d	over 21 d	
1.5–2.0				1–10 d	over 10 d	
2.0–2.5				1–2 d	over 2 d	over 21 d
Over 2.5					1–2 d	over 2 d

d = days

until the baby is ready to go home. Creams, lotions and soaps should not be used routinely as they may all affect the pH of the skin and alter its natural harmless bacterial flora. If a procedure requiring sterilisation of an area of skin is performed, only the smallest suitable amount of antiseptic solution should be used, to reduce the risk of absorption into the circulation or chemical burning of the skin. It is the authors' policy to use 0.015% aqueous chlorhexidine (rather than 0.05%) following a 'burn' in one infant.

Temperature regulation (see also p. 80)

Because of their small size and physiological immaturity, temperature regulation is more difficult in preterm infants. Heat production is low because of limited physical activity and a lack of brown fat (p. 80), heat losses are high because of a large surface area in proportion to weight and a lack of insulating subcutaneous fat. In addition, the immaturity of the responses in the preterm infant's skin blood vessels limits the infant's ability to retain heat, and the increased permeability of the infant's skin to water can result in both hypothermia from excessive evaporative heat loss and dehydration. Low glucose and glycogen reserves also limit the heat-producing metabolic response to these losses and the risk of hypoglycaemia is high. To minimise these problems, the infant must be cared for in an ambient temperature which prevents heat loss by reducing energy expenditure to a minimum and high humidity to diminish fluid losses from the skin.

Incubators are the traditional means of providing a controllable microenvironment for preterm infants whilst allowing ready access to them. The temperatures required to minimise energy expenditure and oxygen consumption in naked babies of different birth weights, known as the 'neutral thermal environment', are shown in Table 8.1. Such figures are used to set incubator temperatures, but lower figures should be used for clothed infants. The nurse should monitor the baby's axillary temperature every 2–4 hours and adjust the incubator temperature accordingly.

Precautions against cross-infection

No nurse or doctor with an infection (particularly of skin or bowel) should be allowed to work in a special care unit until clear. However, rigorous barrier nursing of well preterm infants by healthy attendants is generally unnecessary (p. 85). Meticulous attention to hand washing or the use of an alcohol-based antiseptic lotion before and after handling babies is the greatest practical safeguard against transmitting infection. The wearing of individual gowns or polythene aprons for dealing with any possibly infected babies helps to reduce the contamination of the caregiver's clothing, but their routine use and wearing of masks does not reduce cross-infection. Ensuring that equipment such as stethoscopes and tape measures is used exclusively by one baby should reduce the transmission of pathogenic organisms. Babies transferred from another hospital should initially be isolated and surface swabs taken for bacterial culture to reduce the risk of organisms such as methicillin-resistant *Staphylococcus aureus* (MRSA) being introduced into the neonatal unit.

Weighing

It is useful to know of changes in body weight, especially as a guide to the regulation of food intake, for, unlike term infants, immature babies do not readily show their need for more food by crying. In an ill baby with respiratory difficulties, the disturbance of weighing should be avoided, but otherwise it should be done at least twice a week. The accumulation of oedema from renal or cardiac failure (p. 226) may cause an excessive weight gain and there is a relatively big drop in weight when it diminishes, so these changes must be allowed for. The rate of fetal weight gain in the late stages of pregnancy can only rarely be maintained in the first week after birth. Although early feeding or the use of specialised premature baby formula milks helps to minimise this fall-off, it is often 2 or 3 weeks before adequate weight gain begins, particularly if the baby is sick.

Feeding the preterm infant

Recent advances in our understanding of the nutritional needs of preterm infants have significantly improved the prognosis for these infants, though there is as yet no clear consensus on the most appropriate feed to give them. Gastric feeding from the first day carries a slightly increased risk of regurgitation and inhalation of milk, but this is outweighed by the benefits of preventing hypoglycaemia, dehydration and undernutrition, all of which can have adverse effects on the developing brain. Even providing very small ('non-nutritive') quantities of gastric feed from the start, known as 'trophic feeding', enhances the functional maturation of the gut and reduces the severity of both jaundice and metabolic bone disease (Williams 2000). So long as the baby is well, gastric feeds are usually tolerated and the first one may be given 2–3 hours after birth. Subsequently, the frequency will depend upon the maturity of the baby and the method used (King 1998). It may be given as a continuous infusion, as hourly or 2-hourly bolus feeds in the smaller infants, or, for the larger babies, 3-hourly. The mother's colostrum provides some protection against infection and should be given to the infant wherever possible. However, most very small immature babies need the majority of their fluid and calorie requirements intravenously for at least the first 48 hours. If enteral feeding beyond this period cannot sustain adequate nutrition, total parenteral nutrition will be needed. This involves giving the infant a balanced mixture of amino acids, glucose, fats, electrolytes, minerals and vitamins in solution intravenously, and is described in detail in Chapter 9 (p. 128).

Methods of enteral feeding

The method for giving feeds also depends upon the size, maturity and health of the baby. Infants of more than 35 weeks' gestation are usually able to feed from the breast or bottle. Even if the baby takes no milk, the act of putting the infant to the breast enhances milk production and increases the chance of successful breast feeding later. Some less mature babies may also manage to take part of a feed which may be supplemented by cup feeding (p. 100 & Fig. 8.5). This method has the advantage that the parents can learn the technique rapidly and become more involved in the care of their infant at an early stage.

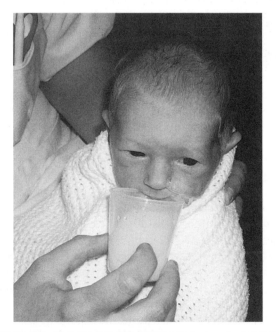

Figure 8.5 Cup feeding with breast milk in a preterm infant.

Oro- and nasogastric feeding, using a narrow disposable polythene tube passed via the mouth or nose into the stomach, are alternative methods for the smaller babies who are unable to suck adequately (Chant 1998). They have the merit of avoiding disturbance, since the tube can usually be left in place for 2 or 3 days, and demand minimal expenditure of the baby's energy. Though normally a nursing task, parents can rapidly become adept at tube and cup feeding and should be encouraged to become involved if they so wish. The length of tube required to reach the stomach is the distance between the nares and the left hypochondrium. The position of its tip can be checked either by aspirating acid from the stomach or by blowing air down the tube and listening with a stethoscope over the stomach.

Type of oral feed

Although there is still much debate about the feeding of the preterm infant (Cooke & Embleton 2000), breast milk remains at present the first choice of milk for both term and preterm babies (King 1998). It has the merit of being well tolerated, better absorbed in the gut and, if not heat treated, provides some protection against infection and necrotising enterocolitis (p. 140). It also contains some long-chain polyunsaturated fatty acids (such as arachidonic and decosahexanoic acids) which are essential for optimal brain development but are not present in some formula milks, and bile salt lipase, which enhances fat absorption.

The mother's early breast milk usually provides between 3 and 5 g of protein per kilogram body weight per day, which is adequate for growth for all but the most growth-retarded infants, but it is very variable in its other constituents, especially its fat content. Milk collected by hand or mechanical expression and drip milk are largely composed of fore-milk, which contains little fat, and the calorie content is often inadequate for the preterm baby. It is essential that the nurse teaches the optimal method of manually expressing the breast to ensure that both fore- and hind-milks are obtained.

Occasionally, breast milk alone is not sufficient. Its low sodium content may lead to hyponatraemia, and rickets of prematurity may result from too low a supply of phosphate, and, occasionally, hypocalcaemia occurs. The total calorie content of human milk is closely related to its fat content, and heat treatment may reduce it below the baby's energy needs. Consequently, the baby's growth rate may be diminished and the reduced fat intake may provide an inadequate supply of fatty acids for optimal brain growth.

Supplementation of breast milk with a commercial 'fortifier' containing additional protein, carbohydrate, sodium, calcium and phosphate may overcome these apparent deficiencies and experience so far suggests they improve the nutritional suitability of breast milk for the very preterm infant. However, since individual babies have differing requirements, the blood levels of these minerals need to be measured regularly and the amounts of supplements adjusted accordingly. Fortifiers must be added to the milk as close as possible to feed times, to minimise the possibility of bacterial contamination, and supplemented milks should not be stored.

Breast milk may need to be stored and this can safely be done in a freezer at $-18°C$. To prevent serious contamination with the skin flora or pathogenic bacteria, prior pasteurisation of the stored milk is often recommended. However, this denatures some of the antibacterial substances in breast milk and, provided that strict sterile precautions are taken in the collection of the milk and regular microbiological monitoring is carried out, it is probably not essential.

In some neonatal units it has become possible to maintain a supply of donated breast milk for the babies by careful selection and informed testing of donors for HIV infection and pasteurisation of the milk.

With these uncertainties about breast milk, some neonatologists favour the use of artificial feeds specially adapted for the nutritional needs of the very low birth weight infants, using the guidelines for composition laid down by the European Society for Paediatric Gastroenterology and Nutrition. A number of such preparations are available for use in the first few weeks of life, each 100 mL providing about 75 kcal for energy purposes and containing approximately 1.8 g protein, 7.5 g carbohydrate in mixed form, and 4.5 g fat – mainly as polyunsaturated fatty acids (Table 7.3, p. 102). The sodium content is also increased over the levels occurring in breast milk. The initial growth rate of well preterm infants is greater when they are fed on these special milks than on unmodified breast milk, though it is comparable when fortifier is added to the latter. Comparative studies of the later developmental progress of infants have not shown a clear-cut advantage for preterm formula milk and some even favour the breast milk groups (Cooke & Embleton 2000). Long-chain polyunsaturated fatty acids (LCPs) are included in certain formula milks, as some evidence exists to suggest that they are essential for retinal and brain structure and function. Modifications are made to specialised preterm baby milks to include these LCPs to rectify these deficiencies. Manufacturers have also added nucleotides, which are essential for the formation of new cells, though at present the amounts in preterm formulae do not match those in breast milk (Leach et al 1995). The addition of the amino acid glutamine, which is important for development of the immune system, is being investigated (Neu et al 1997).

Despite the apparent advantages of preterm formulae, there is real value in allowing the mother to contribute her milk to her baby for at least part of the feeds, supplementing this with fortifier or preterm formula to ensure an adequate calorie intake. This should make the mother feel more involved in her infant's care and that she is contributing to her infant's wellbeing, and will increase the chance of successfully breast feeding the baby later on (Fig. 8.6).

The amount of feed necessary is dependent upon the baby's size, maturity and age, modified by individual variation in requirement which can only be judged by experience. When no initial period of parenteral nutrition is necessary, the first feed should be the mother's expressed colostrum, supplemented, if the blood glucose is low, by some formula milk. Preterm infants need more per unit of body weight than those who are fully mature and an energy value of between 105 and 150 kcal/kg is required to maintain weight gain. It will be seen, therefore, that requirements will vary considerably from one infant to another,

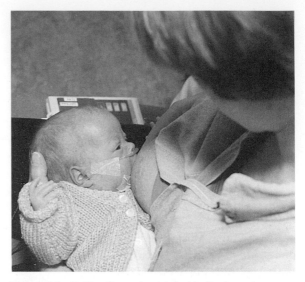

Figure 8.6 Putting the preterm infant to the breast increases the likelihood of successful breast feeding later.

Table 8.2 Average volumes of milk needed by babies under 2000 g birth weight

Day	Volume (mL/kg body weight per day)	Calories (per kg body weight per day)
1	60	50
2	90	70
3	110	90
4	150	120
5	180	130
7	180–210	140

but the figures in Table 8.2 give a guide to average volumes of milk needed by babies under 2000 g birth weight.

Feeds may be given either as hourly boluses infused over 10–20 minutes or as a continuous infusion, but if a syringe pump is used for breast milk it must be sited below the baby to allow the fat to rise and thus reach the infant.

Although little gain in weight will occur in the first 7 to 10 days, thereafter an increase of 15 g/kg body weight per day, in the absence of oedema, indicates an adequate calorie intake and the volume of feeds should be adjusted, within the limits of the baby's tolerance, to achieve at least this rate of growth.

Complications of enteral feeding in preterm infants

Not all preterm infants tolerate gastric feeding initially. If vomiting or abdominal distension occurs, or the gastric aspirate increases in volume or becomes bile stained, the feed should be either temporarily discontinued or reduced in volume and only gradually increased again.

Other feeds

Soya milks are not suitable for preterm infants and should not be used. Elemental feeds, where the constituents of milk have been broken down to basic elements which can be absorbed directly without digestion, are occasionally needed during recovery from necrotising enterocolitis or following surgery for meconium ileus.

Food supplements

Phosphate and vitamin D   The preterm infant below about 32 weeks' gestation has an increased liability to develop rickets after about 3 months of age, and this is particularly related to an inadequate phosphate intake rather than vitamin D deficiency. The blood phosphate level should be measured weekly and breast-fed babies with low values should receive a phosphate supplement of 1 mmol/kg/day and 400 IU/day of vitamin D to ensure good bone mineralisation. Preterm artificial milk formulae are supplemented with adequate amounts for initial feeding but their mineral content is too high for use after the baby has reached 1800 g. Preterm baby follow-on milks (p. 102) have a reduced mineral content, while supplying the phosphate and vitamin D the baby needs, and an enhanced protein and calorie content. Studies have shown an increase in growth of preterm infants fed on this formula.

Other vitamins   Preterm infants require vitamin supplementation due to poor absorption of vitamins from their diet once they are on full gastric feeds. They digest fat poorly in the gut and all fat-soluble vitamins are therefore poorly absorbed. As a result, they have limited stores of these vitamins in their body fat. Deficiency of vitamins results in poor growth. All preterm infants should receive vitamin D 400 IU, vitamin A 500 IU and vitamin C 50 mg daily. Vitamin B supplements are probably not essential but the evidence for this is conflicting, so, for convenience, a multivitamin preparation is usually prescribed from the third or fourth week. Vitamin E deficiency may, rarely, cause a haemolytic anaemia and some authorities recommend supplements of 10 mg daily to prevent it. The doses of supplementary vitamins A and D given must be adjusted according to the amounts already incorporated in the milk preparation used, as this varies from one brand to another – both vitamins can cause serious toxic effects if excessive doses are given.

Iron and folic acid   The second phase of anaemia of prematurity (p. 122) is prevented by giving an iron supplement to breast-fed infants from 4 to 6 weeks of age until full mixed feeding is established. Ferrous sulphate 2.5 mg/kg daily is generally satisfactory, though if it causes constipation some babies may tolerate another preparation of iron better. Some authorities suggest that giving iron reduces the anti-infective properties of unsaturated iron-binding proteins in breast milk but the risk from this effect is small. No iron supplementation is needed for formula-fed infants. Preterm babies of very low birth weight require a small folic acid supplement of 100 µg daily to prevent a later macrocytic anaemia.

The important parental link

In spite of what has been said about the need for specialised nursing care for these small infants, the role of the baby's parents as part of the caring team must be recognised. The initial separation is liable to strain any parent–child relationship and much can be done to reduce this. They should be given encouragement to be involved in the baby's care at every opportunity and their opinions and needs, particularly where decisions will affect other family members, must be taken seriously, for what happens at this early stage will increase their confidence in their parenting skills and thus affect the child's future development.

COMMON DISORDERS OF THE PRETERM INFANT

Most of the conditions described in other sections of this book may affect these babies. When illness occurs, the many disdvantages from immaturity of the infant's organ systems diminish her ability to deal with it and the diagnosis may be delayed since the clinical signs are often non-specific and can be difficult to interpret. The immaturity of the central nervous system, gastrointestinal tract, lungs, liver and immune system lies behind many of the disorders encountered.

Respiratory problems

Periodic respiration

Periodic respiration with repeated short spells of very shallow breathing or complete cessation lasting 3–10 seconds is a commonly observed phenomenon which is almost normal for small preterm babies. The pattern reflects diminished responsiveness of the respiratory centre in the brain stem to changes in the oxygen and carbon dioxide levels in the blood. This varies with the state of consciousness and is therefore more common during sleep. More regular respiration may be achieved by slightly raising the oxygen content of the surrounding air, though it is important to avoid high oxygen levels in the blood by careful saturation monitoring.

Apnoeic attacks

True apnoeic attacks are different and potentially more serious. Breathing stops suddenly, the apnoea usually lasts for more than 20 seconds and may be accompanied by bradycardia and cyanosis. The attacks may not always have a clear predisposing cause but they are often associated with:

- respiratory distress syndrome (p. 132)
- anaemia (p. 122)
- gastro-oesophageal reflux (p. 121)
- hypoglycaemia (p. 54)
- cerebral haemorrhage (p. 150)
- electrolyte imbalance (p. 128)
- sepsis (p. 122).

Treatment of the underlying cause may prevent the attacks, but, if not, the possibility that they are seizures should be considered (p. 156).

During an attack, the infant should be encouraged to breathe by gentle stimulation. Additional oxygen will be needed if the oxygen saturation does not return promptly to normal.

The infant should be continuously monitored until the episodes of apnoea with bradycardia have ceased. After this, apnoea alarm devices are useful in alerting nursing staff to the need for action. The baby lies on a pressure-sensitive pad or has a similar sensor attached to the skin, which automatically activates a buzzer after breathing has ceased for more than a selected period.

Raising the oxygen content of the inspired air is ineffective in more prolonged apnoeic attacks and may be dangerous if the baby is left in a high-oxygen environment after breathing restarts (p. 133). Administration of caffeine is an effective treatment where the infant has no treatable cause for the attacks. It is reliably absorbed after oral administration and blood level monitoring is not often needed. It is given as an initial dose of 20 mg/kg intravenously over 5–10 minutes, or as two oral doses of 25 mg/kg 1 hour apart, followed by 5 mg/kg orally as a daily maintainance dose, increasing to 10 mg daily if periods of apnoea persist (Comer et al 2001). Alternatively, aminophylline can be given intravenously or as a suppository of 2.5–5 mg at 6-hourly intervals, but the blood level should be measured to confirm that a therapeutic dose is being given. When simple measures fail to maintain adequate respiratory function, continuous positive airways pressure (CPAP) is often successful. Only rarely is continued artificial ventilation needed.

The respiratory distress syndrome

Difficulty with breathing soon after birth is very common in preterm infants. An increased respiratory rate, grunting, or recession of the sternum or rib margins may indicate one of a number of possible conditions amongst which are pneumothorax, congenital heart disease with cardiac failure, septicaemia and pneumonia (especially from group B beta-haemolytic streptococcal infection), meconium aspiration and cerebral birth injury. However, by far the commonest cause in the preterm infant is hyaline membrane disease, the familiar clinical picture of which led to the use of the term 'respiratory distress syndrome' (RDS). It occurs in almost all infants under 30 weeks' gestation but is less frequent in more mature babies. This is the main condition requiring artificial ventilation in the newborn period and is described in detail in Chapter 9.

Alimentary tract problems

Gastro-oesophageal reflux

Regurgitation of gastric contents into the lower oesophagus between feeds occurs in most preterm infants. Occasionally, more major degrees of this reflux result in vomiting or posseting, which may be associated with aspiration of milk or acid into the lungs and a consequent respiratory infection. This gastro-oesophageal reflux can be confirmed by a barium swallow X-ray, by ultrasound or by measuring the pH (acidity) of the lower oesophagus continuously, using an indwelling naso-oesophageal electrode. It is treated by keeping the infant tilted head up and using an antacid and alginate mixture to thicken the feed.

Abdominal distension

Distension of the abdomen caused by gaseous dilatation of the immature gut is often troublesome, especially in the second week, and may be severe enough to interfere with respiration by restricting diaphragmatic movement. Whilst it is often benign and relieved by a modification of the feeding schedule, it can also be a manifestation of more serious disorders such as septicaemia or due to a congenital malformation of the intestine. Intestinal obstruction from inspissated milk curd is a rare cause when formula milk is used for feeding and can sometimes necessitate surgical intervention. Hard faeces in the lower colon and rectum may also be a problem but can often be relieved by the use of small rectal suppositories or saline washouts.

Jaundice

Immature liver function renders the baby slow to deal with bilirubin by conjugation and excretion (p. 188). Kernicterus, with its later consequences of nerve deafness, athetoid cerebral palsy and learning difficulties, is more likely to follow in a preterm infant with a lower level of serum bilirubin than in a term baby. Opinions differ about the level of serum bilirubin at which the pigment is likely to pass the blood–brain barrier, but in the smallest infants more than 250 µmol/L (15 mg/ 100 mL) may be a danger whilst 300–340 µmol/L (18–20 mg/100 mL) can be regarded as a hazard for those over 34 weeks' gestation. Phototherapy (p. 195) has reduced the need for exchange transfusion, but it must be employed at an early stage to be effective and charts indicating the levels at which it should be applied are available (Fig. 12.1).

Oedema

The shiny 'full' appearance of the skin of the preterm infant at birth is due to water retention and is lost within a few days, but it should not be regarded as pathological. True oedema with pitting on pressure, due probably to increased capillary permeability, is, however, a common finding in the first week and usually affects the feet, hands, face and external genitalia, subsiding gradually without apparent harm. More serious generalised oedema is seen in conjunction with the respiratory distress syndrome, congestive cardiac failure or severe haemolytic disease. This can be controlled by giving a diuretic such as chlorothiazide or furosemide (frusemide) together with the potassium-retaining drug spironolactone. Fluid restriction is the treatment of choice if the baby is hyponatraemic.

Sclerema

Sclerema is now rare and affects mainly preterm or debilitated infants, particularly those who have suffered prolonged asphyxia, septicaemia or chilling. There is hardening of the skin and subcutaneous tissue, often starting over the buttocks and spreading to the whole body, but no pitting oedema. The skin becomes tight over the underlying tissues and makes the baby feel very stiff and the joints immobile. This pattern has given rise to the apt description of the baby being 'skin-bound'. It has a poor prognosis but exchange transfusion using fresh blood has sometimes been found to be effective when the condition has resulted from severe infection. Systemic steroids are ineffective.

Anaemia

There are several causes of anaemia following preterm birth. The initial high haemoglobin (Hb) slowly falls over the first few weeks, reaching an average of 9 g/dL by 2 months of age (compared with 11 g/dL in a term infant). This early anaemia is largely due to a reduced rate of red cell production in the bone marrow, which occurs in all babies (p. 184), but is accentuated by taking blood samples for laboratory testing. Treatment with iron or folic acid does not alter its progress. If the infant is unable to feed adequately because of breathlessness from the anaemia, a small blood transfusion should be given to raise the Hb level above 12 g/dL (Andersen 2001). The amount of blood, in millilitres, to be given is calculated using the following formula:

- Whole blood: Weight (kg) × required Hb increase (g) × 6
- Packed cells: Weight (kg) × required Hb increase (g) × 4

Treatment with a combination of intramuscular erythropoietin and oral iron can restore the Hb level but it is expensive and rarely justified.

Some 4–6 weeks after the expected birth date the Hb level begins to rise as erythropoietin secretion restarts from the kidney, but there may be a second fall at 3 to 4 months of age in the breast-fed infant, which is associated with iron deficiency and is preventable by oral iron supplements (p. 119). Macrocytic anaemia is occasionally seen in the second or third month and routine administration of folic acid, 100 μg daily, to babies of less than 34 weeks' gestation is advised.

Haemolytic anaemia in the second month, caused by vitamin E deficiency, has also been reported.

Infections

Minor infections found in term infants are described in Chapter 11. These may all occur in the preterm infant but are less easily detected because of the immature infant's poorer immune responses.

Severe infections are much more common than in the term infant (Berger et al 1998) but are much less easy to recognise. The body temperature is more likely to drop than to rise; the infant may develop an increase in oxygen requirements or periods of apnoea or bradycardia may occur. Other signs are non-specific, such as:

- lethargy
- refusal to feed
- vomiting
- pallor
- persistent mild jaundice.

In any baby showing such signs, full septic screening and treatment with intravenous antibiotics should be started while awaiting the results of the bacterial cultures (p. 168).

Other minor disorders related to preterm birth

Umbilical hernias, undescended testes and multiple strawberry marks are all more common in babies born prematurely. None requires treatment in the newborn period, though orchidopexy may be needed in infancy. On the other hand, a third of inguinal hernias (Fig. 8.7) will strangulate and require emergency surgery if untreated and therefore early elective surgical correction should be carried out.

Routine immunisations in preterm infants

Preterm babies should receive the recommended schedule of immunisations at 2, 3 and 4 months after the birth date irrespective of the extent of prematurity. They are able to produce adequate antibody responses at this time and adverse reactions are no more common than in term infants.

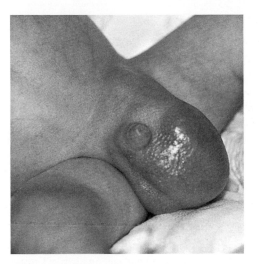

Figure 8.7 Inguinal hernias are more common in preterm infants and are likely to strangulate.

THE OUTLOOK FOR SURVIVING PRETERM BABIES

Great improvements in the quality of life of preterm babies have resulted from improving obstetric and perinatal care in the last few years. Because changes are taking place continuously, it is impossible to give accurate statistics applicable to the present time. The outlook for development depends upon the cause of the prematurity, and it is often more affected by factors operating during intrauterine life than by complications in the neonatal period. Accompanying major congenital malformation may also influence developmental progress. Poor maternal fertility and low socio-economic status also greatly affect the outcome. Male babies tend to have a worse outcome than females (Stevenson et al 2000).

The prospects for survival and normal development in preterm infants are now good, especially if they are more than 1500 g at birth and do not have any associated congenital abnormalities. Over the last two decades, there has been a steady increase in survival, especially in infants under 1500 g birth weight, but it has been accompanied by a small increase in the number of children with cerebral palsy. Those most at risk have a gestation period of well under 28 weeks or are less than 750 g birth weight, especially if they are also undernourished in utero (Wood et al 2000). The outcome for babies under 1000 g is that about 10% of survivors will have a measurable and lasting disability, including impaired growth and retinopathy of prematurity (Vyas et al 2000) (p. 142), and a smaller number will have a more severe handicap. With good obstetrics and the best neonatal care, well over 80% of all babies under 1500 g can now be expected to survive and only some 5% will suffer a handicap sufficient to interfere seriously with their lives. A rather greater number will be found to have some degree of learning difficulties or disorders of behaviour, but perinatal events may have less bearing on this than socioeconomic and genetic factors.

Spastic diplegia, which used to be the predominant form of cerebral palsy seen in preterm babies, is now relatively uncommon. The incidence of other forms such as quadriplegia and athetosis has not significantly diminished and has even shown a slight rise in recent years, particularly in babies of over 1500 g birth weight.

As methods of care improve, the risk of complications – both of prematurity and of its treatment – should reduce. However, even for intact survivors, there is an increased risk of sudden infant death syndrome during the first year of life and this is greater still if the baby has bronchopulmonary dysplasia (p. 143). For this reason, parents should be taught the preventive measures which can be recommended (p. 88).

Prematurity often creates emotional stress in the parents during the initial illness and continued anxiety about the baby after discharge. This is one reason for an increased rate of admission to hospital in the first year of life. Many neonatal units now have community neonatal nurses, who follow up these infants at home to offer support and information to parents to increase their confidence in caring for their child.

REFERENCES

Andersen C 2001 Critical haemoglobin thresholds in preterm infants. Archives of Disease in Childhood Fetal and Neonatal Edition 84:F146–F148

Baker S F, Smith B J, Donohue P K et al 1999 Skin care practices for premature infants. Journal of Perinatology 19(6):426–431

Ballard J L, Khoury J C, Wedig K et al 1991 New Ballard score, expanded to include extremely premature infants. Journal of Pediatrics 119(3):417–423

Berger A, Salzer H R, Weninger M et al 1998 Septicaemia in an Austrian neonatal intensive care unit: a 7 year analysis. Acta Paediatrica 87(10):1066–1069

Blackburn S, Patterson D 1991 Effect of cycled light on activity state and cardiorespiratory function in preterm infants. Journal of Perinatal Nursing 4(4):47–54

Bond C 1999 Positive touch and massage in the neonatal unit: a means of reducing stress levels. Journal of Neonatal Nursing 5(5):16–19

Brocklehurst P, Gates S, McKenzie-McHarg K et al 1999 Are we prescribing multiple courses of antenatal steroids? A survey of practice in the UK. British Journal of Obstetrics and Gynaecology 106(9):977–979

Brocklehurst P, Gates S, Johnson A et al 2000 Effects of multiple courses of antenatal steroids are uncertain. British Medical Journal 321(7252):47

Chant T 1998 Oro- and nasogastric feeding techniques for very low birthweight infants: selecting an appropriate feeding regime. Journal of Neonatal Nursing 5(1):23–25

Comer A M, Perry C M, Figgit D P 2001 Caffeine citrate: a review of its use in apnoea of prematurity. Paediatric Drugs 3(1):61–79

Cooke R J, Embleton N D 2000 Feeding issues in preterm infants. Archives of Disease in Childhood Fetal and Neonatal Edition 83:F215–F218

Darmstadt G L, Dinulos J G 2000 Neonatal skin care. Pediatric Clinics of North America 47(4):757–782

Dubowitz L 1969 Assessment of gestational age in newborn: a practical scoring system. Archives of Disease in Childhood 44(238):782

King C 1998 Enteral feeds for preterm infants: nutrition and therapy. Journal of Neonatal Nursing 4(5):6–10

Leach J, Baxter J, Molitor B et al 1995 Total potential nucleosides of human milk by stage of lactation. American Journal of Clinical Nutrition 61:1224–1230

Neu J, Roig J, Meetze W et al 1997 Enteral glutamine supplementation for very low birth weight infants decreases morbidity. Journal of Pediatrics 131(5):691–699

Rutter N 2000 Clinical consequences of an immature barrier. Seminars in Neonatology 5(4):281–287

Stevenson D K, Veiter J, Fanaroff A A et al 2000 Sex differences in outcomes of very low birthweight infants: the newborn male disadvantage. Archives of Disease in Childhood Fetal and Neonatal Edition 83:F182–F185

Vause S, Johnston T 2000 Management of preterm labour. Archives of Disease in Childhood Fetal and Neonatal Edition 83:F79–F85

Vyas J, Field D, Draper E S et al 2000 Severe retinopathy of prematurity and its association with different rates of survival in infants of less than 1251 g birthweight. Archives of Disease in Childhood Fetal and Neonatal Edition 82:F145–F149

Williams A F 2000 Early enteral feeding of the preterm infant. Archives of Disease in Childhood Fetal and Neonatal Edition 83(3):F219–F220

Wood N S, Marlow N, Costeloe K et al 2000 Neurologic and developmental disability after extreme preterm birth: EPICure Study Group. New England Journal of Medicine 343(6):378–384

Chapter 9
Intensive neonatal care

CHAPTER CONTENTS

Categories of care for newborn infants   125
Requirements for neonatal intensive care   126
  Medical and nursing staff   126
Principles of intensive care   127
  Monitoring   127
  Fluids and nutrition   128
  Enteral feeds   128
  Total parenteral nutrition   128
  Prevention and management of infection   130
  Respiratory care   130
Hyaline membrane disease (respiratory
distress syndrome)   131
  Pathogenesis   131
  Clinical features   131
  Management   132
  Surfactant therapy   133
  Oxygen therapy   133
  Blood gases   133
  Principles of neonatal mechanical ventilation   134
  Other methods of respiratory support   137
  Management of a ventilated baby   137
  Complications of ventilator care   138
  Weaning off ventilation and extubation   138
  Other complications of RDS   139
  Later complications and prognosis   142
Surgical problems and intensive care   144
Some wider implications of neonatal
intensive care   144
  Pain control   144
  Emotional care   144
  'Kangaroo care'   145
  Dying babies   146

CATEGORIES OF CARE FOR NEWBORN INFANTS

The progressive development of skilled neonatal intensive care, particularly for those babies under 1500 g birth weight, has contributed significantly to the falling perinatal mortality rates in developed countries. Not only has there been an increase in survival of these infants but the risk of serious handicap in the survivors is small and diminishing except for a minority with a birth weight below 750 g.

Several books have been written which describe intensive care in detail, but it is our intention only to introduce the subject, outlining the main requirements for its provision and the general principles involved.

The amount of nursing and medical expertise required to provide newborn babies with the care they need varies markedly from one infant to the next. Levels of care are as follows:

- *Normal care* can be defined as that given by the mother, with access to medical and nursing advice at her request.
- *Special care* exceeds normal care but can be provided at the mother's bedside or in a separate unit. It requires qualified neonatal nursing skills and access to paediatric medical care, and involves teaching and supporting the baby's parents.
- *Intensive care* requires a fully equipped unit with skilled neonatal nursing and medical staff on hand at all times. This category is sometimes subdivided to include high-dependency care.

Guidelines for categorising levels of care are shown in Box 9.1.

Box 9.1 Categories of care

Intensive care:
- <1000 g birth weight
- <27 weeks' gestation
- Mechanically assisted ventilation
- RDS requiring >60% O_2
- Severe recurrent apnoea
- Requiring inotrope infusion
- Exchange transfusion
- Emergency surgery

High dependency:
- Total parenteral nutrition
- Seizures
- Moderate RDS (40–60% O_2)
- Serious infections
- Moderate recurrent apnoea
- Respiratory disease requiring additional O_2
- Postoperatively

Special care:
- Requiring continuous monitoring for respiratory disease
- Intravenous infusion
- Tube-fed babies
- After minor surgery
- Barrier nursing
- Monitoring of bilirubin or blood glucose
- Illicit drug withdrawal symptoms
- On antibiotics

REQUIREMENTS FOR NEONATAL INTENSIVE CARE

In Britain, the facilities for long-term intensive respiratory care are mainly situated in major regional hospitals, often many miles from the parents' home. Such care is complex and requires a full range of support for it to be safe and effective. Ideally, all infants likely to require intensive care should be born in a hospital which can provide it, by transferring the mother to that hospital for delivery. However, it is not always possible to achieve this and, all maternity units offering care for higher-risk deliveries should have the equipment and skills to ventilate the baby effectively until he can be transferred to an intensive care unit.

The intensive care unit should be as near as possible to the delivery suite or maternity operating theatre to minimise the hazards during transfer. It must be possible to vary the temperature of each section to suit the needs of the individual infant; there must be hand-washing facilities, good lighting and piped oxygen, and air and suction outlets for each baby. There must be a section to isolate babies with transmissible infections and a place where parents may be reasonably private if, for instance, their baby is dying. Facilities must be available to enable parents to spend as much time with their baby as they wish.

The unit must have support from the full range of laboratory services to provide rapid and accurate haematological and biochemical tests results throughout the day and night using only small blood samples. Apparatus to perform arterial blood gas analysis and bilirubin measurements should be available on the ward itself so that the results are immediately available. It must be possible to X-ray the baby with minimum disturbance and undertake ultrasound examination of the brain or heart within an incubator and without disrupting ventilation. Pharmacy services must be able to provide emergency supplies of drugs and materials for intravenous nutrition at all times, and a dietician should be able to advise on the nutritional requirements of the infant. Since many such infants develop cardiac or surgical complications, there must be rapid access to the relevant departments for advice, investigation and intervention when needed. Much of the equipment used in intensive care is complicated and highly technical and requires maintenance for which expert advice and support must be available.

Medical and nursing staff

The best survival rates of very immature babies without serious handicap are reported from units with an adequate number of fully trained nursing and medical staff who have had long experience in treating the conditions encountered and are familiar with the complex equipment and techniques involved. There must be provision for continuing professional development to ensure staff are updated on evidence-based practices and for giving in-service training on the range of equipment used, particularly when new or updated models are introduced. The emotional costs are also high – parents, other relatives and staff all being likely to feel stressed at times. Some units have a system to ensure that this is recognised so that those feeling the strain can be counselled and supported.

PRINCIPLES OF INTENSIVE CARE
Monitoring

Whatever the underlying condition for which a baby requires intensive care, there are certain general principles which govern how such infants are treated. In general, since they are unable to maintain their normal physiological activities adequately, each needs to be evaluated regularly, deviations from normal detected and corrective measures applied. Routine nursing observations of the infant are the basis of such an evaluation, but, for a more continuous assessment, specific electronic apparatus is needed.

The best equipment is able to monitor several body functions simultaneously, giving an alarm signal when one function strays outside the limits of the normal range to warn the staff that action is needed to remedy it. It can also retain the information gained in its memory and display graphically the variation in the baby's progress over a specified period of time (Fig. 9.1).

The monitor should be able to give continuous display of the following parameters from the infant:

- heart rate and ECG pattern
- central (abdominal skin) and peripheral (toe) temperature
- respiration rate
- blood pressure – invasive and non-invasive
- oxygen and carbon dioxide levels in the blood.

All this can be achieved using electrodes or apparatus attached to the skin of the infant. Most incubators used in intensive care display air temperature, level of humidity and inspired oxygen within the incubator. Other information can be obtained only by testing the baby's blood directly, taking samples from catheters placed in an artery or vein, or by collecting capillary blood from a heel-stab.

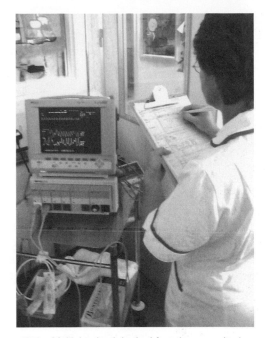

Figure 9.1 Multiple physiological functions monitoring apparatus using both numerical and graphical displays.

Box 9.2   Common recordings in intensive care

Continuously measured parameters:
- Heart rate
- Respiratory rate
- Blood pressure – invasive and non-invasive
- Transcutaneous oxygen saturation
- Transcutaneous pO_2 and CO_2
- Skin and axillary temperature
- Ventilator settings
- Temperature, humidity and oxygen concentration in the incubator

Nursing observations and measurements:
- Skin colour
- Skin perfusion
- Baby's level of activity
- Presence of grunting or costal recession
- Position of the baby
- Care of invasive lines
- Type and volume of infused fluids
- Output of urine, stool, gastric aspirate and respiratory secretions

---

All this information must be recorded on an intensive care chart designed to show it in such a way as to demonstrate the changes which occur and when they do so.

A summary of commonly recorded information is shown in Box 9.2.

Attention to small details of changes in such observations is often the key to a successful outcome for the infant and the importance of careful recording cannot be overstated.

Fluids and nutrition

Correct management of fluid and electrolyte balance is vital for sick preterm infants. In general, more harm is done by giving too much fluid than too little, for it can cause pulmonary and cerebral oedema, cardiac failure and persistent shunting of blood through a patent ductus arteriosus. Sodium depletion or overloading must be recognised and corrected by adjusting sodium intake. Hypocalcaemia is not uncommon and may require correction with 10% calcium gluconate.

The plasma albumin level may fall due to impaired synthesis and can contribute to hypotension and oedema. This can be treated by an infusion of human albumin. Daily measurements of blood electrolytes and protein levels are essential to enable adjustments to be made to the infant's fluid and electrolyte intake.

Fetal bradycardia and hypotension can cause acute renal tubular necrosis from birth. The renal failure which follows causes oliguria, a raised blood urea, and disturbance of electrolyte and acid–base balance. Measurement of urine output can be achieved by weighing nappies or using urine collection bags, and catheterisation is seldom needed. Fluids should be restricted until the urine flow recommences, and adjustment of electrolyte intake is required to correct the biochemical abnormalities. For prolonged failure, renal dialysis may be needed.

In view of the almost inevitable respiratory disorders, oral or nasogastric fluids are seldom tolerated well at first. The baby's fluid requirements in the first few days can be satisfied by giving 10% dextrose intravenously, starting at a rate of 50–70 mL/kg per day and gradually increasing to 150–180 mL/kg per day over 5–7 days. Sodium and potassium additions are necessary after the first 24 hours, which can be provided by using standard neonatal dextrose and electrolyte mixtures. These mixtures also contain appropriate

---

> **Box 9.3** Benefits of non-nutritive feeding
>
> - Promotes gut maturation
> - Increases gut hormone levels
> - Increases tolerance of feeds
> - Decreases gastric residuals
> - Reduces number of days requiring total parenteral nutrition and phototherapy
> - Does not increase the risk of necrotising enterocolitis
> - Reduces the risk of cholestatic jaundice

maintenance quantities of calcium, magnesium, sulphate, gluconate and chloride.

Enteral feeds

Management of enteral feeds in the intensive care area varies from unit to unit, particularly in relation to very small and premature babies (Chant 1998). Recent studies suggest that early small-volume gastric feeding within the first 7 days has many benefits, as outlined in Box 9.3.

This non-nutritive feeding is also referred to as trophic, hypocaloric, gut priming or minimal enteral feeding (McClure & Newell 2000). It involves giving the baby small volumes of either breast milk or preterm formula, e.g. 1 mL every 4 hours, while providing the majority of the infant's nutrition parenterally. The frequency and volume of feeds can be increased depending on how well the baby tolerates them (King 1998) (p. 116). Once enteral feeds have increased to 1 mL hourly and above, the intravenous fluids should be reduced by an equivalent amount until the whole of the fluid requirement is being administered into the gastrointestinal tract.

Total parenteral nutrition

When the nutritional requirements of a sick, preterm infant cannot be met by enteral feeds, a regimen of intravenous feeding must be commenced. Sometimes it will be combined with trophic feeding but occasionally it will be the sole means of feeding the baby. There is no standard regimen for total parenteral nutrition (TPN) for preterm infants, but the components listed in Table 9.1 will provide for all the infant's nutritional needs. It will normally be started on the

Table 9.1 Ingredients in total parenteral nutrition

Amino acids	Enables the baby to make proteins
Glucose	Energy source; provides calories
Lipid emulsion	Provides essential fatty acids for brain growth; also an energy source
Vitamins	A, B group, C, D, E
Electrolytes	Sodium, potassium, chloride
Minerals	Calcium, magnesium, phosphorus
Trace elements	Zinc, copper, iron

Box 9.4   Complications of total parenteral nutrition

Metabolic:
- Electrolyte imbalance
- Phosphate depletion
- Cholestatic jaundice

Infusion:
- Infection – including *Candida albicans* and *Staph. epidermidis* septicaemia
- Thrombosis around the tip of the central catheter
- Tissue necrosis and skin sloughing from extravasation of parenteral nutrition fluids

second or third day of life with small quantities of the major ingredients, the remainder of the baby's fluids being provided by saline and dextrose solutions. The amounts of lipid, amino acids and dextrose are progressively increased until adequate amounts are provided. The vitamins given in the infusion are photodegradable and hence the solution should be shielded from light.

Because there is a risk of introducing infection, the mixtures are made up in the pharmacy under strict sterile conditions.

Administration and monitoring

TPN is best administered through an indwelling intravenous catheter with its tip in the superior or inferior vena cava. If a peripheral catheter is used, the site of entry of the catheter must be inspected frequently for signs of inflammation or oedema which could indicate that extravasation has occurred. The solutions are hypertonic and very irritant and may cause local tissue necrosis, including the overlying skin, if they are allowed to accumulate in the subcutaneous tissues.

Regular blood sampling is necessary to monitor levels of a number of components such as sodium, potassium, calcium and lipids. Adjustments are made to the TPN mixture according to the results of these tests. Measurement of blood albumin and packed cell volume is essential daily, and other investigations such as serum bilirubin, transaminases and triglycerides should be checked at longer intervals. It is essential to monitor lipid levels in the serum regularly, since high values may result in pulmonary, hepatic and possibly retinal damage. If TPN is prolonged, additional vitamin K and B_{12} may need to be given as intramuscular injections.

Complications

These are common and can be divided into metabolic disturbances and those related to the infusion itself, as outlined in Box 9.4.

These complications can mostly be avoided by regular blood tests, care during the siting of intravenous catheters and close observation afterwards. Aseptic technique must be used at all times when the line needs to be disconnected, to avoid introducing infection.

It can be appreciated from this brief account that TPN should not be undertaken lightly and requires both experience and close cooperation between medical, nursing, laboratory and pharmacy personnel to be safe and successful.

Technique of insertion of intravenous cannulae and central venous catheters

Suitable veins for setting up intravenous infusions are found in the antecubital fossae, the back of the hand, the dorsum of the feet and on the side of the scalp. Sometimes, in a thin baby, the saphenous vein at the ankle can be used. If the baby is likely to need a central line, the larger veins, such as those in the antecubital fossae, should be left for this purpose. Attention must be paid to the comfort and safety of the baby throughout the procedure, including:

- use of strict aseptic technique
- comfortable positioning of the limb to be used and the baby
- amethocaine local anaesthetic gel may be used to reduce the pain of the procedure,

though its value in babies under 32 weeks' gestation is uncertain (p. 144)

- careful sterilisation of the skin with weak chlorhexidine solution
- avoiding already bruised areas
- avoiding sensitive areas, e.g. inner aspect of the wrist
- careful taping and splinting of cannulae to minimise skin trauma (p. 114)
- limiting the number of attempts made by one person.

The skin must be sterilised to avoid introducing infection but only the smallest suitable amount of antiseptic solution should be used, to reduce the risk of absorption into the circulation. The limb is then gently squeezed above the chosen site, to distend the vein, and secured below it. For scalp veins, compression below the entry site makes the vein prominent. The cannula is gently advanced into the vein until the blood flows well and samples are collected if needed. The outer cannula is then pushed further up the vein and the stilette withdrawn. Either an infusion is set up or, if not required, the patency of the cannula is maintained by intermittent flushing with normal saline.

In babies where prolonged use of TPN or high concentrations of dextrose solution are likely, a central venous catheter is preferable to avoid damage to smaller veins, tissue necrosis and frequent resiting of peripheral cannulae. A relatively large cannula is inserted into the vein and either a silastic catheter is threaded through it or a fine guidewire inserted into the vein and the catheter subsequently passed over it. When the tip of the catheter is in the central veins, the guidewire is withdrawn and the tube secured with a small transparent occlusive dressing. The position of the tip of the catheter should be confirmed by contrast X-ray before fluids are administered through the line (Reece et al 2001).

Umbilical venous catheters are often used as short-term access in very sick or premature babies but are unsuitable for parenteral nutrition. The umbilical vein can be cannulated at or soon after delivery for the administration of emergency drugs or fluids. In the intensive care area, these lines may be used initially for administration of maintenance dextrose and, particularly, for inotrope, e.g. dopamine, infusions.

Prevention and management of infection

Natural protection against infection is limited in the newborn infant and especially so if the baby is born prematurely (p. 122). Intensive care inevitably involves invasive procedures, such as insertion of cannulae and endotracheal intubation, which give increased opportunity for organisms to gain entry, thus all the precautions to prevent infection must be employed rigorously (p. 115). If, despite this, the baby shows general signs of infection (p. 122), samples of blood, urine and usually cerebrospinal fluid (CSF) should be sent for bacterial culture, together with swabs from suspected infected sites. Broad-spectrum intravenous antibiotics must be started while awaiting the results of the investigations. A combination of gentamicin (or netilmicin) and flucloxacillin, or cefotaxime alone would be suitable initial antibiotics.

In many situations, such as the respiratory distress syndrome, infection enters the differential diagnosis of the baby's symptoms. In such cases, antibiotics should always be given until infection has been excluded by a combination of an improvement in the baby's condition and the results of the initial investigations.

Respiratory care

Many very preterm infants and some sick but more mature babies either cannot breathe adequately or their lungs are unable to maintain normal gaseous exchange. Oxygenation and removal of carbon dioxide from the blood are impaired, which results in abnormal blood gas values and acidaemia. In these circumstances it is often necessary to provide artificial mechanical ventilation for the baby.

Although it is not the only disease for which ventilation is needed, the respiratory distress syndrome is by far the commonest disorder in preterm infants who require this intervention and thus it is described in detail as one example of neonatal intensive respiratory care.

HYALINE MEMBRANE DISEASE (RESPIRATORY DISTRESS SYNDROME)

By far the commonest respiratory disease in preterm infants is hyaline membrane disease. It is often called respiratory distress syndrome (RDS), which reflects the clinical picture seen in the first few hours of life. It is the major underlying cause of death in the preterm infant and constitutes the most common reason for requiring intensive care. It occurs occasionally in mature neonates, particularly in the infants of diabetic mothers, those born after caesarean section or following any illness causing hypotension in the mother in labour. The condition varies greatly in intensity, causing severe problems in some infants, yet, surprisingly, some extremely immature babies do not develop it at all, particularly if there has been prolonged stress or poor nutrition in utero. Pre-eclampsia, maternal hypertension, retroplacental bleeding and prolonged rupture of the membranes all reduce the risk or severity of RDS, as, curiously, does narcotic addiction. Administering intramuscular corticosteroids to the mother 48 hours prior to delivery also diminishes the risk. Currently, the balance of evidence does not favour multiple courses of steroids, though studies are still in progress (Brocklehurst et al 1999). Conversely, acute stress just prior to delivery, or placental abruption may increase the severity of RDS.

Pathogenesis

The pathogenesis of the condition is complex but relates both to the immaturity of the cells lining the alveoli and the inadequate amount of surfactant they produce. Although the bronchi have been completely formed by about the mid trimester, the cells lining the alveoli are thick and cuboidal rather than the thin flattened cells of the mature lung. This reduces the rate of both oxygen transfer from the alveoli to the blood and the loss of carbon dioxide from it. As they mature, some

of the cells lining the alveoli, known as type II alveolar cells, produce surfactant, a phospholipid substance which reduces the surface tension in the alveoli. This prevents the air sacs from collapsing at the end of expiration and enhances their expansion during inspiration. In the absence of surfactant, the surface of the lung available for gas exchange progressively diminishes as more and more alveoli collapse, oxygenation of the blood becomes impaired and carbon dioxide cannot be exhaled adequately. If untreated, the lungs become unable to sustain adequate exchange of oxygen and carbon dioxide and, in the most severe cases, death from respiratory failure will result. In this situation, the postmortem histology of the lungs shows an exudate of hyaline material in the collapsed alveoli and the terminal bronchi, which gives the condition its name.

Before birth, an indication of the amount of surfactant, and thus the maturity of the lungs, can be obtained by measuring the lecithin-to-sphingomyelin ratio in the amniotic fluid. If the level is greater than 1.5:1, severe RDS is unlikely to occur.

As well as the immaturity of the lungs, the pulmonary arterioles do not dilate as rapidly after birth as they do in the mature baby. As a result, the pulmonary vascular resistance remains high, causing shunting of deoxygenated blood through the foramen ovale in the heart, the open ductus arteriosus and through the intrapulmonary capillaries in unventilated portions of the lungs back into the systemic circulation.

Clinical features

Respiratory distress is the major symptom of the condition. It may be present from birth or develop slowly over the next few hours. The respiration rate increases and, if the disease is severe, an increasing concentration of inspired oxygen is needed to prevent cyanosis. There is retraction of the sternum and the lower ribs on inspiration (Fig. 9.2 A & B) and a marked expiratory grunt. Auscultation is often unhelpful but occasionally fine crackles are heard and breath sounds are reduced and often inaudible.

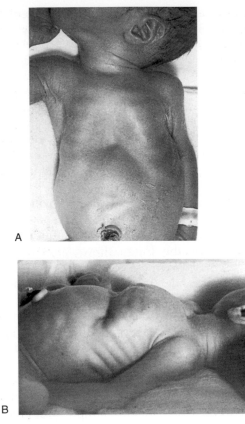

Figure 9.2 Respiratory distress syndrome in preterm infants. A: Sternal recession. B: Subcostal recession.

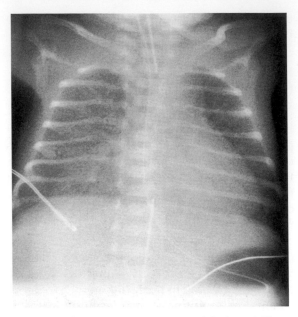

Figure 9.3 Ground-glass appearance of the lungs with a superimposed air bronchogram in a chest X-ray in respiratory distress syndrome.

The baby usually lies still, though he sometimes develops cerebral irritation from birth asphyxia.

Although typical of RDS, these features are common to many respiratory conditions and a chest X-ray will usually establish the correct diagnosis. In hyaline membrane disease, the X-ray shows diffuse 'ground-glass' mottling of the lung fields against which the bronchial tree shows up prominently as an air bronchogram (Fig. 9.3). Even this appearance is not specific to RDS, since the same pattern is seen in congenital group B beta-haemolytic streptococcal pneumonia. This infection is excluded by negative blood cultures, and transient tachypnoea of the newborn (p. 43) by rapid resolution of the respiratory signs within 48 hours. RDS itself persists for much longer, being at its worst between 24 and 72 hours with gradual resolution thereafter.

Management

The severity of RDS varies widely, being mild and resolving rapidly in some but becoming profound, life threatening and requiring mechanical respiratory support in others. In general, the more preterm the infant, the more likely is he to require assisted ventilation. For those infants below 28 weeks, it is usual to assume the condition will be severe and to apply assisted ventilation from the start (Table 9.2).

Treatment starts in the labour ward, where any infant who may develop RDS should be actively resuscitated at birth by giving respiratory support to those infants who do not breathe adequately. Ensuring rapid initial oxygenation and expansion of the alveoli, preventing hypothermia and maintaining a normal blood glucose level all reduce the severity of the subsequent RDS.

The objectives of treatment thereafter are:

- to maintain the oxygenation of the blood at a safe level
- to ensure the elimination of carbon dioxide from the blood
- to maintain a normal body temperature

Table 9.2 Incidence of respiratory distress syndrome (RDS), mechanical ventilation and the administration of surfactant in preterm infants

	Gestation (weeks)					
	24	26	28	30	32	34
RDS (%)	46	66	55	36	24	14
Ventilated (%)	74	96	80	48	23	19
Surfactant administered (%)	50	68	50	29	16	11

From Osborn 2000.

- to keep the baby's biochemical status within normal limits
- to provide adequate nutrition to ensure optimal growth.

In all cases, the baby's vital signs should be continuously monitored and recorded. The baby should be handled with the minimum of disturbance consistent with obtaining the necessary observations.

Surfactant therapy

Several natural and synthetic surfactant mixtures are available for administration directly into the bronchi in RDS. They incorporate a substance to ensure dispersion of the phospholipid mixture throughout the bronchi and alveoli. Surfactant is best given prophylactically – for example, within 15 minutes of birth – before the serious consequences of the disease are apparent, but is effective also as rescue therapy, given after RDS is established. It is usually administered as a suspension in water, injecting the liquid down the endotracheal tube during active ventilation as rapidly as the baby will tolerate it (Lal & Kotecha 2000). It may take only a few minutes to achieve this, and surprisingly little distress is caused to the infant. The tip of the endotracheal tube should be just beyond the vocal cords to allow for equal distribution of the surfactant to both lungs, though it is not necessary to do a chest X-ray first. Lung function and blood oxygenation may improve rapidly, particularly when natural surfactant is used, and it is often necessary to reduce the ventilator pressures shortly after it is given,

to prevent alveolar rupture from overinflation. Synthetic preparations work more slowly. It is usual to give two doses between 50–200 mg of surfactant depending on the preparation used, 12 hours apart, though additional doses are sometimes indicated (Soll 2000). Endotracheal suction should be avoided, as far as possible, for 12 hours after surfactant has been given. It has been shown conclusively that the use of surfactant substantially reduces the mortality from RDS in babies between 24 and 34 weeks' gestation, shortening the duration of artificial ventilation in many cases (Soll & Morley 2000). The incidence of chronic lung disease and retinopathy of prematurity are also diminished (Halliday 1997). Surfactant may benefit babies with meconium aspiration.

Oxygen therapy

The prevention of hypoxia is the primary reason for administering supplementary oxygen and the aim should be to maintain an arterial oxygen saturation of between 92% and 95% or an arterial pO_2 between 6 and 9 kPa. Too much oxygen is as dangerous as too little and may cause a deterioration in lung function or retinopathy of prematurity (ROP) (p. 142). Skin colour is a misleading indicator of significant hypoxia. If a concentration of greater than 30% inspired oxygen is needed, it indicates significant lung dysfunction and both oxygen and carbon dioxide levels should be measured. Transcutaneous oxygen saturation and pO_2 and pCO_2 recorders are useful in showing trends in the levels of blood oxygen, but regular arterial blood gas measurements should be undertaken to obtain accurate figures as monitoring by oxygen saturation measurement alone does not protect the infant from ROP as effectively as following the arterial pO_2 values (Tin et al 2001).

Blood gases

The maintenance of acid–base balance in a baby involves both respiratory and renal function, each adjusting constantly to keep the pH of the arterial blood within the narrow range of 7.33–7.47. If the lungs are normal, the amount of CO_2 exhaled will be adjusted to keep the arterial pCO_2 between

4.4 and 6.0 kPa. A pCO_2 which rises above this level reduces the blood pH. The mature kidney will excrete hydrogen ion (acid) and bicarbonate (alkali) appropriately, to maintain the pH within the normal values. Since renal function is limited in immature infants and respiratory function is diminished by RDS, a reduced pH (acidosis) is common and may be partly respiratory and partly metabolic in origin. A high pCO_2 suggests inadequate lung function, and a low bicarbonate, or an increased base deficit (more than -5 mmol/L), indicates a metabolic cause, especially if the pCO_2 is normal. Persistent hypoxia also results in increasing metabolic acidosis. The most common reason for this is poor perfusion of peripheral organs and muscles and the anaerobic metabolism which results from inadequate oxygen availability.

An arterial pH of less than 7.25, whether respiratory or metabolic, is harmful and requires correction. If the acidosis is metabolic, an infusion of 10–20 mL/kg body weight of normal saline or 4.5% human albumin solution over 30 minutes will improve peripheral perfusion by increasing the blood volume and blood pressure, and usually corrects it. Rapid infusion of bicarbonate has been shown to lower the intracellular and CSF pH, which may be harmful, and it is only occasionally used. Trometamol (THAM) can be used when all other methods fail to correct a serious metabolic acidosis.

A respiratory acidaemia can only be rectified by reducing the carbon dioxide level in the arterial blood by increasing the efficiency of breathing, if necessary by mechanical ventilation.

The most accurate way of analysing blood gases is by using arterial blood samples obtained from the descending aorta via an umbilical arterial catheter (UAC), though peripheral arterial lines are also suitable. Once the UAC has been inserted, the position of the catheter tip should be checked by X-ray, preferably using contrast to confirm its position. If the tip is sited above the diaphragm, there is a lower risk of circulatory complications (Barrington 2000). Blanching, cyanosis or coldness of the legs or oliguria suggests vascular obstruction below the catheter tip and should be regularly checked. Strict aseptic technique when sampling or changing the line will reduce the risk of infection. Careful securing of the catheter and avoiding lying the baby prone helps to prevent displacement. Very fine sensors are now available which are threaded through a UAC, allowing continuous monitoring of all blood gas parameters. This new innovation has many benefits for the baby, including reduced blood taking, lower infection risk, less handling and continuous visualisation of acid–base status.

If an arterial line cannot be inserted, arterialised capillary samples from heelpricks can be used. This causes disturbance to the baby, which may alter the blood gas result, particularly the oxygen level. Results from capillary samples must be interpreted with care.

Principles of neonatal mechanical ventilation

If the baby's respiratory efforts are unable to maintain normal blood gases, some form of mechanical respiratory support is needed. The purpose of mechanical ventilation is to deliver oxygen to the alveoli in sufficient concentration to allow adequate transfer to the blood in the pulmonary capillaries, and, by increasing the amount of air displaced in expiration, to promote the removal of carbon dioxide which has accumulated in the alveoli. There are several makes of neonatal ventilators with different ways of functioning, but most rely on sophisticated electronic devices to provide rapid and precise control of the delivery of gases to the baby while allowing for the monitoring of all aspects of the machine's function. Until recently, all ventilators were designed so that the duration of inspiratory and expiratory air flow can be altered and maximum and minimum pressures set (Fig. 9.4). The volume of air delivered at each breath was determined by the settings chosen and the degree of compliance of the lungs. Newer devices, known as volume-guaranteed ventilators, deliver a specified volume of gas, varying the other parameters breath by breath to achieve this. Most machines allow for several different methods of ventilation, including intermittent mandatory and patient-triggered ventilation. Other modes enable varying degrees of synchronisation of mechanical breaths with the baby's own respiratory efforts, or simply produce a continuous positive airway pressure (CPAP) without pulses of positive pressure ventilation. Since different modes of ventilation may be needed at different times in a baby's treatment, the ventilator must be able to alter many functions independently without disturbing the infant too much. The methods of ventilation are constantly being evaluated and developed to improve outcomes and reduce risk. The most widely used are:

- CPAP
- intermittent mandatory (or positive pressure) ventilation (IMV; IPPV)
- high-frequency positive pressure ventilation (HFPPV)/patient-triggered ventilation (PTV)/synchronised intermittent mandatory ventilation (SIMV)
- high-frequency oscillatory ventilation (HFOV).

CPAP

CPAP provides a continual flow of gases to the baby's respiratory tract through close-fitting cannulae which are placed within the nasal airway (Fig. 9.5). A flow driver maintains a constant elevated pressure in the airway, which reduces the baby's work of breathing, prevents alveolar collapse and restores and maintains functional residual capacity. It is useful in cases of mild to moderate RDS and is usually given at pressures of +4–6 cmH$_2$O. In order to maintain these pressures, there must be a good seal between the prongs and the baby's nose (Goggin 2001). Appropriate-sized prongs and hats must be used

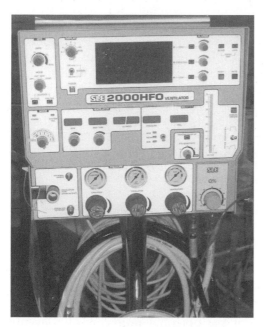

Figure 9.4   Neonatal ventilator including a breath pattern monitor.

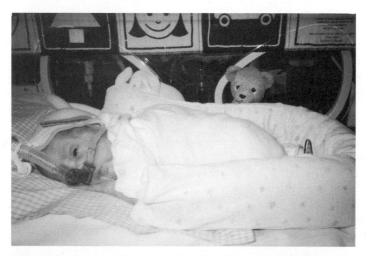

Figure 9.5   Nasal continuous positive airways pressure for mild respiratory distress syndrome. Note the flexed posture of the infant in the restraining nest.

and care must be taken to avoid excessive pressure on the baby's face or nostrils, which may cause skin breakdown. CPAP may also be used when weaning a baby off mechanical ventilation (p. 138). Studies are underway to assess whether CPAP combined with prophylactic surfactant as first-line management of RDS can reduce the number of babies with RDS requiring mechanical ventilation.

Intubation

When CPAP alone is not sufficient to maintain adequate respiration and acid–base balance, the baby will require endotracheal intubation and some form of mechanical ventilation (Greenough 1997). An endotracheal tube is passed through either the nose or mouth and fixed to prevent accidental displacement and to minimise laryngeal trauma. One method of fixation is to put the tube through a modified tracheostomy tube holder which is then tied to a close fitting bonnet (Fig. 9.6). The tube can be secured using sticky tape, but this method should be avoided if possible to prevent skin trauma. Some units have a policy of giving the baby an analgesic such as morphine prior to intubation as the procedure does cause the baby significant discomfort. The correct positioning of the tip of the endotracheal tube can be confirmed by listening for equal air entry in both lungs or by X-ray.

IMV/IPPV

Conventional ventilation involves automatic mechanical ventilation at a rate and pressure determined by the ventilator settings, irrespective of the baby's breathing efforts. The terms IMV and IPPV are used depending on the rate of breaths given, generally IMV being used when the rate is around 20 or below. In this method, a variable level of peak inspiratory pressure (PIP) is used to inflate the lungs and a positive end expiratory pressure (PEEP), which is equivalent to CPAP, is applied to prevent the alveoli from collapsing during the expiratory phase. Although neonatologists vary in their practices, the following figures give an indication of the range of settings commonly used at the start of ventilation:

- ventilator rate: 30–60/min
- PIP: 18–24 cmH_2O
- PEEP: 3–5 cmH_2O
- inspiration/expiration ratio: between 1:1 and 1:1.5
- oxygen concentration: 40%.

HFPPV

One of the potential problems of conventional ventilation is that the respiratory effort made by the baby may counteract the action of the ventilator. For example, the baby may attempt to breathe

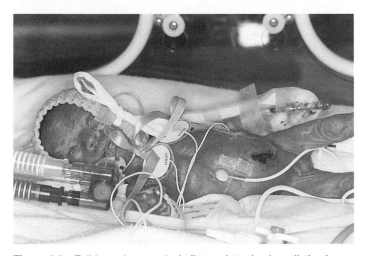

Figure 9.6 Full intensive care including endotracheal ventilation in a 25-week gestation preterm infant of 720 g birth weight.

out against a positive pressure inflation (active expiration). This may raise the intra-alveolar pressure and increase the risk of pneumothorax from alveolar rupture. By using fast inflation rates, up to 120 breaths per minute, it may be possible to synchronise the ventilator with the baby's breathing and reduce the risk of air leaks.

SIMV/PTV

Some neonatologists favour the use of the baby's own respiratory drive and rhythm to determine the rate of the ventilator, allowing the responses of the respiratory centre to modify the rate of breathing to keep the blood gases normal. The baby's own inspiratory effort is detected by the ventilator, which coordinates breaths with the baby's own respiration. In PTV, every spontaneous breath triggers the ventilator, whereas in SIMV, only a set number of positive breaths will be given. Studies suggest that PTV is less suitable for babies less than 28 weeks' gestation, compared with more mature babies. Recent evidence shows no advantage over conventional IPPV (Baumer 2000, Beresford et al 2000).

High-frequency oscillatory ventilation (HFOV)

This mode of ventilatory support has been used in some neonatal units in the UK for the last 5–10 years. It differs from conventional ventilation in that it provides active expiration as well as active inspiration. The technique involves delivering small tidal volumes at very fast frequencies against a constant mean airway pressure (MAP). The frequency is usually set at between 7 and 15 Hz (7 to 15 per second or 420 to 900 per minute). This creates a marked shake of the baby's chest, which may cause anxiety to the parents until an explanation is given. Oxygenation is controlled by the MAP and the inspired oxygen concentration. Elimination of carbon dioxide is controlled by the size of oscillations and their frequency. Typical settings which may be used at the start of oscillation are:

- MAP – 8 cmH$_2$O, or 2 cm higher than the MAP used during conventional ventilation
- Hz – 10

- Amplitude – 35 cm, or until an adequate 'shake' is achieved.

The settings required will vary depending on the oscillatory device used. A chest X-ray should be taken soon after starting HFOV to ensure that the lungs are not overdistended, as this may cause a reduced cardiac output. The high MAP recruits collapsed alveoli, increasing lung volume. An important nursing consideration is that the MAP will be lost if the ventilator circuit is disconnected. This will cause alveolar collapse, which may take some time to re-establish. The baby should be repositioned without being disconnected and endotracheal suction should be performed cautiously (p. 138). Generally, HFOV is used as a rescue therapy where conventional ventilation has failed. However, there is an increasing interest in using HFOV as first-line management of RDS (Hunt & Milner 1999). It is thought that HFOV causes less barotrauma to the lungs and studies are underway to determine whether it lowers the incidence of chronic lung disease.

Other methods of respiratory support

Certain babies who do not respond to these methods may benefit from inhaled nitric oxide (NO) therapy. It is not yet widely used in the UK. NO is a 'selective' pulmonary vasodilator and is of great value in the treatment of persistent pulmonary hypertension of the newborn but its role in RDS is not as yet established (Thomson & Vyas 1998, The Inhaled Nitric Oxide Study Group 2000).

Extracorporeal membrane oxygenation (ECMO) is a process in which blood is diverted from the body through a membrane oxygenator and back to the circulation again in a manner similar to bypass oxygenation circuits used in cardiac surgery. It is mainly used in very severe meconium aspiration pneumonia or when recovery of the lung disease can be reasonably expected in a short time (Davis and Shekerdemian 2001).

Management of a ventilated baby

The necessary monitoring and documentation has been previously described (p. 127). Providing optimal respiratory support can be a challenge to the neonatal team. The following guidelines are worth noting:

- Arterial oxygen saturation is largely maintained by the concentration of oxygen in the inspired gas, although areas of pulmonary atelectasis may also contribute to poor oxygenation. It can be improved by increasing the PIP, the PEEP and prolonging the inspiratory time on the ventilator settings.
- Carbon dioxide levels in the alveoli and therefore in the arterial blood are affected by the volume of gas exchanged each minute (the minute volume), which relates closely to the rate and pressure of the ventilator. Increasing the PIP or ventilator rate, or decreasing the PEEP, will improve carbon dioxide elimination.
- Keeping the inspiratory time to less than half of the respiratory cycle and limiting PIP reduces the risk of pneumothorax.
- Every ventilated baby must be monitored by frequent blood gas measurements and the ventilator settings altered accordingly.
- The air/oxygen mixture must be fully humidified and warmed to prevent drying of the bronchial tree and cooling of the infant.
- If the baby is fighting the ventilator, it can cause pulmonary hypertension and cyanosis from right-to-left shunting of blood. Opiate analgesia often counteracts this, but if it is not adequate, a paralysing agent, e.g. pancuronium, may be added. Careful attention must be made when positioning paralysed babies as they will not be able to move themselves out of an uncomfortable position. Artificial tears should be instilled regularly to prevent drying of the corneas.
- Removal of secretions by endotracheal tube suction can cause adverse effects, including increased blood pressure, bradycardia, hypoxia and mucosal trauma (Wallace 1998). The neonatal nurse should be aware of the hazards and assess the need for suction before performing it. A 'closed' suction system is available which does not disrupt ventilation and is beneficial to babies on HFOV.
- Decreased or unequal air entry, diminished chest movement and reduced chest 'shake' during HFOV are important indicators of complications of mechanical ventilation.
- All ventilated babies should have an orogastric tube in situ, left on free drainage, and aspirated every 4 hours. This is to reduce the risk of aspiration of gastric contents and to prevent gastric distension by air, which may limit movement of the diaphragm.

Complications of ventilator care

If the baby fails to respond to, or deteriorates during, ventilation, one or more of the following complications should be suspected and urgent treatment given if found:

- equipment failure – the ventilator and circuit should be checked for leaks
- displaced or blocked endotracheal tube – the position of the tube should be confirmed and suction given if necessary
- pneumothorax
- pulmonary interstitial emphysema
- intraventricular haemorrhage
- hypoglycaemia
- hypotension
- metabolic acidosis
- shunting through a patent ductus arteriosus
- persistent pulmonary hypertension.

Weaning off ventilation and extubation

As the baby's condition improves, the amount of ventilatory support needed will reduce. The plan for extubation must include stopping any sedation and loading the baby with caffeine as a respiratory stimulant before the tube is taken out.

It is thought that the PIP causes the most barotrauma and it is this parameter that should be reduced first. As ventilation is weaned, regular measurements of blood gases must be taken to assess tolerance of new settings. Practices will vary but, generally, when the ventilator is on low settings – for example, PIP 14 cmH$_2$O, rate of 15/min – and the inspired gas contains 30% oxygen or less, the baby can be extubated. A trial of CPAP alone through the endotracheal tube for up to an hour prior to extubation may be used, though immediate extubation is thought preferable. Where HFOV is used, it is possible to wean and extubate the baby without changing to conventional ventilation first. Intravenous dexamethasone is usually only needed if the baby has had repeated or prolonged intubation (Davis & Henderson-Smart 2001).

Timing of the extubation should be considered and necessary equipment and personnel must be on hand if the baby cannot maintain respiration without help. Most babies will be given a period on nasal CPAP after extubation, but some may cope with increased environmental oxygen alone. An arterial blood gas measurement should be made 1–2 hours after extubation to confirm the adequacy of spontaneous breathing. The baby's parents must be kept informed of these changes and advised of the possibility of reintubation.

Other complications of RDS

Other complications associated with RDS are outlined in Box 9.5.

Pulmonary air leaks

Pneumothorax, pneumomediastinum and pulmonary interstitial emphysema are caused by the leakage of air from the alveoli into the pleural space or the interstitium of the lung. They are particularly common where high inflation pressures have been required or the infant has been fighting the ventilator. Pneumothorax results in a partial collapse of the lung and, in more severe cases, the mediastinum is shifted across to the opposite side of the chest. Rapid deterioration of the infant, hypotension and cyanosis may occur, requiring urgent attention. In less severe cases, there may be an increase in oxygen requirements with associated reduction of breath sounds on one side and asymmetrical chest movement. The diagnosis can be made either by cold-light transillumination or by a chest X-ray (see Fig. 3.5, p. 42). A tension pneumothorax will often respond initially to the insertion of a sterile open needle into the affected pleural space, which allows the escape of the air, and reinflation of the lung, but it is usually necessary to insert an indwelling pleural drain connected to a one-way valve or underwater seal to prevent its recurrence until it is clear the air is not reaccumulating.

Technique of insertion of an indwelling pleural drain   After localisation of the pneumothorax, the baby is placed with the affected side uppermost and the arm fully abducted. The skin is sterilised with an antiseptic lotion and a point in the mid-axillary line in a suitable intercostal space infiltrated with 1% lidocaine (lignocaine). An incision of about 3–4 mm is made in the anaesthetised area and the pleural catheter bored gently between the ribs. Resistance to the pressure suddenly reduces as the pleural space is entered. The tip is then pointed towards the head and advanced until it reaches the apex of the pleural space. The trochar is withdrawn, the cannula attached to an underwater seal and the tube fastened in place with a purse-string suture, which also prevents air from leaking in, and taped to the skin.

Box 9.5   Common complications of respiratory distress syndrome

Early:
- Pneumothorax, pneumomediastinum
- Pulmonary interstitial emphysema
- Persistent pulmonary hypertension
- Necrotising enterocolitis
- Periventricular leucomalacia
- Intraventricular haemorrhage
- Patent ductus arteriosus
- Hyporegenerative anaemia

Later:
- Bronchopulmonary dysplasia
- Oxygen dependency
- Cerebral palsy and learning difficulties
- Retinopathy of prematurity
- Growth failure
- Repeated minor infections
- Rickets of prematurity
- Iron-deficiency anaemia

Circulatory problems

Persistent pulmonary hypertension of the newborn (PPHN)   The pulmonary vascular resistance remains labile in any baby with RDS and rises whenever the infant is disturbed. This results in increased resistance to blood flow through the pulmonary arteries and a rise in right ventricular and pulmonary artery pressure. If this pulmonary hypertension persists and the pressure rises above the aortic blood pressure, cyanosis results from shunting of deoxygenated blood from the pulmonary artery to the aorta through the ductus arteriosus. A similar shunt may occur through the foramen ovale from the right atrium to the left. Management of this condition depends on improving the effectiveness of the ventilation, increasing the concentration of the inspired oxygen, and infusion of plasma to correct the acidosis caused by systemic hypotension. Inhaled NO therapy (p. 137) is effective in the treatment of PPHN but the equipment required to administer it is not generally available and intravenous drug therapy is still in common use. Continuous infusions of tolazoline or epoprostenol, a prostaglandin drug, both potent vasodilators, may be used to dilate the pulmonary vessels and improve oxygenation. The drawback of these drugs is that they also cause systemic vasodilation, sometimes to an extent that infusions of inotropes (e.g. dopamine) are required to counteract it.

Hypotension A mean arterial blood pressure equivalent to the baby's gestational age in weeks can be regarded as a minimum value for preterm infants. Thus, for example, 30 mmHg is the lowest acceptable figure in a 30-week infant. Hypotension commonly occurs and often results from a low blood volume, which may be revealed by finding a low peripheral (toe) temperature compared with the central (rectal) temperature. The most accurate measurement of blood pressure is direct measurement through an umbilical arterial catheter and this is the preferred method in ventilated babies. Initial treatment is to restore circulatory volume with human albumin solution or normal saline but cardiac stimulant drugs may be needed if this is not sufficient.

Necrotising enterocolitis

The cause of this serious complication is still poorly understood, but established predisposing factors include the presence of umbilical catheters, sepsis and hypotension. Part of the gut becomes necrotic, allowing bowel organisms entry to the circulation, and it is often fatal. It occurs mostly in ventilated preterm infants who are fed on formula milk, but breast milk does not protect the infant completely. The baby appears pale and ill with bile-stained vomiting or gastric aspirate, rectal bleeding, loose stools and abdominal distension. An X-ray of the abdomen reveals distended loops of gut, sometimes with air in the bowel wall. Treatment is by stopping enteral feeding, performing frequent gastric aspiration and giving intravenous fluid and broad-spectrum antibiotics. If the baby fails to respond or perforation of the gut is confirmed by finding gas in the peritoneal cavity on an abdominal X-ray (Fig. 9.7), surgical resection of the affected bowel is required (Coit 1999, Badowicz & Latawiec-Mazurkiewicz 2000).

Infections

Infants undergoing intensive care are additionally very susceptible to infection (Ronnestad et al 1998) (p. 167) particularly when an endotracheal tube or intravascular catheters are in place. Coagulase-negative staphylococci (*Staphylococcus epidermidis*) and *Streptococcus viridans,* which are not pathogenic in the older child, frequently infect such tubes and the infection may become generalised. Intravenous antibiotics should be given to cover these organisms (p. 169). Other organisms commonly encountered include *Staph. aureus, Escherchia coli,* group B streptococci and anaerobic organisms. Infected intravenous catheters must be removed, as antibiotics alone cannot eradicate such infections. Parenteral nutrition is commonly complicated by bacterial or fungal (*Candida* spp.) septicaemia and may need to be interrupted until the infection is controlled.

Periventricular ischaemia and haemorrhage

Intracranial bleeding in babies with RDS is not an uncommon occurrence. Hypoxia and hypotension are two preventable contributing factors. The risk can also be reduced by preventing wide fluctuations of heart rate and blood pressure through gentle handling of the baby and minimising pain and discomfort. Certain drugs such as ethamsylate have been disappointing in trials and do not reduce the risk of haemorrhage or its consequences (Elborne et al 2001). Bleeding limited to the immediate periventricular germinal matrix region (grade 1) or confined to the ventricle (grade 2) usually has a good prognosis. Symptomatic haemorrhage associated with ventricular dilatation or extension of the bleed into the brain substance (grade 3) has a high chance of producing permanent brain damage (Fig. 9.8).

Periventricular leucomalacia (PVL) (Fig. 9.9), which results from ischaemic damage during episodes of perinatal hypotension, is more likely to be associated with later brain damage (p. 155) (Pierrat et al 2001). It is seen on the ultrasound scan as an area of echodensity around the lateral ventricles and, in the more advanced cases, cystic

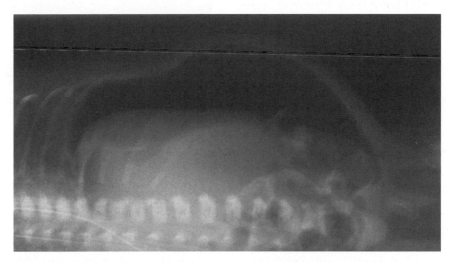

Figure 9.7 Peritoneal free gas confirming perforation of the gut in necrotising enterocolitis.

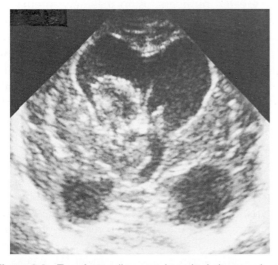

Figure 9.8 Transfontanelle coronal cerebral ultrasound scan showing intraventricular haemorrhage and ventricular dilatation. (By kind permission of Dr Stephen Chapman.)

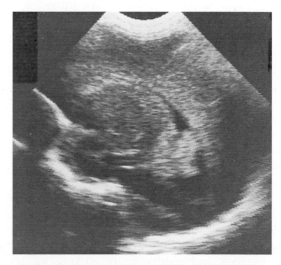

Figure 9.9 Periventricular leucomalacia. Parasagittal ultrasound scan shows increased periventricular echoes. (By kind permission of Dr Stephen Chapman.)

areas can develop, sometimes several weeks after birth. Repeated ultrasound scans performed through the anterior fontanelle can accurately show the extent of the lesions and follow their progress and are thus useful in assessing the outlook for the baby's subsequent development (p. 152). They are most predictive at the equivalent of 40 weeks' gestation. Mild PVL results in cerebral palsy in a third of cases, rising to 70% where the disease is more severe. If the ventricles are dilated by PVL, learning difficulties and cerebral palsy are likely, though these occur less frequently if the dilatation is caused only by haemorrhage. Because of the potentially serious implications of these findings, the baby's parents must be kept informed about the results and be made aware of the neurological problems which may follow.

Persistent ductus arteriosus

Delay in closure of the ductus arteriosus is common in preterm infants and often causes no symptoms, though it may make it difficult to wean a baby with hyaline membrane disease from a ventilator. As the pressure in the pulmonary artery slowly falls below the aortic pressure, blood flows from the aorta through the ductus into the pulmonary vessels, increasing the amount of blood in the pulmonary circulation. The lungs become stiffer, leading to increasing dyspnoea and CO_2 retention. The signs of an open ductus are a tachycardia and an audible systolic murmur in the second left intercostal space. Peripheral pulses are unusually prominent as a result of the high pulse pressure. A chest X-ray may show an enlarged heart and pulmonary plethora. Echocardiography can demonstrate the size of the ductus (Fig. 9.10) and Doppler colour flow mapping readily demonstrates blood flowing through it from the aorta to the pulmonary artery.

Diuretic treatment, for instance furosemide (frusemide), fluid restriction and alterations to management of ventilation may hasten functional closure of the ductus. If these measures are ineffective, indomethacin, 0.1–0.3 mg/kg body weight, given intravenously once daily for 6 days is often effective and can be repeated if the first

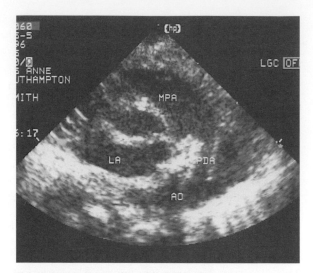

Figure 9.10 Short-axis parasternal echocardiogram showing a persistent ductus arteriosus (PDA) between the aorta (AO) and the main pulmonary artery (MPA) in a ventilated preterm infant. (By kind permission of Dr Elspeth Brown.)

course fails to close the duct. Very occasionally, surgical closure is needed.

Later complications and prognosis

Retinopathy of prematurity (retrolental fibroplasia)

As greater numbers of increasingly premature babies are now surviving, there has been an increase in the incidence of this disorder. It is a condition affecting the retinal blood vessels (Plate 14A & B). In the early stage, proliferative changes in the retinal vessels are seen, followed by haemorrhages and peripheral separation of the retina. Most cases do not progress beyond this stage and there is little effect on the child's eyesight. In a minority of more severe cases, the changes progress to fibrosis and opacity behind the lens, but treatment with cryotherapy can often halt the disease and prevent the progression to blindness. The condition is related to high arterial oxygen levels and is mostly seen in babies below 28 weeks of gestation. Examination of the retina of all preterm babies less than 1500 g birth weight or under 31 weeks of gestation should be carried out between 32 and 40 weeks, the age at which the condition appears, in order to allow timely intervention if it is needed. In general, it is unlikely to occur if the oxygen content of the inspired air is kept below 40%. However, this should not prevent the use of higher concentrations to correct the effect of respiratory insufficiency since it is high blood oxygen levels that cause the damage. Arterial blood oxygen levels (PaO_2) should be carefully monitored to prevent a rise above 10 kPa (80 mmHg). Oxygen saturation monitoring is less effective in keeping the blood oxygen at safe levels (Tin et al 2001).

Chronic lung disease (CLD; chronic pulmonary insufficiency of prematurity [CPIP], or bronchopulmonary dysplasia [BPD])

This condition, which is known by several names, is the progressive destruction of lung tissue and subsequent fibrosis which follows mechanical ventilation in RDS. Many survivors go on to develop CLD which is probably due to persistent inflammation within the lungs. This may be related to intrauterine exposure to chorioamnionitis but high oxygen levels in the alveoli are also thought to trigger the inflammatory process. Barotrauma from positive pressure ventilation seems to play a part but CLD can occur after only a brief period of ventilation. Once the disease is established, a long period of dependence on supplementary oxygen usually follows. More encouragingly, since the introduction of surfactant therapy and new methods of ventilation, the incidence of CLD has fallen (Manktelow et al 2001).

The disorder should be suspected when there is difficulty in weaning a baby off the ventilator and X-rays show progressive widespread lung opacities with patchy translucent areas (Fig. 9.11), followed later by fibrous scarring. Treatment consists in reducing the peak pressure of ventilation while maintaining some PEEP, and measures to close a persistent ductus arteriosus if needed. A course of dexamethasone for established disease may enable earlier extubation and reduce the severity of CLD and the need for long-term oxygen supplements, but the complications of steroids – such as hyperglycaemia, glycosuria and hypertension – occur commonly (Halliday & Ehrenkranz 2001a). Current evidence suggests

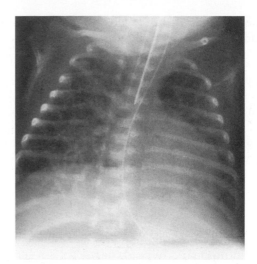

Figure 9.11 Chest X-ray in chronic lung disease (bronchopulmonary dysplasia) following respiratory distress syndrome. Bilateral patchy shadows are interspersed with areas of hyperinflated lung.

that inhaled steroids are ineffective in this situation (Shah et al 2000). The benefits of steroids in the early stages of the disease do not outweigh the risks and are not recommended (Halliday & Ehrenkranz 2001b). Almost complete recovery of lung function can occur but takes several months. However, there is a much higher incidence of sudden infant death syndrome in the first year of life and the infants have an increased susceptibility to respiratory infections. Bronchiolitis, caused by the respiratory syncitial virus (RSV), can be much more serious in babies with CLD, who may need to be ventilated again.

Handicap following RDS

Neurological handicap occurs in less than 10% of survivors of RDS (International Neonatal Network 2000). It occurs largely, though not exclusively, in those in whom periventricular leucomalacia or intracerebral bleeding or ventricular dilatation is seen on ultrasound scans and in babies who have fits or signs of severe cerebral irritability (p. 152). Ventilation for RDS alone and without complications does not cause persisting neurological handicap, and the appropriate use of surfactant and steroids does not affect the risk.

SURGICAL PROBLEMS AND INTENSIVE CARE

Some of the more serious congenital malformations require urgent neonatal surgery. Intensive care is necessary for many, especially when they are born prematurely or are of low birth weight. The complex problems associated with most of these cases make it imperative that only a paediatric surgical team experienced with neonates should undertake this work. Special techniques in radiology, anaesthetics and laboratory back-up are often required.

Respiratory support in the form of assisted ventilation is frequently needed – for example, in the case of diaphragmatic hernia with its associated pulmonary hypoplasia. After surgery for gastroschisis, exomphalos and gut atresia, there is often respiratory difficulty, and a prolonged period of parenteral nutrition may have to follow. The surgery of congenital heart disease is another field in which intensive care facilities and specialised medical support are mandatory.

SOME WIDER IMPLICATIONS OF NEONATAL INTENSIVE CARE
Pain control

It has been thought that newborn infants do not suffer pain, discomfort and distress, but it is clear, both from observational studies and from investigation of metabolic responses in stressful situations in preterm infants, that they do (Sparshott 1998). Many procedures used during intensive care are painful, and preventing or relieving such discomfort should be a high priority. The following methods can be recommended for painful procedures:

- Using a spring-loaded mechanical lancet considerably reduces the pain of heelpricks.
- Giving the baby oral sucrose before painful procedures seems to have an analgesic effect (Stevens & Ohlsson 2001).
- Lidocaine (lignocaine) 1% should be infiltrated into the skin and subcutaneous tissues before chest drain insertion.
- Gentle massage significantly reduces stress reactions in preterm infants.
- Use opiates for analgesia prior to intubation.

Oral or injected analgesics can be used for more prolonged pain relief and control. Paracetamol 15 mg/kg may be given up to 4 times a day, either orally or rectally, for moderate pain. Opiates are widely used to relieve the distress of endotracheal ventilation. Morphine is given as a loading dose of 50–100 μg/kg over 30 minutes followed by a continuous intravenous infusion of between 10 and 30 μg/kg/hour. The equivalent doses of intravenous diamorphine are 50 μg/kg over 30 minutes followed by 15 μg/kg/hour.

Respiratory depression from an acute overdose of opiates can be reversed by giving intravenous naloxone 30 μg/kg, but if they have been used over a prolonged period, naloxone may cause a severe withdrawal reaction (p. 18) and should not be given. Doses should be slowly decreased over several days.

The application of amethocaine local anaesthetic gel has some beneficial effect in the preterm newborn in reducing the pain of venepuncture and other procedures, though it is certainly less effective than in older children (Jain and Griffin 2000).

Emotional care

The provision of intensive neonatal care can generate much emotional tension for parents and for caring staff. Physical stress during exceptionally busy periods and emergencies also takes its toll. Those who organise intensive neonatal care should take this into account and be ready to understand why staffing levels and standards of training have to be very high for it to succeed. It is not enough that medical and nursing staff should be efficient technicians. The baby's survival is initially paramount but the needs of the parents and family should also be part of the treatment plan, since the nature of the hospital care will affect their attitude to the baby. Quite apart from the possible physical sequelae, the incidence of emotional family problems such as non-accidental injury and over-anxiety leading to frequent hospital admissions and behaviour disturbance is known to be increased.

The involvement of the family in the child's care should be recognised as being vitally important from the start. Ideally, the involvement of the parents should start before their baby is born. If a premature delivery is anticipated, the paediatrician should explain in outline what problems the baby might face and the care he may require. If possible, a visit to the unit will help to prepare the parents for the intense environment. If a visit is not possible, a booklet or photograph album showing pictures of small babies and pieces of equipment in common use should alleviate some of their anxieties.

On admission to the neonatal unit, an instant photograph should be taken of the baby and given to the mother. If the baby has been delivered by caesarean section, this may be the mother's first contact with her new baby and it is often a great comfort until she is well enough to visit. The parents should be given an explanation of all aspects of the baby's condition and the care, provided in language they can understand, by an experienced member of the unit staff, especially when changes in treatment or big decisions are to be made. They should be encouraged to have as much physical contact with their baby as is compatible with the infant's condition (Fig. 9.12). At first, this may only amount to touching the baby in the incubator (p. 114), but later, as they gain confidence, they can be involved with other aspects of care such as mouth and nappy care and gastric tube feeding.

'Kangaroo care'

The parents desire to touch and cuddle their baby is very strong but they will assume that their tiny baby, surrounded by tubing, must remain in the safe confines of the incubator. However, it is often possible for these babies – provided their condition allows – to have close physical contact with the parents. This skin-to-skin or kangaroo care involves placing the baby prone on the bare chest of the mother or father inside their clothing (Fig. 9.13). Research suggests its benefits include enhanced parental bonding, improved weight gain and earlier discharge (Bohnhorst et al 2001, Furman & Kennell 2000). Even intubated babies can sometimes be safely held in this way, provided their condition is sufficiently stable and adequate nursing supervision is available.

The needs of other children in the family should be remembered. Ideally, a supervised play area should be available to occupy younger children. Most units have a policy of open visiting and accommodation for parents of seriously ill babies, those with transport difficulties or for discharge preparation. Making the intensive care unit look more appealing by means of a friendly décor is desirable, but understanding and responding to the needs of the family is of much greater importance.

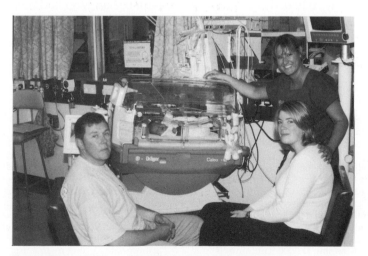

Figure 9.12 Making prolonged intensive care more friendly.

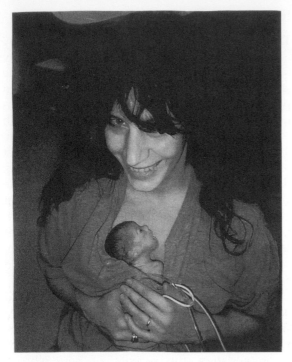

Figure 9.13 'Kangaroo care' of a very preterm infant.

Dying babies (see also p. 244)

The death of a baby undergoing intensive care is not a rare event and giving effective help to parents at this time and afterwards is another heavy responsibility for medical and nursing staff to carry, particularly when a decision to withdraw treatment has been made (Doyal & Larcher 2000). Occasionally, a dying baby will be a suitable organ donor and this will need sensitive discussion with the parents. The opportunity also should be given for the expression of grief and fulfilment of any religious or ceremonial custom that may be important to the particular family.

Often, and particularly when the baby has been involved in a clinical trial, a postmortem examination will be requested. This will involve the temporary removal of internal organs from the body for close visual inspection and to take small samples of relevant tissues for histological assessment. This should be explained to the parents by a doctor with an understanding of the information that may be obtained. If organs or significant amounts of tissue are to be retained for research or for additional analysis, this too should be explained. Some parents may find this final examination too hard to bear and in many cases these feelings should be respected. If they so wish, the parents should be offered a date to return for a discussion about:

- the cause of the baby's death
- the results of the autopsy (if performed)
- the baby's illness
- any questions the parents may have
- any implications there may be for the future.

This discussion should be carried out in an unhurried and sympathetic way by the senior paediatrician who had responsibility for the care given to the baby.

REFERENCES

Badowicz B, Latawiec-Mazurkiewicz I 2000 Necrotising enterocolitis (NEC) – methods of treatment and outcome: a comparative analysis of Scottish (Glasgow) and Polish (Western Pomerania) cases. European Journal of Pediatric Surgery 10(3):177–181

Barrington K J 2000 Umbilical catheters in the newborn: effects of position of the catheter tip. Cochrane Database of Systematic Reviews (2):CD000505

Baumer J H 2000 International randomised controlled trial of patient triggered ventilation in neonatal respiratory distress syndrome. Archives of Disease in Childhood Fetal and Neonatal Edition 82:F5–F10

Beresford M W, Shaw N J, Manning D 2000 Randomised controlled trial of patient triggered and conventional fast rate ventilation in neonatal respiratory distress syndrome. Archives of Disease in Childhood Fetal and Neonatal Edition 82:F14–F18

Bohnhorst B, Heyne T, Peter C S et al 2001 Skin-to-skin (kangaroo) care, respiratory control, and thermoregulation. Journal of Pediatrics 138(2):193–197

Brocklehurst P, Gates S, McKenzie-McHarg K et al 1999 Are we prescribing multiple courses of antenatal corticosteroids? A survey of practice in the UK. British Journal of Obstetrics and Gynaecology 106:977–979

Chant T 1998 Oro and nasogastric feeding techniques for very low birthweight infants: selecting an appropriate feeding regime. Journal of Neonatal Nursing 5(1):23–25

Coit A K 1999 Necrotising enterocolitis. Journal of Perinatal and Neonatal Nursing 129(4):53–66

Davis P G, Henderson-Smart D J 2001 Intravenous dexamethasone for extubation of newborn infants (Cochrane Review). Cochrane Database of Systematic Reviews 4:CD000308

Davis P J, Shekerdemian L S 2001 Meconium aspiration syndrome and extracorporeal membrane oxygenation. Archives of Disease in Childhood Fetal and Neonatal Edition 84:F1–F3

Doyal L, Larcher V F 2000 Drafting guidelines for the withdrawal or withholding of life sustaining treatment in critically ill children and neonates. Archives of Disease in Childhood Fetal and Neonatal Edition 83:F60–F63

Elbourne D, Ayers S, Dellagrammaticas H et al 2001 Randomised controlled trial of prophylactic ethamsylate: follow up at 2 years of age. Archives of Disease in Childhood Fetal and Neonatal Edition 84(3):F183–F187

Furman L, Kennell J 2000 Breast milk and skin to skin kangaroo care for premature infants. Avoiding bonding failure. Acta Paediatrica 89(1):1280–1283

Goggin M 2001 Developments in Ncpap fixation. Journal of Neonatal Nursing 7(2):centre insert

Greenough 1997 Ventilation in the NICU. Journal of Neonatal Nursing 3(2):centre insert

Halliday H 1997 Surfactant therapy: questions and answers. Journal of Neonatal Nursing 3(3):28–36

Halliday H, Ehrenkranz R A 2001(a) Early postnatal (<96 hours) corticosteroids for preventing chronic lung disease in preterm infants. Cochrane Database of Systematic Reviews 2:CD0001146

Halliday H, Ehrenkranz R A 2001(b) Delayed (>3 weeks) postnatal corticosteroids for chronic lung disease in preterm infants (Cochrane Review). Cochrane Database of Systematic Reviews 2:CD001145

Hunt A, Milner A D 1999 High frequency oscillation. Journal of Neonatal Nursing 5(3):centre insert

International Neonatal Network 2000 Risk adjusted and population based studies on the outcome for high risk infants in Scotland and Australia. Archives of Disease in Childhood Fetal and Neonatal Edition 82:F118–F123

Jain A, Griffin N 2000 Does topical amethocaine gel reduce the pain of venepuncture in newborn infants? A randomised controlled trial. Archives of Disease in Childhood Fetal and Neonatal Edition 83:F207–F210

King C 1998 Enteral feeds for preterm infants: nutrition and therapy. Journal of Neonatal Nursing 4(5):6–10

Lal M, Kotecha S 2000 Surfactant therapy. Journal of Neonatal Nursing 6(2):centre insert

Manktelow B N, Draper E S, Annamalai S et al 2001 Factors affecting the incidence of chronic lung disease of prematurity in 1987, 1992, and 1997. Archives of Disease in Childhood Fetal and Neonatal Edition 84:F33–F35

McClure R J, Newell S J 2000 Randomised controlled trial of clinical outcome following trophic feeding. Archives of Disease in Childhood Fetal and Neonatal Edition 82:F29–F33

Pierrat V, Duquennoy C, van Haastert I C et al 2001 Ultrasound diagnosis and neurodevelopmental outcome of localised and extensive cystic periventricular leucomalacia. Archives of Disease in Childhood Fetal and Neonatal Edition 84:F151–F156

Reece A, Uhbi T, Craig A R et al 2001 Positioning of long lines: contrast versus plain radiography. Archives of Disease in Childhood Fetal and Neonatal Edition 84:F129–F131

Ronnestad A, Abrahamsen T G, Gaustad P et al 1998 Blood culture isolates during 6 years in a tertiary neonatal intensive care unit. Scandinavian Journal of Infectious Disease 30(3):245–251

Shah V, Ohlsson A, Halliday H L et al 2000 Early administration of inhaled corticosteroids for preventing chronic lung disease in ventilated very low birth weight preterm neonates. Cochrane Database of Systematic Reviews (2):CD001969

Soll R F, Morley C J 2000 Multiple versus single dose natural surfactant extract for severe neonatal respiratory distress syndrome. Cochrane Database of Systematic Reviews (2): CD000141

Sparshott M 1998 Pain and the fetus: the case for analgesia during invasive procedures. Journal of Neonatal Nursing 4(4):21–23

Stevens B, Yamada J, Ohlsson A 2001 Sucrose for analgesia in newborn infants undergoing painful procedures (Cochrane Review). Cochrane Database of Systematic Reviews 4:CD001069

The Inhaled Nitric Oxide Study Group 2000 Inhaled nitric oxide in term and near term infants: neurodevelopmental follow up of the Neonatal Inhaled Nitric Oxide Study Group (NINOS). Journal of Pediatrics 136:611–617

Thomson S, Vyas J 1998 Is NO good news? Update on the efficacy of inhaled nitric oxide. Journal of Neonatal Nursing 4(3):23–27

Tin W, Milligan D W A, Pennefather P et al 2001 Pulse oximetry, severe retinopathy and outcome at 1 year in babies of less than 28 weeks gestation. Archives of Disease in Childhood Fetal and Neonatal Edition 84:F106–F110

Wallace J L 1998 Suctioning: a two edged sword. Reducing the theory–practice gap. Journal of Neonatal Nursing 4(6):12–17

USEFUL WEBSITES

www.pedinfo.org – Pedinfo, an access database to many other websites in all aspects of neonatal care

www.rcpch.ac.uk – Royal College of Paediatrics and Child Health

Chapter 10
Neurological disorders

CHAPTER CONTENTS

Introduction   149
Physical injury to the head at birth   149
Intracranial haemorrhage   150
Encephalopathy in the newborn baby   150
   Origins of birth asyphxia   151
   Clinical features of cerebral injury   151
   Investigation in cerebral injury   152
   Management of hypoxic-ischaemic
   encephalopathy   154
   Prognosis of cerebral injury   155
   Physiotherapy   155
Neonatal fits   155
   Diagnosis   156
   Management of fits   157
   Pertussis immunisation following
   neurological illness   157
   Prognosis of neonatal fits   158
Hypotonia – the floppy infant   158
   Generalised hypotonia   158
   Spinal injury   159
Nerve injuries   159
   Brachial plexus injuries   159
   Facial nerve palsy   160

INTRODUCTION

There are many ways in which a baby's future development can be impaired through damage to the brain or nervous system. In some cases, congenital disorders, either structural or metabolic (p. 212), are responsible. It may result from complications of prematurity (p. 143) or an accident or illness after birth. This chapter describes the range of neurological disorders occurring around the time of birth, how they present, how they are best investigated and managed, and the likely outcomes. It is important for all involved in the care of newborn babies to be able to distinguish those conditions with a good prognosis from those likely to result in handicapping disability. With such information, sound guidance can be given to the parents about the future for their baby.

PHYSICAL INJURY TO THE HEAD AT BIRTH

Superficial abrasions and bruising are common and almost all are benign. Head moulding during normal birth, scalp contusion resulting from forceps delivery, the bruising or subaponeurotic haemorrhage associated with vacuum extraction and cephalhaematoma (p. 63) are only rarely associated with intracranial pathology. Occasionally, a difficult forceps delivery will result in a linear skull fracture where the blades are applied, but it is rarely diagnosed without an X-ray and is only infrequently associated with underlying brain injury. A depressed skull fracture is less common still, and even then, surgical treatment is rarely needed and full recovery is the rule.

INTRACRANIAL HAEMORRHAGE

Intracranial bleeding is not uncommon and has several causes. Haemorrhage can follow marked deformation of the skull from compression of the head or the sudden re-expansion after rapid delivery of the head. This may cause bleeding either into the cerebrospinal fluid (CSF) in the subarachnoid space from ruptured veins communicating with the sagittal sinus, or into the subdural space from a tear of the sinuses in the edge of the tentorium or falx or from rupture of the small veins which bridge the subdural space. More commonly, bleeding results from perinatal asphyxia, is a complication of hyaline membrane disease in the preterm infant (p. 141) or is associated with a disorder of the blood clotting mechanisms. In all cases, blood clotting factors should be measured and restored appropriately (p. 186).

Subdural haemorrhage is best confirmed by computerised tomography (CT) or magnetic resonance imaging (MRI) scanning, as it is often located over the surface of the cerebral hemispheres (p. 153). Surgical removal of subdural blood may be required to reduce the pressure on the brain, though the skull and fontanelle will normally expand to accommodate the blood clot. Occasionally, tubes may need to be inserted surgically to drain the liquefying blood from the intracranial cavity.

Intraventricular haemorrhage into the lateral ventricles of the brain arises most commonly after birth in preterm babies as a complication of severe respiratory distress syndrome. There may be extension of the bleed into the brain substance in more severe cases, which often results in a poor neurological outcome for the baby (p. 141).

Subarachnoid haemorrhage may cause acute cerebral symptoms and often a full fontanelle from raised intracranial pressure. The diagnosis is confirmed by finding blood in the CSF taken at lumbar puncture. Sometimes the blood will impair the reabsorption of the CSF by the arachnoid granulations and external hyrocephalus will result, requiring insertion of a pressure-relieving valve and tube system to drain the excess fluid into the peritoneum (p. 232).

ENCEPHALOPATHY IN THE NEWBORN BABY

The clinical symptoms which result from disordered brain function are known as encephalopathy and have many causes. They occur in 4 babies in every 1000 born and in 9% of these the underlying damage is serious enough to cause the death of the infant. The brain injury may occur before, during or after birth and in the majority of cases asphyxia plays a large part in its aetiology. Often other factors operating before or during the pregnancy will have made the baby's brain more vulnerable to the effects of hypoxia and these are listed in Box 10.1.

The greatest risk is in those who have suffered intrauterine growth retardation from placental insufficiency or who are postmature. Though it is often not clear precisely why a particular baby has symptoms of an encephalopathy, several mechanisms have been identified which predispose the baby to them. It seems likely that one or

---

Box 10.1 Factors increasing the risk of newborn encephalopathy

Before conception
- Social deprivation
- Unemployment
- Unskilled work
- Family history of neurological disability or epilepsy
- Treatment for infertility

During pregnancy
- Maternal thyroid disease
- Severe pre-eclampsia
- Moderate or severe bleeding during the pregnancy
- Viral infection requiring medical attention
- Abnormal placenta
- Late or no antenatal care
- Abnormal cardiotochograph recording

Factors relating to the baby
- Low birth weight for dates
- Weight below the 3rd percentile
- Intrauterine growth retardation
- Birth beyond 41 weeks' gestation
- Male sex
- Presence of congenital malformation

more of the following mechanisms are involved in causing neonatal encephalopathy:

- cerebral hypoxia from placental insufficiency
- ischaemia from reduced cerebral blood flow
- circulating inflammatory mediators
- hyperthermia from viral infection or reduced placental blood flow
- teratogenic effect of maternal viral infection.

Similar antecedents have also been found in children with cerebral palsy and epilepsy, even if neonatal encephalopathy was not recognised.

Unless they have caused diminished placental function, maternal smoking and excess alcohol consumption do not appear to increase the baby's risk.

In all these circumstances, there is a risk of the baby suffering from cerebral palsy, learning difficulties, hearing loss or cerebral sight impairment. Identification of at-risk babies during pregnancy may provide the opportunity for earlier delivery, to minimise the impact of the fetal hypoxia, but since the baby's oxygen requirements rise substantially at birth, ongoing hypoxia after delivery can significantly worsen its impact on the brain. It is therefore important to have an experienced paediatrician at every delivery where antenatal or intrapartum asphyxia is thought likely, to minimise its impact by prompt and effective resuscitation of the baby.

Origins of birth asphyxia

Even during normal labour, each uterine contraction reduces placental blood flow, resulting in temporary fetal hypoxia. So long as placental function is normal, this does no harm, since oxygenation resumes as the contraction ceases. If, however, the fetus has suffered prolonged mild asphyxia and malnutrition in utero as a result of placental insufficiency, then the risk of cerebral damage from these repeated bouts of hypoxia is increased. Identification of poor fetal growth is sometimes possible by repeated ultrasound examinations, and in such babies, prenatal Doppler ultrasound studies of the fetal arterial blood flow patterns can identify some infants with poor cardiac output and therefore reduced cerebral blood

flow. Often, however, such tests have not been indicated earlier and it is only by being aware that a predisposing condition is present that intrapartum asphyxia can be anticipated. The asphyxiated baby can often, but not always, be identified during labour by characteristic abnormal patterns of heart rate on the fetal cardiotocograph recording (p. 34).

Clinical features of cerebral injury

It is not always possible to predict from the baby's condition immediately after birth – e.g. as shown by the Apgar score – whether signs of cerebral injury will develop. Most infants with low scores at birth will show no permanent abnormal cerebral sequelae, whilst some who initially seem in good condition develop signs of brain dysfunction. The clinical features which follow significant asphyxia are known as hypoxic-ischaemic encephalopathy.

Mild hypoxic-ischaemic encephalopathy

In most cases when the asphyxial insult to the baby has been mild, a recognisable pattern of symptoms known as cerebral irritation emerges. In this condition, the baby will lie quietly most of the time but minor disturbances result in excessive jittery muscular activity. There may also be a shrill high-pitched persistent cry which is recognisably different from the normal cry of a hungry baby. Often there is abnormal wakefulness, the eyes remaining constantly open with an anxious or frowning expression. Rapid eye and tongue movements may occur and short myoclonic twitching movements are sometimes seen. Head retraction and hyperextension of the limbs is a less common feature. Occasionally, rhythmical alternating extension and flexion of the limbs may occur, resembling bicycling or boxing movements. These movements are readily distinguishable from fits because they persist for long periods whereas fitting movements are less complicated and usually brief. Where there is any doubt, an electroencephalogram (EEG) recording may help.

More severe asphyxia results in reduced responsiveness, depressed respiration abnormalities

---

Box 10.2 Clinical features of significant neonatal encephalopathy

Moderate
- Seizures alone
- Abnormal consciousness
- Difficulty maintaining respiration (central)
- Difficulty feeding of central origin
- Hypertonia
- Hypotonia
- Abnormal reflexes

Severe
- Central respiratory depression requiring ventilatory support
- Seizures requiring repeated anticonvulsant treatment
- Coma
- Such disordered cerebral function that death results

---

of muscle tone, difficulty with feeding and, sometimes, brief fits. Occasionally, seizures are the only indication of cerebral asphyxial insult (Box 10.2).

Severe hypoxic-ischaemic encephalopathy

After more profound asphyxia, the baby has a diminished level of consciousness, and respiration may be depressed or periodic from birth. Repeated seizures may occur and these may be clonic (repeated rhythmical jerking), myoclonic (single sudden major jerks) or tonic (e.g. stiffness of a limb) (p. 156). There is usually profound hypotonia (see Fig. 10.3) and immobility, which may last from a few hours to several days and results from brain stem dysfunction. The infant is unresponsive to handling and most reflex responses are lost. An inability to suck, low body temperature, vomiting, abnormal crying and cyanotic attacks are also features of more severe cerebral dysfunction. A tense or bulging fontanelle is common and reflects raised intracranial pressure, but papilloedema is rarely seen.

Over the next 24 hours, a period of cerebral irritability occurs, with increased extensor tone causing back arching, which results from rising intracranial pressure associated with cerebral oedema. The head is retracted, the trunk and limbs tend to extend, and reflex responses are brisk. The asymmetric tonic neck response (p. 74) is consistently obtainable and may be initiated through spontaneous movements of the body. This exaggerated extension posture makes feeding difficult and, because the baby arches away from the mother, development of the normal emotional attachment between them may be impaired. The symptoms gradually subside and there is a slow return to a more normal pattern of behaviour unless the cerebral injury has resulted in permanent damage.

Investigation in cerebral injury

An increasing number of techniques can now be applied to the investigation of cerebral conditions. In cerebral injury from trauma or hypoxic-ischaemic encephalopathy, these can give useful information for the management of the infant but they have only limited value in predicting whether a baby will have a long-term neurological handicap or its type.

Cerebral ultrasound examination or CT or MRI scanning can distinguish between intracranial haemorrhage, cerebral oedema and cerebral infarction (Blankenberg et al 2000, Marret et al 2001). A lumbar puncture seldom clarifies the diagnosis and should be avoided unless meningitis or subarachnoid haemorrhage is suspected.

Ultrasound

Ultrasound scanning through the open anterior fontanelle can identify haemorrhagic lesions in the periventricular white matter and intraventricular haemorrhage. It can also reveal localised and generalised areas of ischaemic damage in the brain substance, but it is often not possible to find subdural haemorrhage over the surface of the brain with this technique. Its great virtue is that it can be carried out in the infant's cot or incubator, involves no radiation, does not require the baby to be sedated or anaesthetised and frequently it alone provides the information necessary for correct treatment and for assessing the prognosis. Scans can be performed from day 3 and it is often by following the changes in the images obtained at weekly intervals that the real nature and extent of the pathology becomes evident and its prognostic significance clear.

CT and MRI scanning

Computerised tomography (CT) and *magnetic resonance imaging* (MRI) require the baby to be motionless for around 20 minutes and for this an anaesthetic is often needed. Both can show more accurately than ultrasound the distribution of hypoxic-ischaemic changes in the brain parenchyma (Fig. 10.1), particularly the more diffuse lesions which are associated with a higher

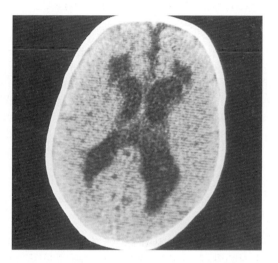

Figure 10.1 Cerebral oedema and ventricular dilatation in hypoxic-ischaemic encephalopathy demonstrated by CT scan.

incidence of permanent brain damage (Martin & Barkovich 1995). They can also visualise the subdural space, which is often difficult to locate with ultrasound. MRI can, in addition, reveal recent infarcts in the brain and is superior to other techniques in examination of the spinal cord.

As the results of these scans will only occasionally affect the immediate management of the infant, they are not usually appropriate until the baby is stable enough for transfer to the imaging department and for receiving an anaesthetic.

Electroencephalography

The standard EEG pattern has limited value in the neonate, though continuous recordings may have more prognostic significance (Connell et al 1989). It can confirm that abnormal movements are fits if they are associated with epileptic features on the recording. In severe cerebral injury, a pattern of low-voltage activity with bursts of high-voltage sharp waves, known as burst suppression (Fig. 10.2), indicates a poor prognosis with residual brain damage. If repeated recordings are made, the more rapidly any abnormalities resolve, the better the prospects for full recovery of the infant. A normal EEG pattern in a baby with cerebral symptoms is often an indication of a favourable prognosis (Pressler et al 2001).

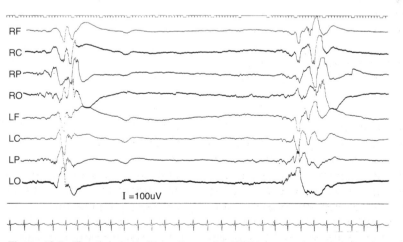

Figure 10.2 'Burst-suppression' pattern on an EEG in severe hypoxic-ischaemic encephalopathy – an indication of a poor prognosis for later cerebral function. (With kind permission of Dr Christian Wulff.)

Cerebral blood flow

Cerebral blood flow measurements using Doppler ultrasound techniques can give some indication of the adequacy of perfusion of the brain but the usefulness of this investigation remains uncertain at present.

Management of hypoxic-ischaemic encephalopathy

Mild hypoxic-ischaemic encephalopathy

The most important aspect of management is prevention. Monitoring of the fetal heart rate changes during labour (p. 34), particularly where fetal growth retardation has been identified, will identify many, but not all, asphyxiated infants. Delivery by emergency caesarean section may be required if an unfavourable pattern occurs.

It is difficult to tell initially how severe the consequences of asphyxia will be and affected babies dislike being handled or disturbed. All infants with early cerebral symptoms should therefore be nursed in quiet surroundings with subdued lighting in an incubator to maintain body temperature and for close observation of vital signs. The baby should be handled only as much as is needed for essential observations, feeding and changing the nappy, but the parents should be encouraged to help with the baby's nursing care. The blood glucose level should be maintained by small frequent feeds, if necessary by nasogastric tube. Temporary sedation may be needed if the baby is distressed and, provided the baby does not vomit, chloral hydrate 30 mg 6-hourly may be given to a term infant while restlessness persists. Normal oxygen saturation levels should be maintained by transcutaneous monitoring, since both too much and too little oxygen can cause additional damage.

Severe hypoxic-ischaemic encephalopathy

The management of severe hypoxic-ischaemic encephalopathy is outlined in Box 10.3. As cardiac function is often compromised by severe hypoxia, and CO_2 retention from hypoventilation may cause a further rise in intracranial pressure,

---

Box 10.3 Management of severe hypoxic-ischaemic encephalopathy

- Avoid unnecessary disturbance
- Prevent hypoxia and hyperoxia
- Prevent hypercapnia
- Maintain normal blood pressure
- Maintain normal blood glucose level
- Control seizures
- Restrict fluids
- Monitor fluid and electrolyte balance

---

regular blood gas analysis is essential to assess whether assisted ventilation will be needed and to ensure normal blood gas values are maintained. The blood pressure should be monitored closely and hypotension treated by increasing the blood volume with transfusions of human albumin solution. The blood glucose values should be kept in the range 4–5.5 mmol/L (75–100 mg/dL) with intravenous 10% glucose infusions since both hypoglycaemia and hyperglycaemia can accentuate existing brain injury.

If seizures occur, they should be treated with intramuscular phenobarbital followed by daily oral maintenance doses (p. 157), since persistent fits can reduce cerebral blood flow and exhaust brain glucose even in the presence of normal blood glucose levels. (See also page 157 for a fuller discussion of the treatment of neonatal fits.)

Fluid intake should be restricted to minimal maintenance levels with close monitoring of the electrolytes and osmolality of both blood and urine. This prevents fluid overload and electrolyte imbalance, both of which frequently occur. Measurement of urine output and urinalysis will assist in maintaining fluid balance, especially if hypotension has impaired renal function.

There is little evidence to support the use of steroids or hyperosmolar solutions to reduce intracranial pressure, though their occasional use in severe cerebral oedema may be justified.

Chronic subdural haematoma is a rare sequel which develops over several months and causes vomiting, failure to thrive, fits and enlargement of the head. It can be treated by repeated subdural taps if strict attention is paid to aseptic technique.

Research using magnetic resonance spectroscopy has shown some of the biochemical changes which occur in the brain cells as a result of asphyxia, and studies are underway to assess whether keeping the infant mildly hypothermic (Wagner et al 1999) or the use of drugs such as magnesium sulphate or allopurinol can protect the brain and reduce the risks of long-term damage (Volpe 2001).

Prognosis of cerebral injury

Infants who have shown signs of what is thought to be traumatic cerebral injury and who survive the neonatal period only exceptionally have permanent damage. Neurological disability only occurs in approximately 1 in 10 severely affected babies treated with the intensive management described above. Such disabilities range from a specific learning difficulty with clumsiness of movement and poor attention span to more serious forms of cerebral palsy, epilepsy or mental retardation. The great majority of more mildly affected babies fully recover without sequelae.

Cerebral injury from prolonged asphyxia, as opposed to trauma, is much more likely to result in permanent ill-effects, particularly if the baby's growth in utero was impaired or the baby was of low birth weight (Badawi et al 2001). It is very difficult to tell from the clinical features in the newborn period alone which babies will fail to make a full recovery (Box 10.4). Attempts have been made to develop objective methods of neurological assessment to evaluate progress and assess prognosis but these have remained largely research tools rather than clinically valuable methods. On the other hand, the occurrence of cerebral infarction, periventricular leucomalacia, haemorrhagic necrosis or cyst formation on imaging investigations are usually followed by the development of cerebral palsy, developmental delay or epilepsy (Doyle et al 2000, Pierrat et al 2001). The occurrence of repeated fits in the first few days, continued failure to suck requiring ongoing tube feeding, and the persistence of other neurological signs of cerebral injury for more than about 4 days are also features often associated with long-term neurological disability. Failure to establish normal respiration within 30 minutes of birth despite adequate artificial ventilation makes full recovery

---

Box 10.4 Indicators of a poor prognosis in hypoxic-ischaemic encephalopathy

Imaging features
- Cerebral infarction
- Periventricular leucomalacia
- Haemorrhagic necrosis
- Parenchymal cyst formation

Clinical features
- Repeated seizures
- Persisting failure to suck
- Persisting neurological signs
- Persisting symptoms of cerebral injury
- Failure to breathe for more than 30 minutes at birth

---

extremely unlikely; however, the absence of such features gives no guarantee of a good prognosis and only prolonged follow-up will show the full extent of any neurological deficit.

Physiotherapy

After the acute stage of cerebral injury is over, the baby may have persistence of abnormal tone and motor responses which can be indicators of an emerging neurological deficit. Although the eventual degree of handicap is not known at this time, a paediatric physiotherapist with understanding of neurological development can advise the parents on ways of positioning the baby during sleep and handling the infant while awake to modify the progression of the neurological signs and enable the baby to follow a more normal sequence of development. Not only can this improve the outlook for the baby but also it increases parental confidence in handling the infant and gives the opportunity to identify and treat at an early stage any deviations from normal development. Such specialised physiotherapists can also advise parents after discharge of the baby if difficulties with feeding occur or the infant requires tube feeding.

NEONATAL FITS

It is important to recognise fits in the neonatal period since, in contrast to fits in older children, they are frequently a manifestation of an underlying condition whose treatment may materially affect the infant's prognosis. They occur in 2.6 per 1000 live births, but in up to 8% of babies in intensive care units, and are most common in the preterm infant (Ronen et al 1999, Sheth et al 1999). Seizures themselves can cause injury to the neonatal brain (McCabe et al 2001, Volpe 2001) and may continue unrecognised for some time. Occasionally they result from an inherited metabolic disease which, if diagnosed early, may affect the family's decision on having further children.

Fits in the first few weeks of life have a different pattern from the common seizures of later infancy and childhood. Instead of the generalised 'grand mal' type of convulsive fit, the most usual pattern is one of brief jerking or twitching of a single limb, which rapidly moves from one part of the body to another. Sometimes these movements change site so rapidly that they appear to be generalised, whilst at other times a repetitive twitching of one limb or side of the face is all that is seen. Generalised tonic seizures with hyperextension of the trunk, neck and limbs are another variation. More difficult to recognise as fits are momentary changes of respiratory pattern (perhaps apnoeic attacks), flickering of the eyelids, tonic deviation of the eyes to one side, drooling or lipsmacking. Focal fits do not necessarily signify a localised brain lesion but may occur even when the cerebral involvement is diffuse, as in metabolic disorders such as hypoglycaemia or hypocalcaemia. Sometimes the diagnosis of fits can only be established for certain by a continuous EEG recording (Connell et al 1989).

The causes of neonatal fits can broadly be classified as follows:

- Common causes
  - —hypoxic-ischaemic encephalopathy
  - —intracranial haemorrhage or oedema from birth trauma
  - —infection, particularly meningitis
  - —metabolic disturbances, including hypoglycaemia, hypocalcaemia and hyponatraemia
- Less common causes
  - —structural abnormalities such as hydrocephalus or an arteriovenous malformation

- —withdrawal of drugs, e.g. heroin, barbiturates, alcohol
- —inborn errors of metabolism, e.g. phenylketonuria, organic acidaemias or pyridoxine dependency
- —benign familial neonatal seizures
- —toxicity from local anaesthetics or theophylline.

Diagnosis

Fits in any neonate must always be regarded as potentially serious and their cause investigated thoroughly. In some cases the baby will have a diagnosed condition in which fits are not unexpected. If the baby has a poor colour, is lethargic, hypotonic, is feeding poorly or having periods of apnoea, she needs an urgent lumbar puncture to exclude meningitis, and immediate blood glucose and blood gas measurements. Such symptoms can also occur with certain rare metabolic disorders, and urinary chromatography for amino acids or organic acids should be performed.

If the baby's condition is more stable, the investigations will include estimation of blood glucose at the cotside and laboratory measurement of calcium, electrolytes and urea. A skull X-ray may show calcification from intrauterine infection and a cerebral ultrasound scan may identify haemorrhage, dilatation of the ventricles or a space-occupying lesion. Occasionally a CT scan will be required, particularly if a lesion on the surface of the cortex such as a subdural haemorrhage or arteriovenous malformation is suspected. MRI scanning may show a cerebral infarct. Phenylketonuria should be excluded by the routine neonatal screening test for the condition (p. 211).

In some cases no cause can be found despite extensive investigation. Occasionally a baby may have many fits without apparent cause and be surprisingly well between them. If there is a family history of neonatal fits of similar type, it is likely that the infant has the syndrome of benign familial neonatal fits. The fits subside spontaneously and there is a normal neurological outcome in the majority of cases.

Management of fits

Because fits are potentially so serious, the blood glucose and gases should be checked immediately and an intravenous infusion set up to give the appropriate drugs while an urgent search is made for the underlying cause. If the blood glucose is below 2.5 mmol/L (45 mg/dL), hypoglycaemia should be assumed and the term baby given 5–10 mL/kg of 10% glucose (0.5–1.0 g/kg) intravenously immediately, followed by an infusion of 10% dextrose at a rate suitable to maintain a blood glucose level of 4–8 mmol/L (75–150 mg/dL). A response to this regimen suggests that a low blood glucose is the cause but other conditions should be sought if no improvement is obtained.

Hypoxaemia, hypercapnia or acidaemia should be corrected using enhanced inspired oxygen, mechanical respiratory support for high CO_2 levels, and intravenous correction for metabolic acidosis (p. 134).

Hypocalcaemia is confirmed if the serum calcium level is below 1.7 mmol/L. In most cases this condition occurs towards the end of the first week of life and is associated with a high phosphate load in the milk. Most modified cow's milk formulae now have low levels of phosphate, hence the condition is becoming increasingly uncommon. If the hypocalcaemic infant is simply hypertonic and irritable with increased tendon reflexes (the condition known as hypocalcaemic tetany), oral calcium gluconate 200 mg/kg per day or 50% magnesium sulphate 0.1–0.2 mL/kg intramuscularly will raise the calcium level and improve the condition. If fits occur, 0.3 mL/kg of 10% calcium gluconate should be given by slow intravenous injection over at least 10 minutes while monitoring the electrocardiogram for T-wave changes or arrythmias. Babies suffering from hypocalcaemia in the newborn period have been found to suffer from dental enamel hypoplasia in the milk teeth. It seems probable that maternal vitamin D deficiency in late pregnancy may also play a part in its causation.

Anticonvulsant drug treatment

In the absence of an easily treated metabolic cause, anticonvulsant drugs form the mainstay of treatment (Evans & Levene 1998). Continuous fitting is relatively uncommon and drugs are not often needed to terminate an individual fit. However, if the baby has repeated seizures, it is usual to give a loading dose of phenobarbital 20 mg/kg intramuscularly, but this does take time to act. Occasionally, it may be necessary to repeat the dose intravenously to raise the blood level quickly. If fitting continues, phenytoin 20 mg/kg intravenously may be effective. An intravenous injection of clonazepam 100–200 μg/kg over 30 seconds, followed by an infusion of 30 μg/kg per hour, may be needed if even this does not control the fits. However, clonazepam causes respiratory depression and ventilation may be needed to maintain adequate respiration. Diazepam 0.3 mg/kg intravenously can also be used but may cause apnoea and accentuate jaundice by releasing the bilirubin from its binding sites on albumin. It should, therefore, be used with caution.

For longer-term control of fits, phenobarbital remains the drug of choice. The same loading dose (i.e. 20 mg/kg i.m.) is given to achieve a therapeutic blood level of approximately 20 mg/mL, though it may take some hours to reach this. Subsequently, this level can be maintained with daily oral doses of 3–4 mg/kg. The rate of excretion of phenobarbital is slow but very variable and blood level monitoring is desirable to avoid sedation from overdosage.

Phenytoin 20 mg/kg given by slow intravenous injection, followed by 5 mg/kg per day maintenance, is often effective where phenobarbital is not. Sodium valproate is a less effective anticonvulsant in the newborn period than it is at other ages, but may occasionally be used. Anticonvulsant treatment is usually given for only 2–3 months after control of neonatal seizures, since recurrence of the fits is unusual after this time.

If no response is obtained from anticonvulsants, a therapeutic trial of pyridoxine 50 mg daily will reduce fitting in the rare infant with pyridoxine dependency.

Pertussis immunisation following neurological illness

At one time pertussis immunisation was regarded as contraindicated in infants who had

had neurological problems in the neonatal period while research was carried out to determine its level of safety. Although the risk of damage from the vaccine is at worst very slight, it is wise to defer the pertussis fraction for those infants who have had fits or severe hypoxic-ischaemic encephalopathy, until it is clear that they have no progressive neurological disorder. There are no other perinatal contraindications to its use and for all other infants it should be recommended.

Prognosis of neonatal fits

The outcome in later childhood for those babies who have suffered from fits in the first week depends more on the prognosis of the underlying cause than on the fits themselves, though the greater the number of fits, the more likely is there to be continuing neurological damage. When fits are due to transient hypocalcaemia, normal development is the rule. When caused by intraventricular, subdural or subarachnoid haemorrhage or oedema, the outlook is also good in a high proportion of cases (Temple et al 1995). There is a high incidence of subsequent neurological handicap when fits result from cerebral anoxia, persistent hypoglycaemia or meningitis, particularly when this is associated with other neurological signs such as lethargy, hypotonia, apnoea and poor feeding. When an associated structural abnormality of the brain is identified, or when a bleed, ischaemic changes or cyst formation is found within the cerebral cortex, the likelihood of abnormal development is high. If a metabolic disorder is identified as the cause, the outlook is often poor (p. 212).

HYPOTONIA – THE FLOPPY INFANT

Muscular hypotonia is a feature of many conditions in the newborn infant. The preterm infant of less than 34 weeks' gestation is always hypotonic and its extent is used in the estimation of gestational age (p. 110). It is a prominent feature in Down syndrome and often helps to confirm the diagnosis when it is suspected from a dysmorphic facies (p. 207). Cerebral injury from trauma or asphyxia (p. 152), hypoglycaemia (p. 54),

hyponatraemia and any infection, especially with septicaemia or meningitis, are also causes, though in many cases other manifestations of these conditions are present. Certain drugs such as diazepam and opiate analgesics can also cross the placenta and cause sedation or hypotonia. In a baby with a myelomeningocele affecting the lumbar spine, the legs are floppy from incomplete innervation whereas the arms are normal (p. 231).

Generalised hypotonia

More rarely, low muscle tone or weakness of the muscles is found in an otherwise well infant which results from one of a group of neuromuscular diseases that either are present at birth or develop during the first weeks of life. The differentiation of these conditions is difficult. The family history, cytogenetic studies and DNA analysis can be helpful in diagnosing some cases since many are genetically inherited, but often extensive investigation, including biochemical testing, electromyography and muscle biopsy, is needed.

A degenerative process involving the anterior horn cells in the spinal cord is the cause of the muscular weakness in a group of conditions known as Werdnig–Hoffmann disease or progressive infantile spinal muscular atrophy. The condition is recessively inherited. Although weakness and hypotonia become noticeable only after the first few weeks or months, they can be present at birth. Progressive weakness of all muscle groups, particularly the trunk and respiratory muscles, leads to death in infancy in all but a few exceptional cases.

Another group includes the familial myopathies and muscular dystrophies. In these, the rate of progression of the weakness is very variable, but ultimately most have a relentless downhill course with slowly increasing paralysis.

For certain types of muscle disorders there are diagnostic blood tests. For example, with Duchenne muscular dystrophy, a very high blood creatine phosphokinase level in the first few days of life is diagnostic and, with informed consent, the test should be performed on all male infants where there is a family history of the disorder (Dubowitz 1992). The disease can even be

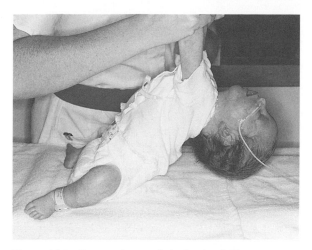

Figure 10.3 Extreme hypotonia in Prader–Willi syndrome.

predicted with some certainty antenatally, using DNA analysis (p. 22). Early diagnosis enables genetic advice to be given so that parents are informed about the risks for future sons.

Hypotonia in a male infant with crypt-orchidism suggests the Prader–Willi syndrome (Fig. 10.3) with the associated development of obesity and mild mental retardation. The diagnosis is confirmed by finding a characteristic gene deletion on chromosome 15 in cytogenetic studies (Plate 15) (Richer et al 2001).

Myasthenia gravis is extremely rare except in the transient form which occurs when the mother has the condition (p. 28), and in myotonic dystrophy one of the parents may show some signs of the condition such as a characteristic tight and rather immobile facies and difficulty in relaxing a clenched hand.

In many 'floppy infants' no specific diagnosis is found despite complete investigation and the baby's muscle power and tone improves gradually. This group probably comprises a mixture of different conditions but the term 'benign congenital hypotonia' has been used to describe it. However, such babies often have learning difficulties in later childhood.

Spinal injury

Injury involving the spinal cord is rare. Dislocation in the upper cervical spine may follow hyperextension of the neck during a difficult delivery. The clinical picture is that of extreme floppiness and immobility together with diminished respiratory effort, but facial movements are spared. Depending on the degree of damage, this injury may result in spastic quadriplegia, though, provided the brain itself is unaffected, the child will not usually have learning difficulties.

NERVE INJURIES
Brachial plexus injuries

Injury to the cervical nerve roots may cause paralysis of the arm which varies in extent and distribution depending on which nerves are involved. Erb's palsy, the commonest abnormality, is due to contusion, or more rarely avulsion, of the fifth and sixth cervical nerve roots from downward traction of the arm or shoulder during delivery. It occurs in larger babies, especially when the delivery is complicated by shoulder dystocia, a situation more commonly seen in poorly controlled maternal diabetes mellitus. The result is paralysis of the abductors of the shoulder, the flexors of the elbow and the supinator. Characteristically, the relatively immobile arm is held to the baby's side, extended at the elbow with the forearm pronated (Fig. 10.4). Loss of movement in the arm can be shown by demonstrating that only the unaffected arm moves when performing the Moro reflex (p. 74). It is very occasionally accompanied by phrenic nerve palsy, causing paralysis of the diaphragm on the same side.

Much less commonly, the eighth cervical and first thoracic nerves are injured by upward traction on the arm. The resultant paralysis (Klumpke's palsy) involves mainly the intrinsic muscles of the hand and the flexors of the wrist and fingers. Sensory loss may be present but is not easily demonstrable with certainty. Rarely, complete paralysis of the whole arm may occur from more extensive plexus injury.

Injury is sometimes caused to the radial nerve in the upper arm or the posterior interosseous nerve in the forearms due to traction or local pressure. Wrist drop is the presenting feature and eventual recovery is usual.

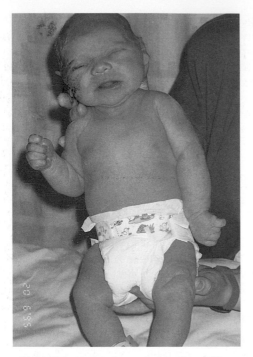

Figure 10.4 Extended and pronated posture of the affected left arm in Erb's palsy.

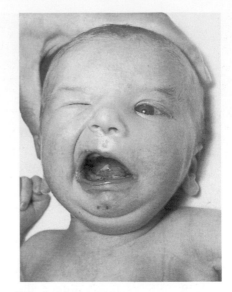

Figure 10.5 Left facial palsy.

Differential diagnosis

The only difficulty lies in distinguishing these brachial plexus injuries from pseudoparalysis caused by a painful lesion in the arm itself, such as osteomyelitis or a fracture of the humerus or clavicle. In these cases, the arm is held limply and no movement can be demonstrated, but there may be tenderness on pressure, and swelling, erythema or bruising. An X-ray will demonstrate a fracture but a bone scan would be needed to show osteomyelitis.

Prognosis and treatment

Fortunately, most cervical nerve injuries result from contusion and complete division is rare. Movement gradually returns and improvement continues for up to 18 months. Eventually, around 80% get a reasonable recovery of hand and arm

function. Encouraging movement of the arm and preventing contractures by means of physiotherapy is important, but nerve grafting using microsurgical techniques and later release of soft tissue contractures can improve the outlook when there is little evidence of recovery in the first 3 months.

Facial nerve palsy

Facial nerve palsy is sometimes caused by trauma to the facial nerve by forceps, though more often it occurs after normal delivery and is due to compression of the side of the face on the maternal sacrum during delivery. Unilateral facial weakness becomes obvious as the baby cries, the eye on the affected side failing to close and the mouth being pulled across to the opposite side (Fig. 10.5). There is no interference with feeding, and recovery is usually complete within a few weeks. When bilateral, there is just a remarkable lack of facial expression when crying, but this is rarely due to pressure and other causes such as nuclear agenesis (Moebius syndrome) have to be investigated.

REFERENCES

Badawi N, Keogh J M, Dixon G 2001 Developmental outcomes of newborn encephalopathy in the term infant. Indian Journal of Pediatrics 68(2):527–530

Blankenberg F G, Loh N N, Bracci P et al 2000 Sonography, CT and MR imaging: a prospective comparison of neonates with suspected intracranial ischemia and hemorrhage. American Journal of Neuroradiology 21(1):213–218

Connell J, Ozeer R, de Vries L et al 1989 Continuous EEG recording of neonatal seizures: diagnostic and prognostic considerations. Archives of Disease in Childhood 64(4):452–458

Doyle L W, Betheras F R, Ford G W et al 2000 Survival, cranial ultrasound and cerebral palsy in very low birthweight infants: 1980s versus 1990s. Journal of Paediatrics and Child Health 36(1):7–12

Dubowitz V 1992 The muscular dystrophies. Postgraduate Medical Journal 68:500–506

Evans D, Levene M 1998 Neonatal seizures. Archives of Disease in Childhood Fetal and Neonatal Edition 78:F70–F75

Mc Cabe B K, Silveira D C, Cilio M R et al 2001 Reduced neurogenesis after neonatal seizures. Journal of Neurosciences 21(6):2094–2103

Marret S, Lardennois C, Mercier A et al 2001 Fetal and neonatal cerebral infarcts. Biology of the Neonate 79(3):236–240

Martin E, Barkovich A J 1995 Magnetic resonance imaging in perinatal asphyxia. Archives of Disease in Childhood Fetal and Neonatal Edition 72:F62–F70

Pressler R M, Boylan G B, Morton M et al 2001 Early serial EEG in hypoxic-ischaemic encephalopathy. Clinical Neurophysiology 112(1):31–37

Pierrat V, Duquennoy C, van Haastert K et al 2001 Ultrasound diagnosis and neurodevelopmental outcome of localised and extensive cystic periventricular leucomalacia. Archives of Disease in Childhood Fetal and Neonatal Edition 84:F151–F156

Richer L P, Shevell M I, Miller S P 2001 Diagnostic profile of neonatal hypotonia: an 11-year study. Pediatric Neurology 25(1):32–37

Ronen G M, Penney S, Andrews W 1999 The epidemiology of clinical neonatal seizures in Newfoundland: a population-based study. Journal of Pediatrics 134(1):71–75

Sheth R D, Hobbs G R, Mullett M 1999 Neonatal seizures: incidence, onset, and etiology by gestational age. Journal of Perinatology 19(1):40–43

Temple C M, Dennis J, Carney R et al 1995 Neonatal seizures: long-term outcome and cognitive development among 'normal' survivors. Developmental Medicine and Child Neurology 37:109–118

Volpe J J 2001 Perinatal brain injury: from pathogenesis to neuroprotection. Mental Retardation and Developmental Disability Research Review 7(1):56–64

Wagner C L, Eicher D J, Katikaneni L D et al 1999 The use of hypothermia: a role in the treatment of neonatal asphyxia? Pediatric Neurology 21(1):429–443

Chapter 11

Infections

CHAPTER CONTENTS

Mechanisms of protection from infection   163
   Immunoglobulins (antibodies)   163
   Complement   164
   Cellular immune systems   164
   Colostrum   164
Sources and routes of fetal and neonatal infection   164
Minor infections   165
   Infections of skin and subcutaneous tissues   165
   Eye infections   166
   Upper respiratory tract infections   166
   Infections of the alimentary tract   167
Serious acute infection   167
   Clinical signs of bacterial sepsis   168
   Investigation in suspected bacterial septicaemia   168
   Organisms causing neonatal infection   168
   Septicaemia   169
   Meningitis   169
   Congenital pneumonia   171
   Urinary tract infections   172
Interpreting the laboratory results   173
   Acute gastroenteritis   174
   Acute osteomyelitis and septic arthritis   174
Use of antibiotics in the newborn period   174
   General principles   174
   Dosage   175
   Prevention of antibiotic resistance   175
Viral and protozoal infections   175
   Antenatal infection   175
   Specific transplacentally acquired infections   176
   Other viral infections   177
Chronic infections   178
   Tuberculosis   178
   HIV infection   178
   Hepatitis B infection   180
   Hepatitis C infection   180
   Herpes simplex   180
   Congenital syphilis   181
   Malaria   181

MECHANISMS OF PROTECTION FROM INFECTION

Full-term newborn babies are more vulnerable to attack from bacteria, viruses and fungi than are older infants because their defence mechanisms are immature and some organisms which are non-pathogenic in the older child can cause serious infection in the neonatal period. In the preterm infant, these defences are even less mature, so that serious consequences of infection are more likely. Male babies are more susceptible to infection than are females. Some protection, however, is afforded through the following immune responses.

Immunoglobulins (antibodies)

Until about 3–4 months of age, the baby has only a limited capacity to produce antibodies in response to infection. Some passive immunity is gained by transfer of some immunoglobulin G (IgG) antibodies from the mother in the last weeks of pregnancy, but the infant has no maternal IgM or IgA antibodies since neither is able to cross the placenta. If the mother has formed antibodies following infection with viruses such as measles, mumps, chickenpox and rubella, her IgG antibodies give the infant protection from such infections for 4–6 months. However, antibodies formed against most bacteria, including *Escherichia coli*, group B streptococci, *Haemophilus influenzae* and *Streptococcus pneumoniae*, are not usually transferred, which may partly explain why these organisms in particular are more likely to infect the newborn baby.

Complement

Complement is a group of substances which damage the cell membranes of invading organisms and enable their further destruction by phagocytes. These are present in reduced amounts at birth.

Cellular immune systems

Lymphocytes

Lymphocytes which produce immunoglobulins are immature at birth and those which recognise invading organisms or have cytotoxic activity have only limited function in the term infant.

Polymorphonuclear leucocytes

Polymorphonuclear leucocytes, which accumulate at the site of infection under the influence of the complement system and phagocytose or kill bacteria, migrate less well in the neonatal period, but their killing capacity is mature once the baby approaches term. With overwhelming infections, the bone marrow becomes unable to keep up an adequate production of white cells and neutropenia may result, causing a reduction in the infant's capacity to eradicate bacteria.

Colostrum

Colostrum from breast feeding affords some protection against infection by providing the infant with substances such as IgA, lysozymes, lactoferrin and lymphocytes. Later on, breast milk reduces the proliferation of organisms in the gut since the acidity produced by the breakdown of the excess lactose in the large bowel favours the growth of harmless lactobacilli and inhibits the more pathogenic *E. coli* organisms.

SOURCES AND ROUTES OF FETAL AND NEONATAL INFECTION

Before birth, infection may take place either across the placenta or by ascending the birth canal. Amongst infections acquired principally by the transplacental route are rubella, cytomegalovirus,

Table 11.1 Maternal infection – the impact on the baby

Maternal infection	Effect on the infant
Rubella	Congenital malformations, growth retardation and mental retardation
Toxoplasmosis	Hydrocephalus, choroidoretinitis, jaundice and mental retardation
Cytomegalovirus	Microcephaly, hepatitis and mental retardation
Genital herpes	Encephalitis
HIV/AIDS	AIDS
Hepatitis B	Hepatitis or chronic carrier of virus
Coxsackie B	Myocarditis
Chickenpox	Chickenpox fetopathy Severe neonatal chickenpox
Chlamydia	Conjunctivitis
Candida albicans	Oral and perineal thrush
Gonorrhoea	Severe conjunctivitis
Syphilis	Snuffles, skin lesions and congenital malformations
Malaria	Congenital malaria
Tuberculosis	Miliary tuberculosis or meningitis

toxoplasmosis, syphilis, tuberculosis and human immunodeficiency virus (HIV). In such cases, the mother must have contracted the infection and the organism is in her circulation (Table 11.1).

Those organisms which reach the fetus via the birth canal, especially after prolonged rupture of the membranes, include the group B streptococcus, *E. coli*, *Listeria monocytogenes and Mycoplasma hominis*, which are usually harmless commensal organisms for the mother. More often they infect the baby during the birth. Gonococci, hepatitis B virus, *Candida albicans (Monilia), echovirus*, coxsackievirus and *Chlamydia trachomatis* all cause maternal infection which may be transmitted to the baby during delivery.

Within the first few days of life, the baby becomes colonised by bacteria which are usually harmless but which can occasionally cause disease, and the pattern of pathogenic organisms changes over the years. The skin and umbilicus are colonised by staphylococci, the lower gut by *E. coli*, and the upper respiratory tract by streptococci. Spread from one baby to another is a constant risk. For instance, a mild staphylococcal 'sticky eye' which is trivial in itself can be a source of much more serious infection like staphylococcal pneumonia or osteomyelitis in other infants at a later stage. Staphylococcal, streptococcal and *E. coli* infections often originate from caregivers carrying the organisms and much less frequently from the mother. Occasionally, breast milk may transmit a virus infection if the mother is viraemic at the time (Michie & Gilmour 2001, Hamprecht et al 2001).

Some mechanical apparatus is easily contaminated and it is essential to ensure adequate sterilisation of incubators, ventilators, suction apparatus, breast-milk pumps and weighing scales after use. Some organisms like *Pseudomonas aeruginosa*, on the other hand, tend to live in moist places such as wash basins and have even been found in some 'disinfectant' fluids and soaps.

Clinical factors predisposing to infection are preterm birth, low birth weight, hypothermia, prolonged rupture of the membranes, and the presence of certain congenital malformations, particularly superficial lesions such as meningomyelocele, and abnormalities of the urinary tract.

MINOR INFECTIONS
Infections of skin and subcutaneous tissues

Isolated superficial pustules caused by staphylococcal infection are common, occurring singly or in crops. They are most troublesome in moist areas like the groins or axillae, though they can arise anywhere. Sometimes the lesion is just a small blister with no surrounding erythema. Although usually trivial in itself and rarely the primary cause of a disseminated staphylococcal infection, it is a source of cross-infection to others, so it should never be passed over casually. The little yellowish-white spots on an erythematous or urticarial base which characterise urticaria neonatorum (p. 62) are sometimes mistakenly diagnosed as pustules.

Paronychia

Reddening of the skin in the nailfold area is also common and may proceed to pus formation, usually involving more than one finger at a time. The usual causative organism is *Staphylococcus aureus* and local treatment with an antistaphylococcal cream is all that is normally required.

Bullous impetigo

Bullous impetigo (pemphigus neonatorum) is an uncommon skin infection caused by *Staph. aureus*. Large vesicles develop containing thin pus, rupturing and leaving raw areas that form scabs. Ritter's disease, or the scalded skin syndrome, is a more serious variety of the same infection in which the lesions rapidly coalesce and large areas of exfoliation of skin result, resembling a scald. These infections can range from mild to very serious and flucloxacillin is the antibiotic of choice, given intravenously if the baby is very sick. Dehydration and hypotension may occur unless careful attention is paid to replacing the fluids lost from the open skin areas.

Periumbilical infection

Infection of the periumbilical skin bears a special risk of spread via the umbilical vein, giving rise to thrombophlebitis and possibly leading to suppuration in the liver itself with severe jaundice. Some cases of portal hypertension with oesophageal varices arising in later childhood have been attributed to this cause.

Treatment of skin sepsis

Culture of material from any skin lesion should always be attempted because information about the type of organism and its sensitivity to antibiotics is of value in minimising its spread. For minor lesions, local application of an antiseptic powder is usually sufficient. Systemic antibiotic treatment is not usually necessary and in general should be avoided since the overenthusiastic use of antibiotics encourages the development of resistant organisms such as methicillin-resistant *Staph. aureus* (MRSA), which is increasing in prevalence in hospitals in the UK and elsewhere. When they are needed, flucloxacillin is a good first choice since the majority of skin infections are caused by staphylococci, most of which remain sensitive to it (p. 175).

Acute mastitis

This infection usually occurs in an engorged neonatal breast and is generally caused by

Staph. aureus. It appears as an inflamed red swelling under the nipple and the infant is usually febrile. Occasionally it may develop into an abscess which requires surgical incision and drainage, but if it is treated early with antibiotics the infection will usually resolve. Flucloxacillin is the drug of choice, given orally if the infection is minor, but systemically if the baby is ill.

Eye infections
Sticky eye

A sticky eye in the first 1 or 2 days of life is often due only to chemical irritation and clears spontaneously. The only treatment necessary is to wipe away the secretions with cooled boiled water when they accumulate. After this age, it is likely to be infective in origin.

Conjunctivitis

Conjunctivitis with a purulent discharge from the eye is relatively common. Staphylococci, *E. coli or* streptococci are frequently grown in culture but it is difficult to be sure that they are the true cause. After taking swabs for culture, treatment should be started immediately with chloramphenicol 1.0% eye ointment applied at least four times a day and should be continued for 5 days or until the infection has resolved.

More persistent infection not responding to routine treatment may be caused by *Chlamydia trachomatis* (Plate 16). This is an organism which silently infects the female genital tract and is increasingly being seen in sexually transmitted disease clinics in the UK. It is usually acquired by the baby from the birth canal, causing a number of infections including conjunctivitis (Jain 1999). The conjunctiva tends to be more 'fleshy' in appearance and is associated with swelling of the eyelids. The organism is difficult to grow in the laboratory and special swabs are needed to capture it. Treatment with tetracycline eye ointment every 4–6 hours is usually effective, combined with oral erythromycin in more severe cases. Topical chloramphenicol suppresses infection with this organism but does not cure it.

Dacrocystitis

Dacrocystitis is occasionally seen as a complication of conjunctivitis, with a reddened swelling over the region of the lacrimal sac at the root of the nose. Pressure over the sac produces a little purulent discharge from the lacrimal duct in the lower eyelid and this can be gently carried out three or four times daily as a therapeutic measure, combined with local instillation of chloramphenicol ointment and systemic flucloxacillin.

Ophthalmia neonatorum

Ophthalmia neonatorum caused by gonococcal infection is uncommon where treatment of sexually transmitted diseases is readily available but is a common preventable cause of blindness world-wide. Prevention can be achieved by giving an infant born to an infected mother a single intramuscular dose of penicillin 50 mg/kg at birth. Maternal gonorrhoea is often asymptomatic but in the infant the effect is dramatic. It is a serious acute infection beginning as a purulent conjunctivitis but liable to involve deeper structures of the eye, causing irreparable damage if left untreated. The diagnosis can usually be made quickly from a direct Gram stain on a smear of pus, which shows the presence of gram-negative cocci, but culture to determine antibiotic sensitivity is essential since penicillin resistance is becoming more frequent throughout the world.

Treatment The eye should be irrigated with chloramphenicol eyedrops as frequently as is needed to reduce the profuse production of pus. In the most severe cases, this may be every 15–30 minutes initially. In addition, benzylpenicillin 50 mg/kg should be given intramuscularly 12-hourly for at least 7 days to clear the infection, though intravenous cefotaxime should be given if the organism is penicillin resistant.

Upper respiratory tract infections
'Snuffles'

An excess of nasal secretion which partially blocks the nasal airway is common in the first few weeks of life. It is sometimes present at birth, when it may be a clear mucoid discharge or, much less commonly, a mucopurulent one. Although included amongst the infections, it is likely that many of these cases are not infective. Respiratory syncytial virus is occasionally the cause of relatively mild upper respiratory tract infection in the newborn, in contrast to the more familiar acute bronchiolitis seen in older infants.

Although congenital syphilis is rare where antenatal screening and treatment are available, it is a cause of purulent or blood-stained nasal discharge, often associated with other features of congenital syphilis (p. 181).

No treatment for the common variety of 'snuffles' is usually necessary, but interference with feeding caused by nasal obstruction justifies a drop of 0.25% ephedrine nasal solution into the nose before feeds. It should be used sparingly since the ephedrine can raise the heart rate and blood pressure of the infant significantly. Otitis media is often missed in the newborn period because it is not suspected or because the eardrum is difficult to see. It gives rise to irritability and failure to feed and thrive. Needle aspiration of the middle ear is the only means of proving the diagnosis, but this is obviously too painful and hazardous a procedure to use in most circumstances and is unnecessary. *Staph. aureus* and streptococci are the commonest infecting bacteria and nearly all cases respond well to a combination of oral ampicillin and flucloxacillin given for 5 days.

Infections of the alimentary tract

Thrush

Thrush, or moniliasis, which is caused by the yeast *Candida albicans*, most commonly affects the mouth but may also involve the oesophagus and gastrointestinal tract, resulting in diarrhoea and vomiting. It is a common cause of rashes in the nappy area at this age (p. 87 and Plate 13). The source of monilial infection is usually the vagina of the mother, but the organism is commonly found on the skin, including that of the breast. Infants who have received broad-spectrum antibiotics are particularly vulnerable to candidal

infection. Oral thrush shows itself as numerous small white plaques (resembling curds of milk) on the tongue and inside of the mouth which are difficult to dislodge. The resulting soreness sometimes causes distress and refusal of feeds. Nystatin suspension, 1 mL (100 000 units) given by a dropper directly into the mouth after each feed, for 7–10 days, is usually effective treatment, but may have to be repeated. Other effective topical preparations include miconazole and clotrimazole.

SERIOUS ACUTE INFECTION

The incidence of serious acute infections in the newborn period is about 3 per 1000 live births in the UK and they include meningitis, pneumonia and urinary tract infection, often with septicaemia. Making a specific diagnosis may be difficult because clinical signs pointing to the site of the infection are often absent (Box 11.1)

Immaturity of the immune responses allows the infection to become rapidly disseminated throughout the body and cause widespread organ damage which can be permanent and handicapping if not treated at the earliest possible moment. For this reason, it is important to recognise the initial clinical signs of serious infection, to investigate rapidly to identify the site of

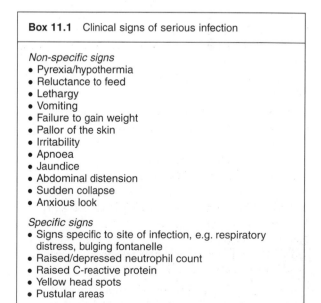

Box 11.1 Clinical signs of serious infection

Non-specific signs
- Pyrexia/hypothermia
- Reluctance to feed
- Lethargy
- Vomiting
- Failure to gain weight
- Pallor of the skin
- Irritability
- Apnoea
- Jaundice
- Abdominal distension
- Sudden collapse
- Anxious look

Specific signs
- Signs specific to site of infection, e.g. respiratory distress, bulging fontanelle
- Raised/depressed neutrophil count
- Raised C-reactive protein
- Yellow head spots
- Pustular areas

the infection and the organisms responsible, and to start antibiotic treatment immediately (p. 169). The earlier the diagnosis is made and the treatment started, the better the prognosis for the infant. Innovative treatments, including the administration of granulocyte colony stimulating factor, show promise but the mainstay of therapy remains the effective use of antibiotics (Modi & Carr 2000). It remains uncertain whether intravenous immunoglobulin improves the prognosis (Ohlsson & Lacy 2001).

These infants are often very sick and the infection can be life threatening. The parents will need great care and support themselves and the mother may blame herself for transmitting the infection to the infant. Explanation and appropriate reassurance should be offered, particularly about the unpleasant procedures such as lumbar puncture which may have to be undertaken.

Clinical signs of bacterial sepsis

The clinical signs of septicaemia are often very non-specific and are summarised in Box 11.1. The emergence of such indicators should trigger an immediate search for a causative organism even though in some cases other diagnoses such as heart failure or metabolic disorders may present in similar ways.

Occasionally, transitory fever can be associated with dehydration alone, but this is not seen in infants fed adequately from birth. The body temperature may reach 39–40°C (103° or 104°F) and it occurs typically on the third or fourth day. It is associated with crying and restlessness, but not with the general signs of infection, and is relieved within 24 hours by giving the baby extra water to drink.

The disseminated intravascular coagulation syndrome may complicate the clinical picture and usually presents as circulatory failure and haemorrhage from one or more sites (p. 187).

Investigation in suspected bacterial septicaemia

In any infant showing the clinical signs of more than a trivial local infection, it is mandatory to carry out the following investigations to confirm the diagnosis and find the causative organism:

- Full blood count – the white cell count may show either a depressed or a raised neutrophil count. The red cells are fragmented and the platelets low in disseminated intravascular coagulation syndrome.
- Blood culture – this must be taken from a peripheral vein because samples from the femoral or umbilical veins are often contaminated and results are unreliable.
- Urine culture – either a clean-catch or suprapubic sample (p. 172).
- Swabs from the throat, nose, ear and any evidently infected site.
- Lumbar puncture and CSF culture – it is good practice to do many lumbar punctures which turn out to be negative to pick up the one case of meningitis at an early stage.
- Chest X-ray – if there are any respiratory symptoms such as tachypnoea, costal recession or grunting.

In addition to these, the blood electrolytes and blood gases may be measured if the infant is particularly ill. Acute-phase reactants such as C-reactive protein are occasionally useful in identifying early infection but are rarely crucial in the diagnosis.

Organisms causing neonatal infection

Although in the past *Staph. aureus* was the commonest cause of serious neonatal infections, more recently in the UK *E. coli* and group B beta-haemolytic streptococci have been the most frequently isolated organisms in cases of septicaemia, pneumonia and meningitis. *E. coli* is a universal bowel organism and between 5% and 20% of mothers carry the group B streptococcus in the birth canal. The latter may be acquired by the infant during vaginal delivery but treatment of the mother with penicillin before and during labour reduces the risk of infection in the baby. Only rarely, however, does either organism cause serious illness. *Staph. epidermidis* (coagulase-negative staphylococcus) commonly causes serious infection in preterm infants, and in term infants it is increasingly causing serious infection later in the first month of life.

Around 10–20% of mothers carry the group B streptococcus harmlessly in the vaginal flora. The organism is acquired from the birth canal by the infant but current attempts to prevent neonatal infection with this organism remain limited. Treating known carriers with antibiotics in preterm labour may be effective, but treating all mothers at term whose membranes rupture well before the delivery or those with a fever would prevent less than half of such infections (Towers et al 1999).

Although it has been traditional to take swabs for bacterial culture from several sites on each infant admitted to neonatal units, they rarely either identify which baby will develop a serious infection or predict the infecting organism. However, the swabs may identify an increasing rate of colonisation by potentially pathogenic bacteria and then show when it is necessary to take additional precautions to prevent cross-infection within the unit – for example, if MRSA is found. Some units restrict routine bacterial culture to infants born after prolonged rupture of the membranes and those transferred in from other hospitals. Although there has been an increase in some virus infections in the newborn, e.g. herpes simplex encephalitis and echovirus 11 infection, most outbreaks have been small and confined to one unit, though each has had its fatalities.

Septicaemia

Infection may originate before birth, during the first few days of life, or later in the first month. The commonest organisms identified in early-onset sepsis are the group B haemolytic streptococcus and *E. coli*. *Listeria monocytogenes* and other organisms may cause an occasional case. In later-onset septicaemia in many industrialised countries in Europe, the USA and Australia, over half the infections are caused by coagulase-negative staphylococci, many of which are resistant to methicillin (Pauli et al 1999, Berger et al 1998). Many other organisms are cultured in individual cases. Increasingly, bacteria are identified which are resistant to commonly used antibiotics

and the pattern seen in each neonatal unit will affect the drugs chosen for treatment.

Treatment

Intravenous antibiotic treatment should start before the causative bacteria have been identified but the antibiotics chosen will vary according to the age at onset of the infection. For early-onset infection, a combination of penicillin or ampicillin and gentamicin is commonly used, though a third-generation cephalosporin such as cefuroxime or cefotaxime is preferred in some units. For later-onset sepsis, the same antibiotics may be used if there is no history of MRSA in the unit. Coagulase-negative staphylococci rarely cause fulminant sepsis and a change of antibiotic when the organism is isolated is usually appropriate. Where resistant staphylococci have been found in other babies, it is more appropriate to start with vancomycin and gentamicin. A positive blood culture enables any necessary change in treatment to be made according to the sensitivity of the organism found and the antibiotics should be continued for 14 days. For *Bacteroides* infections, metronidazole is the treatment of choice.

Attention should also be paid to other aspects of treatment such as maintenance of body temperature, fluid and electrolyte balance, blood glucose values and nutrition. In a meta-analysis, Jenson and Pollock (1997) concluded that adding treatment with intravenous immunoglobulin reduced mortality rates in septicaemia.

Meningitis

Fortunately, this infection is rare, affecting only 1 in 3000 newborn infants. Most neonatal meningitis is due to infection by group B streptococci, *E. coli* or, occasionally, L. *monocytogenes*, *Strep. pneumoniae* and *Neisseria meningitidis*. Many other organisms may cause it, particularly in preterm infants undergoing intensive care, but *Haemophilus influenzae*, which causes meningitis in older infants, is rarely implicated. Occasional outbreaks of enteroviral meningitis are recorded caused by such viruses as echovirus II or Coxsackie B.

Meningitis usually follows a stage of septicaemia and in the early phases of the illness there are no signs to localise the infection to the meninges. The usual clinical features include listlessness, a reluctance to feed, vomiting, pallor and temperature instability, and only later does fullness of the anterior fontanelle become detectable. Convulsions and depressed consciousness are common, but neck rigidity is often completely absent until the late stages of the disease.

Diagnosis should be confirmed by examining the cerebrospinal fluid (CSF) obtained at lumbar puncture urgently, before antibiotics have been started. Early diagnosis, and thus more effective treatment, of one case justifies a lumbar puncture of many which turn out to be negative.

Technique of lumbar puncture

Lumbar puncture is a relatively simple procedure and is not usually hazardous if carried out correctly. However, some very sick babies will not tolerate the procedure well and the nurse holding the infant should watch carefully for cyanosis, bradycardia or apnoea and administer oxygen if required.

The infant should be held gently but firmly either in a sitting or in a lying position so as to flex the spine and enlarge the interspinous spaces (Fig. 11.1). Strict aseptic technique must be employed throughout to prevent the introduction of organisms to the CSF. The operator should sterilise his hands and wear sterile gloves. Sterilisation of the skin should be achieved with a small amount of weak chlorhexidine solution only, as significant amounts of the preparation can be absorbed by the neonatal skin and cause chemical burning, especially in the preterm infant. The baby should be covered by sterile towels. A small lumbar puncture needle with a stilette is inserted into a space between the vertebral spines, approximately on a level with the upper border of the iliac crests. After the initial puncture of the skin, the operator waits until the infant remains still and then gently and slowly inserts the needle at a right angle to the surface, not deviating to either side of the midline. Often, a definite click is felt as the dura is punctured, but it is advisable to advance the needle very slowly until spinal fluid flows. If inserted too far, it invariably causes bleeding and it can then be difficult to confirm the high white cell count or see the infecting organisms on Gram staining.

The normal neonatal CSF often contains up to 20 white cells/mm^3, 1.5 g/L of protein and a glucose level of 2.7–4.4 mmol/L. Usually, the white cell count and protein levels are higher and the glucose value lower than these in meningitis,

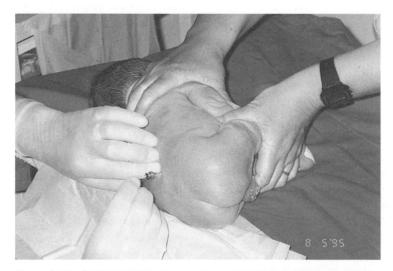

Figure 11.1 Technique of lumbar puncture, showing the position in which the baby should be held.

though the overlap is large and they are not often conclusive in making the diagnosis. A Gram stain of a smear of the fluid will often demonstrate bacteria and guide the choice of antibiotic, but it is essential to culture the CSF to identify the organism and confirm its antibiotic sensitivities. A specific latex agglutination test can be used to confirm group B haemolytic streptococcal infection.

Treatment

All the general measures to treat septicaemia must be instituted and suitable antibacterial therapy started immediately. The chosen antibiotics must pass freely into the CSF and be given intravenously in maximal doses to give adequate bactericidal concentrations to cover the most likely organisms. There is little advantage in instilling the antibiotic directly into the CSF and the amount of trauma this causes to the baby rarely justifies such treatment.

The antibiotics used must penetrate well into the CSF and produce bactericidal concentrations in it. Amoxycillin or ampicillin, to which group B streptococci and *Listeria monocytogenes* are usually sensitive, is often combined with cefotaxime or ceftriaxone, both of which are powerful against *E. coli*. The aminoglycoside antibiotics gentamicin and netilmicin are very effective against gram-negative organisms such as *E. coli*, and are often prescribed even though they do not cross well into the CSF. Other rarer organisms should be treated with the advice of the hospital microbiologist.

Chloramphenicol is occasionally used because it is so well concentrated in the CSF when given systemically, though it is probably not adequate for the treatment of *E. coli* or other gram-negative organisms. It can cause hypotension, cardiac failure and peripheral cyanosis, a condition known as 'grey baby syndrome', if given in excessive dosage and blood levels of the drug must be measured if this is to be avoided.

Whatever antibiotic is chosen initially, it is essential to obtain laboratory confirmation that the causal bacteria are sensitive to it. Monitoring of blood and, if possible, CSF levels of the drug is advised if gentamicin is used, in view of the risk of toxicity at this age (p. 175).

Sometimes lumbar puncture either fails or is thought inadvisable because the baby is too sick to tolerate it. In these circumstances, treatment must be given on an assumption both of the diagnosis and of the organism responsible. Cefotaxime with ampicillin is suitable for this situation as it will cover most causative bacteria.

The duration of treatment depends upon the cause and severity of the meningitis but, in general, systemic treatment should continue for 10–14 days after CSF culture becomes negative. There is some evidence that the administration of steroids to babies with meningitis may reduce the incidence of deafness in survivors.

Outlook

The overall mortality rate for neonatal meningitis treated in the UK has fallen considerably through early diagnosis and improved treatment, from 19.8% in the mid 1980s to 6.6% now (Holt et al 2001). Around 20–30% of survivors have had permanent neurological handicaps in the past, but the incidence with current treatment is not yet determined. The presence of persistent seizures, leucopenia and the need to sustain the circulation with inotrope infusions are predictive of ongoing handicap (Klinger et al 2000), but many babies without these features will not fully recover. Deafness and blindness are frequently seen since complications like hydrocephalus, subdural effusion and ventriculitis are common. As both the infection and the aminoglycoside antibiotics can cause sensorineural deafness, it is advisable to assess the baby's hearing with otoacoustic responses after recovery.

Congenital pneumonia

This is generally part of an acute septicaemic illness acquired prenatally, especially when the membranes have been ruptured for more than 24 hours before the onset of labour. It is most commonly due to the group B haemolytic streptococcus and may be rapidly fatal if not treated immediately.

Prevention is possible only if the organism has been grown from a maternal vaginal swab, in which case the prophylactic administration of penicillin to the mother during labour and to the baby immediately after birth is effective in reducing the risk of serious infection.

Pneumonia of later onset is due to aspiration of infected material or droplet infection, and gram-negative bacilli are the most usual organisms involved. *Staph. aureus* may also cause pneumonia but is much less common.

Clinical features

The clinical features are those of acute septicaemic infection with the signs of respiratory distress. Local signs are generally confined to fine râles on auscultation. A chest X-ray is essential for differentiating infection from the many other causes of respiratory distress. In staphylococcal pneumonia, a lung abscess or the formation of a tension cyst, with or without pneumothorax, may complicate the picture.

Treatment

The baby is best nursed lying prone or on the side but gently moved at intervals to prevent local accumulation of secretions. The head end of the cot or incubator platform should be tipped upwards. Humidified oxygen should be given in adequate concentration to maintain a normal pO_2 or oxygen saturation, which should be continuously monitored along with other vital signs. Antibiotics, always including penicillin, should be started. Often it will be combined initially with a powerful cephalosporin such as cefotaxime, but treatment should usually continue with penicillin alone if cultures identify a group B haemolytic streptococcus. Treatment will continue until the infection resolves. If the infant is only mildly ill, he or she may be given small frequent bottle feeds to avoid compression of the lungs from a full stomach. It is often better to conserve the baby's energy by passing an orogastric tube to administer fluids and nutrients. Nasogastric tubes increase the work of breathing by significantly obstructing nasal airflow and should be avoided. Chest physiotherapy and pharyngeal suction is appropriate when significant amounts of secretions are being produced.

Urinary tract infections

Urinary infection, usually caused by *E. coli* but less often by other gram-negative organisms, varies in severity from a fully bacteraemic illness to one causing little clinical disturbance. It can remain undiagnosed in the newborn baby unless the possibility is borne in mind, since its clinical features can be entirely non-specific. The evidence shows that progressive kidney damage leading ultimately to chronic renal failure often begins in the neonatal period, due to vesicoureteric reflux of infected urine or to severe pyelonephritis associated with septicaemia.

Symptoms and signs

Symptoms and signs are non-specific and consist of reluctance to feed, drowsiness, vomiting, failure to thrive and, sometimes, jaundice. Pyrexia may or may not be present.

Making the diagnosis

Infection will be missed unless urine is cultured in all babies with such clinical features. The diagnostic difficulty lies in collecting an uncontaminated specimen.

It is often possible, with patience, to obtain a 'clean catch' mid-stream specimen after cleansing the external genitalia with sterile water. Sometimes the baby can be induced to empty the bladder when held erect over a container and the lower abdomen is tapped with the finger about once per second. However, although many such techniques have been suggested, most still require much patience.

Suprapubic aspiration of the bladder is achieved by inserting a number 1 needle on a 5-mL syringe, perpendicularly to the skin, about 2 cm deep, midway between the top of the symphysis pubis and the umbilicus (Fig. 11.2). It is a relatively quick and safe procedure provided that it is done with full aseptic precautions and a single needle insertion. The bladder at this age is more an abdominal than a pelvic organ, so the procedure is often successful if attempted about 30 minutes after a feed, but ultrasound imaging

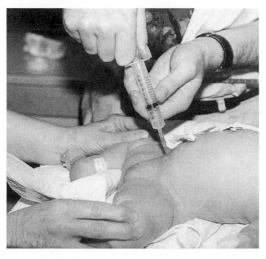

Figure 11.2 Technique of suprapubic aspiration of urine. The needle is inserted half-way between the pubic bone and the umbilicus to a depth of 2 cm.

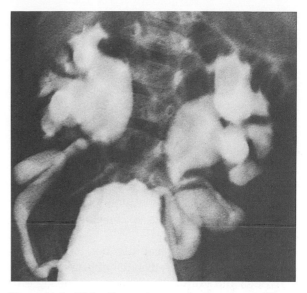

Figure 11.3 Micturating cystogram showing gross reflux and dilatation of the pelves of the kidneys and the ureters in a baby with a urinary tract infection. (By kind permission of Dr Jo Fairhurst.)

of the bladder can improve the success rate of the procedure.

Collection in an adhesive polythene bag appliance frequently results in contaminated urine, making the results of the investigation hard to interpret. Because of the skin trauma from applying and removing the bag and the unreliability of the results obtained, the technique should be used only as a last resort. An alternative of collecting a sample in a cotton-wool ball is better for bacterial culture but a reliable cell count cannot be guaranteed.

INTERPRETING THE LABORATORY RESULTS

As an approximate guide, for a 'clean catch' specimen, 50×10^6 pus cells per litre of uncentrifuged urine in the female and 25×10^6/L in the male suggest infection, and a pure bacterial growth of more than 10^8 organisms per litre confirms the diagnosis. Any growth of pathogenic organisms from a suprapubic aspirate is diagnostic of infection.

Treatment

Antibiotic therapy should be started before the results of the urine culture are obtained if the baby is obviously ill. Intravenous cefotaxime is probably the most effective antibiotic to use at the present time. Alternatively, gentamicin or netilmicin may be given intravenously, but since they are both nephrotoxic and ototoxic, if recommended doses are exceeded, their blood levels must be carefully monitored, especially if renal function is already impaired. The size and frequency of the doses should be adjusted accordingly. If sensitivity tests allow, amoxycillin, trimethoprim or cotrimoxazole may be used after the first week of life and continued for 10–14 days. Subsequent urine checks are essential together with careful follow-up of progress in the first year.

Imaging of the renal tracts after completion of treatment is essential since there is a relatively high incidence of congenital anomalies or vesico-ureteric reflux. An isotope scan can demonstrate evidence of scarring in the renal parenchyma and may show the relative function of the two kidneys, an ultrasound scan any obstructive lesion or malformation, and a micturating cystogram will identify any reflux (Fig. 11.3). If such problems are identified, the baby should be referred for a paediatric surgical assessment.

Acute gastroenteritis

Infective diarrhoea and vomiting are fortunately uncommon in the newborn. Colostrum and breast milk confer some degree of protection against this infection, so it is less common in breast-fed than in formula-fed babies. Outbreaks do occur from time to time in maternity or newborn baby units, and the condition is most commonly due to infection with a rotavirus. Occasionally, bacteria such as *Salmonella*, *Shigella* or *Campylobacter* species are identified in the stools. The disease can be rapidly fatal at this age, especially when it affects either low birth weight infants or those with a severe congenital malformation.

The newborn baby rapidly becomes ill from dehydration and electrolyte imbalance when diarrhoea and vomiting are profuse. The signs of dehydration are an inelastic skin, sunken eyes and fontanelle, dryness of the mouth and oliguria. Later, if left untreated, there is tachycardia, hypotension and a greyish pallor from circulatory impairment.

Treatment

Isolation from other babies is essential since the organisms are highly contagious. In addition to the clinical evaluation of the infant, estimation of blood electrolytes and urea is necessary to assess the effect of the fluid losses and to monitor the infant's progress. Replacement of excess losses of fluid and electrolytes is central to successful treatment. An initial rapid intravenous infusion of 20 mL/kg of albumin solution to improve the blood pressure and restore the circulating volume is needed for the more severely dehydrated infant, but in most cases a rather slower correction with 0.9% saline is sufficient. Once the initial replacement is complete, intravenous fluid volumes should be calculated to provide the normal daily fluid requirements plus the estimated deficit and additional losses from diarrhoea and vomiting, restoring the baby's fluid balance over 48 hours. Regular measurements of blood electrolytes and urea will guide the choice of fluids and indicate in particular whether additional sodium or potassium replacement is required.

Breast feeding should be continued unless the baby is vomiting, though cow's milk formula should not be given during treatment. Antibiotics are needed only when an accompanying septicaemia is suspected.

Acute osteomyelitis and septic arthritis

Although it is an uncommon occurrence, staphylococcal infection in bone or a joint occasionally follows some apparently minor superficial sepsis after a latent period of 2 or 3 weeks. Other organisms such as group B haemolytic streptococci and *H. influenzae* may also cause a similar infection. In the case of a long bone of the arm or leg, attention may be drawn to the condition simply by the fact that the limb is not being used (pseudoparalysis), but there is often local swelling and redness of skin. The general constitutional disturbance is surprisingly slight, though fever is almost always present. Appropriate systemic antibiotic treatment (usually flucloxacillin) is continued for several weeks, and, provided that resistant organisms are not encountered, surgical intervention is seldom needed.

USE OF ANTIBIOTICS IN THE NEWBORN PERIOD
General principles

Widespread indiscriminate use of antibiotics, especially those with a broad spectrum of activity, is to be strongly deprecated for there is evidence that usually harmless organisms can become pathogenic when the normal bacterial flora of the baby is disturbed. Increasing numbers of antibiotic-resistant organisms are emerging throughout the world from inappropriate prescribing. Prophylactic antibiotic treatment should be used only exceptionally, when its value is scientifically proven. Antibiotics are ineffective in preventing colonising organisms from causing serious infection and should not be used when, for example, an organism is cultured from an endotracheal tube but the infant has no clinical sign of sepsis. On the other hand, since the outcome of serious infections at this age is so much better if early treatment is given, the presence of non-specific clinical features of infection do justify the use of appropriate antibiotics before a specific bacterial diagnosis has been reached.

Dosage

The pathways of metabolism and excretion of many antibiotics are immature in the newborn baby. Blood levels of all antibiotics, therefore, tend to be higher and are sustained for longer in the first few days of life on a given dose, particularly if the baby has been born prematurely or is very ill. Diminished renal function will reduce the rate of disposal of drugs which are primarily excreted in the urine and the decline in blood levels of drugs eliminated by hepatic metabolism will be slowed by the immaturity of liver enzyme function in the newborn baby. It is essential to measure the blood levels of gentamicin and netilmicin, both of which are excreted mainly by the kidneys, and adjust the dose accordingly to avoid accumulation in the blood, since high concentrations of these may cause nerve deafness and renal failure.

The recommended doses of the antibiotics most commonly used in the neonatal period are given in the Pharmacopoeia in Chapter 15. The frequency of these doses varies according to the maturity of the baby, and the following dose frequencies are given as a guide to the initial dose intervals:

- For term and post-term infants (37 weeks' gestation and beyond), the dose is given 12-hourly for the first 48 hours, 8-hourly between the 3rd and 14th day, and 6-hourly thereafter.
- For pre-term infants (less than 37 weeks), the dose is given 12-hourly for the first week, 8-hourly for the second, third and fourth weeks, and 6-hourly thereafter.
- For infants of greater immaturity, the interval between doses may need to be increased further. It is not uncommon for doses to be required no more than once every 24 hours. Blood level monitoring is even more necessary, to prevent accumulation of toxic levels of the drugs.

Gut absorption of antibiotic preparations given orally is uncertain and irregular during the first week of life and so intravenous or intramuscular administration is preferable for the more seriously ill baby.

Prevention of antibiotic resistance

Because of the emergence of bacteria resistant to currently available antibiotics, it is the responsibility of all who prescribe them to minimise the risk of creating new resistant strains (Isaacs 2000). If the following guidelines are kept, the likelihood of resistant strains emerging should be reduced:

- The use of antibiotics should be confined to babies with clinical evidence of sepsis and who have had appropriate investigations.
- If bacterial cultures are negative at 2–3 days, antibiotics should be withdrawn.
- Positive cultures should be followed by a reappraisal of the treatment regimen and an antibiotic regimen prescribed appropriate to the identified pathogen. In many cases this will require the use of only a single antibiotic.
- The finding of an organism on cultures of the umbilicus, an indwelling endotracheal tube or a removed intravascular catheter should not be regarded as evidence of infection without clinical signs and requires no treatment.

VIRAL AND PROTOZOAL INFECTIONS
Antenatal infection

Transmission of bacterial infections across the placenta to the fetus is a remarkably rare event, but any infection which produces severe illness in the mother may affect fetal growth by interference with the transplacental supply of nutrients. Certain microorganisms, however, are able to pass the placental barrier, infect the fetus and interfere with its growth, differentiation or development. *Toxoplasma gondii*, rubella, cytomegalovirus, herpes simplex virus and *Treponema pallidum* (syphilis) are the best-known examples, and their effect on the fetus can be devastating. HIV may occasionally infect the fetus. It does not cause malformation of the infant, but has long-lasting effects by means of damage to the immune system after birth. Exceptionally, transplacental infection occurs from Coxsackie and varicella viruses, whilst the bacteria causing tuberculosis and listeriosis have been known to spread to the fetus in this way also. Hepatitis B probably does not cross the placenta but commonly affects the infant during labour.

Specific transplacentally acquired infections

Congenital rubella

When contracted in early pregnancy, rubella virus can cross the placenta and cause serious damage to the developing fetus. In the first 12 weeks there is a 90% chance of fetal infection, which may cause malformation of the eyes (microphthalmia, retinopathy and cataracts), the brain (microcephaly and mental retardation) and the heart (especially between the fifth and eighth weeks), and sensorineural deafness. Infection in the third month causes the deafness alone in up to 30% of cases, the risk diminishing during the fourth month. In addition, maternal infection at any stage up to 20 weeks may result in nonspecific signs at birth such as hepatosplenomegaly, jaundice, thrombocytopenia and growth retardation. X-rays of the long bones may show changes characteristic of rubella osteitis. There appears to be no significant risk if the fetus is exposed after this time. Because of such high rates of damage in the early weeks, termination of pregnancy is often considered if maternal infection can be proved by rising antibody levels.

Confirmation of the infection in the neonate may be made by virus culture from the stools or CSF or by demonstrating IgM antibodies to the virus or a persisting titre of IgG antibody over the first few months of life. Infection in the nervous system is accompanied by a high protein level and an increase in mononuclear cells in the CSF. Despite the presence of antibody, these infants continue to excrete the active virus for many months after birth and may therefore spread the infection, which can be dangerous to women in early pregnancy. Appropriate isolation precautions must thus be taken.

No treatment is available for the infection, but if the woman has antirubella antibodies before pregnancy, infection of the fetus is prevented. National rubella immunisation programmes in teenagers have all but eliminated the risk of fetal infection in their children. However, a small number of adult women are still found to be susceptible to the infection at routine screening at their first antenatal visit and they should be offered immunisation immediately after the birth of the baby. This is particularly important for any immigrants to the UK who arrive at an age beyond that covered by the school immunisation programme. The incidence of congenital rubella is doubled in women of Asian origin for this reason.

Congenital cytomegalovirus infection

Cytomegalovirus (CMV) infection is a trivial and flu-like illness in adults but infection of the fetus can result in spontaneous abortion, stillbirth, serious multisystem disease or intellectual impairment. Unsuspected CMV infection of the brain probably accounts for learning difficulties in about 400 children in Britain each year. About 1% of susceptible women acquire the infection during pregnancy and in 40% of cases it affects the fetus no matter at what stage of pregnancy it occurs. Over half of women of childbearing age have already been exposed to the virus, as shown by the presence of circulating antibodies, but reactivation of the virus during pregnancy can still involve the baby. Occasionally, the infection can be acquired from breast milk postnatally if the mother is viraemic (Hamprecht et al 2001, Golding 1997). Only about 10% of infected infants show clinical evidence of the disease at birth, but many of these infants go on to have serious long-term neurological problems. A minority of asymptomatic infants also may develop nerve deafness or other neurological deficits, though about 90% will develop quite normally.

The liveborn affected infants are often of low birth weight. The full clinical picture is one of widespread involvement of many systems of the body, with early jaundice, purpura, haemolytic anaemia, hepatosplenomegaly, pneumonia with cough and respiratory distress, or, less commonly, fits, rigidity, microcephaly, choroidoretinitis and osteitis. Longer-term complications include hepatitis, leading to cirrhosis of the liver, and progressive neurological disorders with mental retardation and cerebral palsy. The diagnosis is confirmed by isolation of the virus from cultures of the urine and a throat swab together with identification of CMV antibodies in the mother and child. In symptomatic infants, the CSF protein level is raised and mononuclear cells are found in the fluid. The antiviral agent ganciclovir is occasionally used if the baby is seriously affected, though subsequent brain damage is often not prevented by this treatment and the baby may continue to excrete the virus for some years. Prevention is not yet possible as there is no vaccine for the infection.

Congenital toxoplasmosis

Toxoplasmosis is caused by the protozoon *Toxoplasma gondii*, which behaves in a similar way to CMV. Symptomatic infection is very common in childhood and early adult life, and by the age of 20 years about a quarter of the population has acquired the antibody. Primary maternal infection occurs during two pregnancies in every 1000, but in less than half of these does the organism pass across the placenta to the infant. Infection in the first trimester is accompanied by a high risk of fetal damage, fetal death and abortion, but later infection has fewer complications. Although only 10% of babies infected before birth have clinical signs of it in the newborn period, it is these infants who will develop the later problems, the asymptomatic infants probably having no lasting effects.

The incidence of the disease in pregnancy may be partially reduced by recommending the avoidance of undercooked meat and contact with cats, which are the alternative host for the organism. If a maternal acute infection is confirmed, treatment with spiramycin throughout the pregnancy reduces the incidence of congenital disease. If fetal toxoplasmosis is diagnosed in pregnancy, the mother should be treated with spiramycin, though its efficacy in treating the fetus remains uncertain.

Although congenital toxoplasmosis may present as a fulminating type of illness with anaemia, purpura due to thrombocytopenia, jaundice and enlargement of liver and spleen, the more usual presentation is a widespread involvement of the central nervous system (CNS). In this form of the infection, fits and the signs of cerebral irritation are followed by the development of hydrocephalus and choroidoretinitis, which leads ultimately to blindness. Intracranial calcification is a later characteristic radiological finding. The diagnosis is confirmed if the organism itself and antibody to it is found in the CSF; in the absence of CNS disease, the diagnosis relies on finding antibody in the serum of the mother and baby. An affected newborn baby should be treated with alternating courses of spiramycin and a combination of sulfadiazine, pyrimethamine and folic acid for the whole of the first year to reduce the risk of choroidoretinitis.

Other viral infections
Coxsackie virus

Coxsackie B virus may occasionally be responsible for severe illness in the neonatal period, sometimes as an epidemic outbreak in a hospital unit. It is usually manifested as acute myocarditis or meningoencephalitis and no specific treatment is available.

Echoviruses

Echoviruses, usually of type II, have been increasingly recognised as a cause of neonatal illness. Infection arises mainly from the mother during delivery but may also be postnatal from others who come into contact with the baby. Outbreaks have been reported in maternity or special care neonatal units.

The clinical features vary from mild disturbance of general health to a fulminating septicaemia-like illness. Almost any system may be involved but outbreaks of gastroenteritis are perhaps most usual.

Viral cultures are essential for prevention of the spread of the infection in an outbreak, but they only help with treatment to the extent that antibiotics may be omitted. Fortunately, the great majority of echovirus infections are mild and the infant successfully uses his own defence mechanisms to achieve full recovery. Normal human immunoglobulin contains antibody to this virus, which may be of some value in treatment in the early stages of the illness.

Varicella

Maternal infection in the first few weeks of pregnancy may cause fetal varicella syndrome, which results in eye, limb and brain defects. Infection around the time of delivery can pass to the infant either before or just after birth. The chickenpox which results may be more severe than that seen in older children and has a high mortality. For these babies, treatment with intravenous acyclovir together with a dose of zoster immune globulin should be given.

CHRONIC INFECTIONS
Tuberculosis

Neonatal tuberculosis is rare in Britain, though there is a higher risk in some British Asian families where pulmonary tuberculosis is more common. It occurs more frequently in many developing countries, particularly those with a high incidence of HIV infection (Adhikari et al 1997). It can be acquired from the mother before or after birth and the symptoms are non-specific – refusal of feeds, loss of weight, vomiting, a slight pyrexia, and enlargement of the liver and spleen. It usually presents clinically some 6 weeks after birth. Death may occur from miliary tuberculosis within a month if it is not treated. The tuberculin test is of no value in diagnosis at this age since the infant is unable to react to it. The chest X-ray of an infected infant is likely to show miliary shadowing in the lungs. Treatment with rifampicin and isoniazid is likely to be fully successful if started in good time and continued for 6 months to a year.

Protection of the asymptomatic at-risk infant by treatment with isoniazid may be necessary until the immunisation with BCG vaccine has had time to take effect. Almost always, however, the maternal disease is quiescent or cured and BCG alone is sufficient. In communities where the prevalence of tuberculosis is increased, neonatal immunisation using 0.05 mL of BCG vaccine intradermally should be given to those considered at risk, but it should not be used if the baby has HIV infection or is taking steroids.

HIV infection

Although still an uncommon infection during pregnancy in the UK except in some drug abusers, HIV infection is increasing rapidly throughout the world but is particularly common in sub-Saharan Africa (Williams & Gouws 2001), where up to 30% of mothers are infected in some communities. It is wise to consider the possibility of infection in immigrants and refugees from such countries.

The acquired immune deficiency syndrome (AIDS) is a fatal disease caused by HIV. Pregnancy appears to reactivate the virus and in approximately 25% of asymptomatic carriers the baby will be infected either across the placenta or through contact with infected blood at delivery, but this falls to around 8% or less (Deville & Bryson 2001, Gibb et al 1997) if the mother has been treated with AZT during the pregnancy. The rate of fetal infection is higher in women with symptomatic disease and in those who are vitamin A deficient or who suffer from other sexually transmitted diseases. There does not appear to be any increase in the incidence of preterm labour or stillbirth.

Infection of the baby is more likely if the infant is growth retarded or preterm, or there has been prolonged rupture of the membranes or a prolonged second stage of labour.

The diagnosis of true HIV infection in the infant is difficult since maternal antibody readily transfers across the placenta and may persist in the baby's blood for some months. It may in some cases be possible to culture the virus or identify viral antigen in the baby's blood, but it is often only by the emergence of the characteristic clinical picture in the baby that infection is confirmed. Although the affected infant will be well in the

Table 11.2   Immunisation schedule for HIV-infected infants

Vaccine	Age for immunisation
Diphtheria, tetanus and pertussis	2, 3 & 4 months
Polio – inactivated i.m. vaccine[a]	2, 3 & 4 months
Influenza vaccine	6 months
Haemophilus influenzae type B (Hib)	2, 3 & 4 months
Mumps, measles, rubella (MMR)	15 months
Pneumococcal vaccine	2 years
Meningitis C vaccine	2, 3 and 4 months

[a] Oral (live) polio vaccine should *not* be administered.

neonatal period, the characteristic repeated serious infections with opportunistic organisms such as CMV and *Pneumocystis carinii* will begin to appear, leading commonly to the baby's death within the first 2 years of life.

Currently, no specific treatment exists other than that of the infections as they occur, but each potentially infected infant should receive all the vaccines in Table 11.2. Live vaccines must not be given, in view of the infant's diminished immunity. The risk of contracting *P. carinii* infection can be reduced by continuous treatment with cotrimoxazole orally once the baby's immune status is shown to be compromised.

Management

During labour in an HIV-positive woman, it is essential to avoid the use of fetal scalp electrodes or taking fetal blood samples, to prevent the direct innoculation of the virus into the bloodstream of the infant. Delivery by caesarean section significantly reduces the risk of transmission of HIV from mother to infant and it is the recommended mode of delivery where possible.

Since the mother and baby are both potentially infected, there is a risk of transmission of the virus to those caring for the infant, but only from contact with infected blood. It is wise for caregivers to wear protective gloves whenever contact with the infant's blood is likely – for instance, when taking venous or heelprick blood samples – and to wash the hands thoroughly after the procedure. Contact with other body fluids is safe since they are most unlikely to contain the virus. Isolation of the infant is not necessary, though it

is important that the mother is aware of the importance of washing her hands before and after handling the infant.

Postnatal infection through ingestion of infected maternal lymphocytes in breast milk does occur but the risk of this is probably smaller than intrapartum transmission of the virus (Michie & Gilmour 2001, Morrison 1999). HIV-positive mothers should not breast feed their infants when safe bottle feeding can be provided as an alternative. When it cannot, the small risk of transmission of HIV infection through breast milk must be balanced against the known benefits of breast feeding and other medical and social hazards which may affect the infant. The decision to breast feed or not is one which must be made in the light of the circumstances of the individual. In more affluent countries, it is usually safer to recommend formula feeding for the majority; however, where safe water is not available, breast feeding may be preferable.

Prevention of neonatal HIV infection can only be achieved by measures designed to limit spread of the infection to HIV-negative women. Screening by HIV testing at antenatal clinics remains a sensitive ethical issue but is becoming increasingly accepted as the evidence of the benefits of treatment in pregnancy is emerging (p. 178). All these facts must be carefully explained to the parents when counselling them about the risks to the infant in further pregnancies.

Social aspects of HIV infection

HIV-infected mothers have a higher incidence of other sexually transmitted diseases and in the UK are more likely to be drug abusers. Each of these situations may have an independent effect on the health of the baby (pp. 16 & 17). Social deprivation is also common and may result in adverse emotional consequences for the child (p. 16). Serious maternal ill-health from progression to AIDS may occur during the child's infancy and some mothers may die from it. As a result of these circumstances, up to 20% of children will not be living with their natural parents by 1 year of age and many will need support from the extended family and Social Services (Benson 1994).

Furthermore, in some parts of Africa, many children not infected have been orphaned as a result of losing both of their parents to AIDS. However, early follow-up studies show that the health and development are not adversely affected in the majority of uninfected infants.

Hepatitis B infection

Hepatitis B infection or carriage is widespread throughout the world but is particularly common in many developing countries, occurring in up to 10% of the population in some parts of the Far East. It is also more common amongst women who have many sexual partners or are intravenous drug abusers. Although it may cause acute hepatitis in the mother, it more commonly results in asymptomatic chronic carriage of the virus in apparently healthy people. It can be transmitted to the baby through blood and body secretions during birth, or later, by infected mothers. The risk of infection is particularly high if the mother carries the hepatitis B e antigen (HBeAg) or the HB s antigen (HBsAg). If the baby contracts the infection, he may rarely develop fulminant, and often fatal, hepatitis, but otherwise the asymptomatic chronic carrier state develops in the large majority of infants. Immunisation of the infant of a known carrier within 12 hours of birth with hepatitis B vaccine together with 200 IU of hepatitis B immunoglobulin intramuscularly reduces the risk of infection to under 5%. Without immunisation, about 70% of infants born to infected mothers will become carriers with the risk of developing chronic active hepatitis or cirrhosis of the liver in later childhood. The colostrum and milk of HBeAg-positive mothers is always infected and their babies should not breast feed until they are fully protected by the immunisation schedule.

Since the baby's blood may be infectious, the same precautions should be taken to protect the carers of the infant as were described for HIV infection.

Hepatitis C infection

Hepatitis C infection is largely asymptomatic in mothers, about half of whom infected in the UK contract the disease from intravenous drug abuse or contact with blood or blood products. Its incidence in different countries is very variable, from under 0.1% in the UK, USA and Scandinavia to around 20% in Egypt. Transmission to the baby occurs in about 6–7% of cases, but the rate is higher if the mother is also HIV positive and lower after elective caesarean section birth. Most infants have no symptoms from the infection until later life. The virus can be found in breast milk in 20% of viraemic women but the risks of breast feeding are probably small (Gibb et al 2000, Hadzic 2001).

Herpes simplex

Neonatal *Herpes simplex* infection is uncommon, though its incidence seems to be increasing. There is an increased risk of preterm birth, and, very occasionally, intrauterine infection results in microcephaly, choroidoretinitis and microphthalmia. More usually, the infection is acquired from direct contact with infectious vesicles on the mother's genitalia, and infection of the infant is more likely with recently acquired maternal infection.

In the infant, the disease may either be localised as an eye, skin or mucous membrane infection or spread in a generalised and often fatal form. Jaundice, hepatosplenomegaly, meningo-encephalitis, and sometimes haemorrhage as a result of the syndrome of disseminated intravascular coagulation (p. 187) are all features of the more serious form of the disease. Diagnosis is achieved by culture of the virus from any available area, such as a vesicle on the skin, but to be successful, treatment must be given as soon as the possibility of infection is identified, often from birth, and certainly before the disease becomes widely disseminated. Apart from general supportive measures, specific treatment of the baby with intravenous acyclovir can reduce the severity of the disease and hasten the eradication of the virus, but many survivors of the encephalitic form of the disease will remain brain damaged.

When the maternal genital herpes infection is diagnosed antenatally, caesarean section is justifiable to prevent exposure of the infant to the virus, though it is probably only necessary if there are active vesicles on the vulva at the time of delivery. It is not yet clear whether antenatal administration of antiviral agents is beneficial for the baby, but it is not necessary to use them prophylactically in asymptomatic babies after birth.

Congenital syphilis

Syphilis, which is caused by infection with the spirochete *Treponema pallidum*, is common in many parts of the world, but in Britain, only about 10–15 cases of congenital infection are identified each year. One-third of affected infants are stillborn and half are born with active infection. The more recently the mother has acquired the disease, the more likely the baby is to be affected.

Routine early antenatal blood tests for maternal syphilis had almost eliminated congenital syphilis in the UK, but the recorded incidence of the infection in adults is rising and the possibility of congenital infection must again be considered. The infection involves the placenta and is not acquired by the fetus before the fourth month of pregnancy. Thus, to prevent fetal infection, serological testing should be undertaken and the mother treated with penicillin before that time.

The clinical features are sometimes present at birth, but more often they appear between the second and sixth weeks. The classical signs of the condition include the following: purulent rhinitis with a profuse and sometimes bloody discharge; various skin eruptions (generally maculopapular with a copper tinge fading to brown); splenic enlargement which is almost invariable; and jaundice with enlargement of the liver due at first to fatty infiltration and later to pericellular cirrhosis. Anaemia is a usual finding and bone involvement shows radiologically as a thickened dense epiphyseal line at the end of the long bones with a zone of rarefaction proximal to it (Fig. 11.4). The finding of specific IgM antibody in the baby's blood is now the most useful diagnostic test. The Venereal Disease Research Laboratories (VDRL) test on serum may be falsely negative or positive at birth and during the first few weeks. False-positive reactions occur often in those

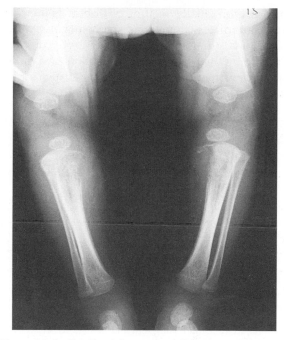

Figure 11.4   Osteitis of the proximal tibiae in congenital syphilis.

whose mother's reaction is positive, so, in the absence of other clinical signs, the test should be repeated at 3 months, before regarding it as a reason to start treatment. The CSF should be examined once the diagnosis is made because involvement of the CNS influences the duration of the treatment. Penicillin 15 mg/kg body weight twice daily by intramuscular injection for a minimum of 10 days is the treatment of choice and most cases respond well to this regimen.

Malaria

This infestation should be considered in any febrile baby whose mother, during the pregnancy, visited a country where malaria occurs. Pregnant women seem more susceptible to infection with malarial parasites in countries where it is common. *Plasmodium falciparum* may infect the placenta, reducing its function and causing intrauterine growth retardation in the fetus. It can also cause premature labour. The organism only rarely crosses the placenta to the fetus; however, if it does, the baby is usually well at birth but develops a fever, jaundice, anaemia and splenomegaly within 10–20 days. Infection is confirmed by finding the parasite by microscopical examination of a blood smear. Treatment with chloroquine 10 mg/kg by mouth immediately, repeated 6 hours later and followed the next day with two doses of 5 mg/kg, should overcome the initial illness. A blood transfusion may be needed if the anaemia is severe.

REFERENCES

Adhikari M, Pillay T, Pillay D G 1997 Tuberculosis in the newborn: an emerging disease. Pediatric Infectious Disease Journal 16(12):1108–1112

Benson M S 1994 Management of infants born to women infected with the human immunodeficiency virus. Journal of Perinatal and Neonatal Nursing 74:79–89

Berger A, Saltzer H R, Weninger M et al 1998 Septicaemia in an Austrian neonatal intensive care unit: a 7-year analysis. Acta Paediatrica 87(10):1066–1069

Deville J, Bryson Y 2001 Perinatal transmission of HIV: recognition and treatment interventions. Current Infectious Disease Reports 3(4):388–396

Gibb D M, MacDonagh S E, Tooley P A et al 1997 Uptake of interventions to reduce mother-to-child transmission of HIV in the United Kingdom and Ireland. AIDS 11(7):F53–F57

Gibb D M, Goodall R L, Dunn D T et al 2000 Mother to child transmission of hepatitis C virus: evidence for preventable peripartum transmission. Lancet 356:904–907

Golding J 1997 Unnatural constituents of breast milk – medication, lifestyle, pollutants, viruses. Early Human Development 49(suppl.):S29–S43

Hadzic N 2001 Hepatitis C in pregnancy. Archives of Disease in Childhood Fetal and Neonatal Edition 84(3):F201–F204

Hamprecht K, Maschmann J, Vochem M 2001 Epidemiology of transmission of cytomegalovirus from mother to preterm infant by breastfeeding. Lancet 357:513–518

Holt D E, Halket S, de Louvois J et al 2000 Neonatal meningitis in England and Wales: 10 years on. Archives of Disease in Childhood Fetal and Neonatal Edition 82:F85–F89

Isaacs D 2000 Rationing antibiotic use in neonatal units. Archives of Disease in Childhood Fetal and Neonatal Edition 82:F1–F2

Jain S 1999 Perinatally acquired Chlamydia trachomatis associated morbidity in young infants. Journal of Maternal and Fetal Medicine 8(3):130–133

Jenson H B, Pollock B H 1997 Meta-analyses of the effectiveness of intravenous immunoglobulin for prevention and treatment of neonatal sepsis. Pediatrics 99(2):E2

Klinger G, Chin C N, Beyene J et al 2000 Predicting the outcome of neonatal meningitis. Pediatrics 106(3):477–482

Michie C A, Gilmour J 2001 Breast feeding and the risks of viral transmission. Archives of Disease in Childhood 84:381–383

Modi N, Carr R 2000 Promising strategems for reducing the burden of neonatal sepsis. Archives of Disease in Childhood Fetal and Neonatal Edition 83:F150–F153

Morrison P 1999 HIV and infant feeding: to breast feed or not to breast feed: the dilemma of competing risks. Breastfeeding Review 7(3):11–20

Ohlsson A, Lacy J B 2001 Intravenous immunoglobulin for suspected or subsequently proven infection in neonates (Cochrane Review). Cochrane Database of Systematic Reviews 2:CD001239

Pauli I, Shekhawat P, Kehl S et al 1999 Early detection of bacteraemia in the intensive care unit using the new BACTEC system. Journal of Perinatology 19(2):127–131

Towers C V, Suriano K, Asrat T 1999 The capture rate of at-risk newborns for early onset group B streptococcal sepsis determined by a risk factor approach. American Journal of Obstetrics and Gynecology 181:1243–1249

Williams B G, Gouws E 2001 The epidemiology of human immunodeficiency virus in South Africa. Philosophical Transactions of the Royal Society of London Board of Biological Sciences 356(1141):1077–1086

Chapter 12
Haematological problems and jaundice

CHAPTER CONTENTS

Haematological values in the healthy term infant   183
Polycythaemia and anaemia at birth   183
Blood transfusion   184
Haemorrhagic disorders and bleeding   185
   Fetal haemorrhage   185
   Haemorrhage in the newborn baby   185
   Haemorrhagic disease of the newborn   186
   Disseminated intravascular coagulation   187
   Hereditary clotting factor deficiencies   187
   Purpura and bruising   187
Haemoglobinopathies   188
Jaundice   188
   Patterns of jaundice   189
   Investigation in neonatal jaundice   189
   Kernicterus and bilirubin encephalopathy   190
   Haemolytic disease of the newborn   191
   Rhesus haemolytic disease   191
   Haemolytic disease due to ABO incompatibility   194
   Inherited causes of haemolytic disease   194
   Jaundice in preterm infants   195
   Evaluation of the severity of jaundice   195
   Treatment of haemolytic jaundice   195
   Other common causes of jaundice   197
   Obstructive jaundice   198

HAEMATOLOGICAL VALUES IN THE HEALTHY TERM INFANT

Large changes take place in the constituents of the blood during the first few hours and days of life; furthermore, the range of variation from one baby to another is relatively wide compared with that in the adult. It is therefore difficult to define normal values for the newborn baby but the values given in Table 12.1 are those commonly seen in healthy term infants.

The blood volume is about 85 mL/kg body weight (40 mL/lb), giving the average 3-kg baby a total blood volume of 240–300 mL. Thus, the loss of 40–50 mL of blood from a newborn infant is roughly equivalent to a loss of 500 mL from an adult.

POLYCYTHAEMIA AND ANAEMIA AT BIRTH

The oxygen tension in the fetal blood is only about 3–4 kPa (20–30 mmHg), as compared with the healthy newborn value of 12–13 kPa (90–100 mmHg), and thus the amount of oxygen available to the fetus is relatively small. To offset this, the fetus produces large numbers of red cells containing fetal haemoglobin (which has a higher oxygen-carrying capacity) to enable them to obtain sufficient oxygen for the fetus direct from the maternal red cells across the placental membrane. Certain antenatal factors – such as intrauterine growth retardation or fetal hypoxia from placental insufficiency, and maternal diabetes – increase the red cell production still further. Haemoconcentration occurs in all babies in

Table 12.1 Haematological values in the newborn baby

Constituent	Value	Comments
Blood volume	85 mL/kg (40 mL/lb)	
Haemoglobin (Hb)	Range: 15–20 g/dL (Average 17 g/dL)	Lower in preterm infants; the value is influenced significantly by the volume of placental transfusion before the cord is cut
Packed cell volume (PCV)	Range: 36–60%	Rises to an average maximum of 70% at about 3 hours of age, then falls to around 50% in 2 days
Red cell count	At birth: 6×10^{12}/L At 4 weeks: 4.5×10^{12}/L	The fall is due to reduced red cell production in the bone marrow, which fails to keep pace with the natural loss of red cells
White cell count	Range: $6–22 \times 10^{9}$/L	The total count falls after the second day, changing from predominantly neutrophils to lymphocytes, which account for about 60% of white cells by 14 days
Platelets	Range: $150–200 \times 10^{12}$/L	Similar to adult values

the first few hours of life, resulting in a small additional rise.

Occasionally in these circumstances, the blood becomes excessively viscous and the circulation sluggish. Whilst this polycythaemia usually causes no obvious trouble, at a packed cell volume (PCV) of over 65% the viscosity of the blood rises steeply and may give rise to respiratory difficulty or cerebral symptoms from slowing of the blood flow within the first few days of life. If the PCV is greater than 70%, cerebral blood flow may be compromised and the blood should be diluted to reduce its viscosity by a small plasma exchange transfusion. Through a catheter placed in the umbilical vein, small volumes of blood are removed and replaced by similar volumes of human albumin solution repeatedly until 20 mL/kg of blood have been exchanged.

On the other hand, a mild degree of anaemia may result from clamping the umbilical cord before the baby has received the full quota of placental blood through the umbilical vein. Holding the baby above the level of the placenta after birth – for instance, by delivering the baby up onto the mother's abdomen – does not prevent this placental transfusion of blood.

During the first 6–8 weeks of life, the haemoglobin level slowly falls, since the bone marrow does not initially replace the expiring red cells. The iron from these cells is stored. At the lowest point, the haemoglobin concentration may fall as far as 9 g/dL, or lower in the preterm infant, and iron supplements do not prevent the fall. When the available haemoglobin is unable to sustain adequate blood oxygen levels, the kidneys restart production of erythropoietin, which increases red cell production in the bone marrow, resulting in a rise in the haemoglobin level in the blood. This usually occurs at around 8–10 weeks of age. So long as there are no symptoms from this 'physiological anaemia', it requires no investigation or treatment. If, on the other hand, the infant becomes tired, breathless or slow to feed, it may be sufficient to check that the number of reticulocytes (immature red cells) in the blood is elevated – which indicates that the bone marrow is actively producing red cells – and follow the rise in haemoglobin level at weekly intervals. It is occasionally necessary to give a small top-up transfusion of blood.

BLOOD TRANSFUSION

Administering blood or blood products is a procedure frequently seen on the neonatal unit but is one which should never be undertaken lightly (McCormack 1998). The need for a transfusion and its risks should be discussed with the parents and they should be enabled to voice their concerns. In some units it is policy to obtain written consent from the parents. Some religions forbid transfusions and in these circumstances the parents' wishes should be noted. It is essential that honest but clear information be given to the parents about the hazard to the baby from not having a transfusion. In many cases, discussion can resolve the situation. Very occasionally it may be necessary to obtain a court ruling on whether the transfusion should go ahead.

The following gives guidance on the management of a blood transfusion intended primarily to raise the oxygen-carrying capacity of the blood:

- Packed red cells, rather than whole blood, are used to treat neonatal anaemia.
- The volume of a packed-cells transfusion can be calculated using the formula: Desired rise of Hb (g) × baby's weight (kg) × 4.
- Blood must be cross-matched against the mother's blood, as the circulating antibodies are all maternal in the neonatal period.
- As the baby has not yet produced his own antibodies, it is essential that transfused blood is free from blood-borne viruses such as cytomegalovirus, hepatitis B and human immunodeficiency virus (HIV).
- Transfusions are generally given over about 4 hours, though the blood is only stable at room temperature for about 6 hours.
- If there is concern the baby may become fluid overloaded, either a diuretic can be given or the maintenance fluids reduced for the duration of the transfusion.
- Baseline recordings of the baby's heart rate, respiratory rate, temperature and blood pressure should be documented and these variables monitored throughout the transfusion.
- The site of the intravenous cannula should be inspected for signs of extravasation of blood during the transfusion.

HAEMORRHAGIC DISORDERS AND BLEEDING
Fetal haemorrhage

Blood loss from the baby may occur before, during or after birth. The antenatal loss of blood from fetal to maternal circulation is a recognised occurrence, though it is rarely diagnosed. It may occur spontaneously across the placental membrane or be a complication of amniocentesis or fetal blood sampling. It can be confirmed, if suspected, by finding red cells containing fetal haemoglobin in the mother's blood (p. 192). Transfer of blood from one twin to another is commonly diagnosable at birth as it can result in substantially different haemoglobin concentrations in the two infants. Occasionally, this may result in heart failure in the baby receiving the extra blood in utero, but it is more usual for one twin to require a top-up transfusion because of a significant anaemia (p. 57).

Bleeding into the liquor or birth canal during delivery, from rupture of vessels on the fetal side of the placental circulation or from the umbilical cord, may cause a serious enough loss to require an emergency blood transfusion to restore the blood volume and haemoglobin level. It is more likely to occur if there is placenta praevia or a velamentous insertion of the cord, and the bleeding can be difficult to distinguish from maternal blood. As the fetal blood volume is only 80 mL for every kilogram of body weight, the loss of as little as 50 mL of blood can rapidly put a newborn baby into hypovolaemic shock, which causes pallor, tachycardia and tachypnoea. Unless blood loss is thought of as a possible cause of these symptoms, they can easily be misinterpreted as asphyxia and the vital blood volume replacement omitted. Transfusion of a minimum of 20 mL/kg body weight should be given immediately the condition is identified, further volumes being given if needed to raise the haemoglobin above 12 g/dL.

Haemorrhage in the newborn baby

Haemorrhage after birth may occur from many sites. The umbilical cord stump may bleed, but this is usually prevented by proper cord clamping. Rarely, enough blood may accumulate in a cephalhaematoma to cause loss of blood volume. Haematemesis and melaena most commonly result either from maternal blood being swallowed during delivery or from blood-contaminated milk being ingested during breast feeding. The maternal origin of the blood can be confirmed by identifying exclusively adult haemoglobin in the vomit or stool. Pulmonary haemorrhage and intraventricular bleeding are almost always complications of severe hyaline membrane disease in preterm infants. Vaginal bleeding, which results from hormonal changes after birth, is common, benign and resolves rapidly without treatment.

These conditions usually cause relatively limited blood loss and treatment is confined to that of the underlying cause. Nevertheless, if it is thought that the blood loss is significant, the haemoglobin level, platelet count and clotting studies should be checked and blood cross-matched against the mother's blood in case a transfusion is needed. All infants who have had a bleed should also be given intramuscular vitamin K, 1 mg, to ensure early treatment if the cause turns out to be haemorrhagic disease of the newborn.

Haemorrhagic disease of the newborn

Vitamin K is derived from food and is also synthesised in the gut by intestinal bacteria. It is essential for the production of blood clotting factors II, VII, IX and X by the liver. If these are deficient, the baby may bleed spontaneously from one or more sites. This condition, known as haemorrhagic disease of the newborn, most commonly occurs between the third and sixth days of life but can occur even several weeks after birth. It is confined to exclusively breast-fed infants, as breast milk contains little vitamin K whereas all formula milks contain sufficient quantities to prevent the condition in all but babies with liver disease.

Most commonly, bleeding occurs from the gastrointestinal tract, either as haematemesis or as melaena. Less often, it presents as an intracranial haemorrhage, haematuria or umbilical stump bleeding. Haemorrhagic disease should be considered likely if the prothrombin time, which measures the vitamin K-dependent blood clotting factors, and the partial thromboplastin time are prolonged and the platelets normal, but it must be remembered that the normal prothrombin time in the newborn is only some 20–50% of the adult value.

Once haemorrhage has occurred, the treatment depends on its severity. In the milder cases with little or no evidence of loss of blood volume, it may be sufficient to give 1 mg of vitamin K intramuscularly. The baby is kept warm and observed half-hourly. Increasing pallor, the development of tachycardia above 160 beats/min and a falling blood pressure are indicators of serious blood loss requiring an urgent replacement of blood. Fresh frozen plasma contains the deficient clotting factors, and rapid intravenous infusion of about 20 mL/kg body weight is sufficient both to stop bleeding and to restore the blood volume. This may have to be followed by a slower transfusion of fresh blood if the loss has been great enough to cause symptomatic anaemia.

Venepunctures for samples for investigation of bleeding and clotting disorders must only be taken from peripheral veins. Puncture of the femoral vein and neck vessels can cause serious bleeding which is difficult to contain (Plate 17). After all other venepunctures and heelpricks, local pressure should be applied to prevent bruising. Intramuscular injections should not be given until a clotting factor deficiency has been excluded by the appropriate tests.

Prevention

Prevention of this form of haemorrhagic disease is assured either by intramuscular administration of 1 mg of vitamin K on the first day of life or by formula feeding from birth, since all such milks are fortified with this vitamin in the UK. A single oral dose of vitamin K at birth to all gives protection from such bleeding for the first week or two but does not completely prevent it occurring later on. A report in 1992 (Golding et al 1992) suggested a link between childhood leukaemia and intramuscular vitamin K administration, but several further studies have failed to either prove or disprove the association (Von Kries 1999). Thus, at present, oral prophylaxis is preferred. Several trials of ongoing oral vitamin K supplementation for breast-fed infants, mostly using oral Konakion, have been carried out. Repeated oral doses at 2-week intervals have been shown to give almost complete protection. In one study (Wariyar et al

---

Box 12.1 Prevention of haemorrhagic disease of the newborn; Recommendations of the Royal College of Paediatrics and Child Health

- All newborn infants should receive vitamin K
- Intramuscular vitamin K ensures adequate prophylaxis in normal term infants
- One dose of vitamin K orally is adequate prophylaxis for the majority of normal term infants; further doses should be considered for breast-fed infants
- Infants with jaundice suggestive of cholestasis and infants with unexplained bleeding should receive further vitamin K, preferably parenterally

---

2000) using a medium-chain triglyceride based preparation (Orakay), the only failures were where the vitamin was not given as recommended or the baby had undiagnosed liver disease. The Royal College of Paediatrics and Child Health recommendations (Box 12.1) also indicate the importance of intramuscular vitamin K for those found to have liver disorders. In the unusual case of a mother taking warfarin, rifampicin or anticonvulsants, all of which interfere with vitamin K metabolism, intramuscular administration of vitamin K 0.1 mg/kg during the pregnancy is advised. Whatever method is chosen to prevent haemorrhagic disease of the newborn, it is prudent for the parent to give consent to its administration after being fully informed about the slight uncertainties which remain about its safety.

Disseminated intravascular coagulation

A more severe haemorrhagic state may arise when the circulating clotting factors and platelets are consumed in a widespread process of clotting in small blood vessels. This uncommon condition, known as disseminated intravascular coagulation, usually occurs as a complication of septicaemia. The bleeding which results from the consequent lack of clotting factors may occur from any site and the falling platelet count may cause purpura to appear in the skin. The diagnosis is made by finding red cell fragmentation on microscopy of blood smears and an increase in fibrin degradation products in the blood.

Treatment is directed primarily towards the underlying condition. The use of heparin, by intravenous infusion, to prevent further intravascular clotting is of little value in the newborn period. Fresh frozen plasma may help by replacing depleted clotting factors, and exchange transfusion may occasionally be needed.

Hereditary clotting factor deficiencies

Disorders such as haemophilia (factor VIII deficiency) and Christmas disease (factor IX deficiency) rarely cause prolonged bleeding in the neonatal period. However, when there is a family history, extra care should be taken to observe sites of potential haemorrhage, such as the umbilical cord stump and the site of heelpricks. These problems may be reduced if the haemophilia has been identified in early pregnancy by DNA analysis of samples of fetal blood.

Purpura and bruising

Bruising into the skin most commonly occurs during delivery, particularly during breech presentation, when the buttocks and genitalia may be affected. In very preterm infants it may result from deficient clotting factors and an excessive capillary fragility, both of which are related to the baby's immaturity. Petechiae from capillary leakage are often seen in term infants due to congestion – as in 'traumatic cyanosis' (p. 62) – asphyxia or a deficiency of platelets.

Platelet numbers vary markedly in the neonatal period. However, the further they fall below 100×10^{12}/L, the greater is the risk of bruising and bleeding, though the risk varies with the underlying cause. Thrombocytopenia may be a consequence of any severe infection, including the antenatal infections (p. 176). It is also found in disseminated intravascular coagulation.

Platelet deficiency also occurs in about 50% of infants whose mothers suffer from idiopathic thrombocytopenic purpura, due to transmission of maternal IgG antiplatelet antibodies across the placenta. The purpura and bleeding may be severe enough to require fresh platelet transfusion, though the thrombocytopenia is usually mild and transient. Corticosteroid treatment is ineffective but infusion of immunoglobulin may raise the platelet count in some cases (Roberts & Murray 2001).

Very occasionally, thrombocytopenia is found to be due to incompatibility of the platelets between the mother and baby in a way rather similar to that of Rhesus haemolytic disease of the newborn (Kaplan 2001). It may be the presenting feature of congenital leukaemia and is also seen in cases of congenital hypoplastic anaemia.

HAEMOGLOBINOPATHIES

Although thalassaemia and sickle cell disease cause few problems in the neonatal period, they are included here since both are inherited as recessive disorders, which makes early diagnosis desirable, particularly for genetic counselling of the parents (p. 213). In both disorders, carriers of the defective gene can be identified, and advice for prospective parents who are carriers has reduced the incidence of the major forms of the disease.

In thalassaemia, defective haemoglobin synthesis causes a severe anaemia after the first few months of life, requiring repeated blood transfusions if the sufferer is to survive. It occurs mainly in people from the Mediterranean countries and those from the Indian subcontinent. Prenatal diagnosis by DNA analysis of chorionic villus samples and termination of affected pregnancies have almost eliminated thalassaemia in Cypriots in Britain, but so far this approach has been less acceptable to the UK Pakistani population (Cao et al 1998).

Sickle cell disease results in crises of haemolytic anaemia throughout childhood and primarily occurs in those originating from Black African countries.

Both these conditions can be identified by haemoglobin electrophoresis from the 'Guthrie' blood spot, and screening for both conditions is now routine in certain parts of the USA where people from many ethnic groups live (p. 76).

JAUNDICE

Jaundice is a yellow discoloration of the skin and is very common in the newborn period. It has

Table 12.2 Bilirubin metabolism and the origins of neonatal jaundice

Metabolism of bilirubin	Pathological mechanisms which result in neonatal jaundice
Haemoglobin breakdown ↓	Excess breakdown of red cells e.g. Rhesus haemolytic disease, ABO incompatibility, G6PD deficiency, congenital spherocytosis
Porphyrins ↓	
Unconjugated bilirubin ↓	
Conjugation by liver enzymes ↓	Diminished activity of enzymes e.g. physiological jaundice, prematurity, urinary infection, breast milk jaundice, hypothyoridism
Conjugated bilirubin ↓	Neonatal hepatitis prevents excretion of conjugated bilirubin
Passes through bile duct ↓	Obstruction to the flow of bile e.g. biliary atresia, choledocal cyst
Excreted in stools	

G6PD = glucose-6-phosphate dehydrogenase.

many causes. In some circumstances, the condition is serious and may threaten life or impair normal development. Consequently, it should always be taken seriously, investigated urgently and treatment instituted without delay when necessary. An understanding of the formation and metabolism of bilirubin should help an understanding of the many causes of neonatal jaundice (Table 12.2).

All red blood cells have a maximum lifespan of 120 days (around 80 days in the preterm baby), after which they release haemoglobin into the circulation as they die. As it is metabolised, the iron from the haemoglobin molecule is stored and reutilised. The protein is broken down and resynthesized. Porphyrin, the molecule which aggregates with the iron, is broken down in the circulation to bilirubin, a yellow pigment which is fat soluble. When produced in normal quantities, the liver metabolises bilirubin by conjugating it with glucuronic acid to yield a water-soluble compound which is also yellow in colour. This is excreted via the bile duct into the gut, causing the yellow colour of the newborn infant's stools. In the gut, the excess bilirubin is broken down by the gut bacteria to urobilinogen, which is reabsorbed and excreted in the urine.

The liver enzyme glucuronyl transferase, which conjugates the bilirubin, becomes effective slowly after birth and so it takes several days for the liver to cope with the amount of bilirubin produced by the normal turnover of haemoglobin. The consequent rise of unconjugated bilirubin concentration in the blood and its deposition in the skin is sufficient to cause visible jaundice in a third or more of healthy term infants and is called 'physiological' jaundice.

More severe jaundice associated with raised levels of unconjugated bilirubin follows an unusually rapid breakdown (haemolysis) of red cells, which is most often the result of incompatibility between the blood groups of the mother and baby. As the bilirubin in this type of jaundice is fat soluble, the kidneys cannot excrete it and the urine is not bile stained. The excess load of bilirubin is excreted as fast as the liver is able in the bile, resulting in an excess of urobilinogen derived from the breakdown of bilirubin in the gut. If there is obstruction to the outlet pathways for bile in the liver or bile ducts, the resultant jaundice is due to an accumulation of bilirubin which has been normally conjugated by the liver. Being water soluble, this form of bilirubin is excreted in the urine, which is thus dark in colour.

When jaundice occurs because of impairment of liver cell function, as in hepatitis, there is usually some intrahepatic obstruction to the flow of bile as well as liver enzyme failure, so the excess bilirubin is partly unconjugated but mainly conjugated. Some will therefore be excreted in the urine because it is water soluble. Jaundice associated with dark yellow or brown urine is never normal and investigation must be undertaken to find its cause (p. 198).

Conversion of unconjugated bilirubin deposited in the skin to a water-soluble product which can be excreted also takes place through the action of daylight or its equivalent. This disposal mechanism is made use of in phototherapy (p. 195).

Patterns of jaundice

Jaundice is a common physiological event, occurring in around one in three full-term infants during the first week of life. Nevertheless, the possibility of a pathological process should always be considered both because of the risk to the infant from the jaundice itself and because of the importance of identifying the cause and instituting treatment. The level of bilirubin is notoriously difficult to gauge clinically, especially in dark-skinned babies, and should always be measured in the blood where there is any clinical suspicion either that the level is high or that the infant has a serious underlying cause for it. Any jaundice with a serum bilirubin level over $200 \, \mu mol/L$ (12 mg/dL) should be investigated to identify the underlying cause.

Jaundice may appear with one of a number of characteristic patterns (Fig. 12.1) (Brown et al 1993). If it occurs within the first 24 hours and the bilirubin level rises at a rate of more than $10 \, \mu mol/L$ (0.5 mg/dL) per hour, the likely cause is a serious haemolytic process (p. 191). When it rises more slowly over 3–4 days and then falls towards normal, it is likely to be physiological and due to immaturity of the hepatic bilirubin conjugation enzymes. The level of bilirubin can be increased by, for example, an excessive load of haemoglobin from a large cephalhaematoma, polycythaemia, dehydration, calorie deprivation or even sepsis. Prolongation of moderately high levels of bilirubin beyond the 10th day of life may be associated with prematurity, urinary infection, hypothyroidism or, most commonly, breast feeding (p. 197). Very rarely, galactosaemia may be a cause. Later-rising jaundice is often associated with the accumulation of conjugated bilirubin due either to obstruction of the bile ducts or to hepatitis (p. 198).

Investigation in neonatal jaundice

It is important to establish at the outset whether the baby's bilirubin is conjugated or unconjugated, since the investigations required are very

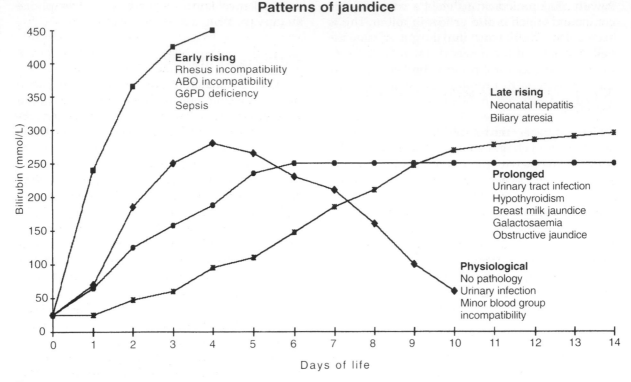

Figure 12.1 Patterns of neonatal jaundice with some illustrative causes.

different. If unconjugated, investigation should seek to exclude a blood group incompatibility between mother and baby, sepsis, red cell enzyme abnormalities and serious metabolic disease such as galactosaemia. If it is conjugated, liver function tests, blood clotting studies (to exclude a deficiency of vitamin K-dependent factors produced by the liver) and specific tests to identify the cause of obstruction to bile flow should be performed (p. 199).

Kernicterus and bilirubin encephalopathy

When unconjugated bilirubin in the plasma rises above a threshold value, it is deposited in the body tissues. The brain is particularly vulnerable since it contains so much fat, and damage from excessive bile pigment there is known as kernicterus, which causes the clinical picture of bilirubin encephalopathy. The infant becomes lethargic, refusing to suck, and may show muscular twitching, eye rolling, rigidity with arching of the back and, finally, respiratory failure. In the absence of treatment, two-thirds of these babies would die at this stage, whilst the remainder would be handicapped in later life by the choreoathetoid form of cerebral palsy, learning difficulties or nerve deafness. The point at which hyperbilirubinaemia becomes a danger to the developing brain is not determined by a critical blood level but is influenced by many other factors. Albumin in the blood binds a proportion of the circulating bilirubin, rendering it innocuous, so kernicterus occurs more readily when the albumin level is low. Partly for this reason, the brain is vulnerable at lower bilirubin levels in preterm infants. The danger is increased by any substance which competes with bilirubin for binding sites with albumin; certain sulphonamide-containing drugs and the benzoate preservative in diazepam injection solution, for instance, have this action. A period of asphyxia, acidosis, hypo-glycaemia, hypothermia or significant dehydration (Bertini 2001) may add significantly to the risk of kernicterus.

At what point is there a serious risk of brain damage?

Taking all these factors into account, it is only possible to give general guidance about the bilirubin level at which brain damage is likely to occur. In the term baby, a level of 425 μmol/L (25 mg/dL) or more of unconjugated bilirubin may be regarded as dangerous. When less than 36 weeks of gestation, or when there has been a period of asphyxia, the blood level must be kept below 300 μmol/L (18 mg/dL), and in the very low birth weight or very preterm infant, below 250 μmol/L (15 mg/dL).

Haemolytic disease of the newborn

Several different processes accelerate the breakdown of red cells in the blood and release greater amounts of bilirubin into the circulation. This is known as haemolysis and is a common cause of significant jaundice in the neonate. It may result from:

- an incompatibility of blood groups between mother and baby
- abnormalities of shape or structure of the red cells
- inherited deficiencies of enzymes in the red cells
- sepsis.

Rhesus haemolytic disease

Development of Rhesus antibodies

This disease arises from a discrepancy between the Rhesus (Rh) blood type of the mother and fetus. Rh-positive people have Rh antigen on the surface of their red cells. Those who are Rh negative have no Rh surface antigen, but when Rh-positive cells enter the circulation IgG antibodies are formed against it, which rapidly destroy the Rh-positive cells. A Rh-negative mother carrying

a Rh-positive baby may receive a transfer of Rh-positive cells across the placenta or during birth and form Rh antibodies. In a subsequent pregnancy, she will transfer these antibodies back across the placenta to the baby. If the infant is Rh positive, the maternal antibodies will attach to the Rh antigen and the red cells will be destroyed more rapidly than usual. It is this rapid destruction of red cells which is the basis of the disease in the baby.

Fortunately, the development of antibodies occurs in only 10% of such pregnancies. In white ethnic groups, around 85% of people are Rh positive and 15% negative, and although 1 in 10 pregnancies will have a Rh-negative mother and a Rh-positive father, only around 1 in 100 pregnancies is affected by the disease. However, the percentage of Rh-negative people varies from country to country and the incidence of this disease also varies. For example, only 1% of West African people are Rh negative, so the disease is rare in that ethnic group.

To fully appreciate this disease and its proper management, it is also important to know how the Rh gene is inherited. There are three pairs of genes, named C, D and E, which endow the red cells of the bearer with Rh C, D or E antigens and these people are called Rh positive. Those who receive a gene which does not produce the Rh antigen are designated c, d or e. Only the D gene causes haemolytic disease, so the discussion will be limited to this, but the same mechanisms apply to the inheritance of C and E antigens and many other genes also. Each parent has either DD, Dd or dd genes. As D is dominant, both DD (homozygous) and Dd (heterozygous) people are Rh positive but those with dd (homozygous recessive) are Rh negative.

Figure 12.2 illustrates the various situations for a Rh-negative mother. If the father is Rh negative, the pair cannot produce a Rh-positive offspring as neither carries the D gene. A DD father will pass to all his children the D gene and all his children will be Rh positive, but half the offspring of a Dd father will be Rh positive and half Rh negative. Thus, the disease occurs only when the father is Rh positive and the mother Rh negative.

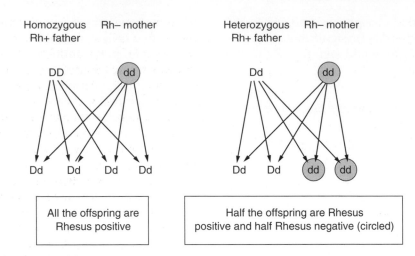

Figure 12.2   Diagram to show the inheritance of the Rhesus blood groups.

Clinical impact of Rhesus antibodies

The amount of antibody transferred from the mother to the baby across the placenta will determine how the baby is affected:

- Transfer of large amounts of antibody will result in severe haemolysis during the pregnancy, which can cause severe anaemia and heart failure. The gross generalised oedema and ascites which results is known as hydrops fetalis. Without treatment, stillbirth is common in this condition.
- Moderate antibody transfer causes jaundice arising during the first few hours after birth associated with a variable degree of progressive haemolytic anaemia; the jaundice is not obviously present at birth because until then the excess of bilirubin has been excreted through the placenta by the mother.
- A smaller antibody load results only in a gradual onset of anaemia during the course of the first few weeks with no more than slight jaundice.

The main threats to an affected liveborn baby are developing severe anaemia or kernicterus from rapidly progressive hyperbilirubinaemia. The bilirubin level reached depends on the balance between the rate of red cell destruction and the rate of bilirubin excretion. The latter varies with the efficiency of liver enzyme function, which may be impaired by this disease. Preterm infants have even less efficient bilirubin conjugation mechanisms, so the shorter the gestation period, the more likely is severe jaundice to occur (p. 121).

Prevention

The appropriate and timely use of anti-D immunoglobulin is an effective method of prevention except where maternal Rh antibodies are already present, failures usually relating to late administration or omission of the dose (Hughes et al 1994, Howard et al 1997). Using the Kleihauer technique of acid elution on maternal blood, it is possible to show immediately after the birth of the first baby whether or not fetal red cells have entered the maternal circulation and, if so, the size of this 'transfusion'. Giving the affected mother anti-D globulin intramuscularly within 48 hours after delivery of the baby destroys the 'transfused' fetal Rh-positive red cells; 100 μg of the immunoglobulin is generally used, but the dose depends on the size of the fetomaternal transfusion.

If the mother and child are ABO incompatible (mother O, infant A or B), the fetal cells are destroyed in the maternal circulation and no sensitisation ensues. Some centres are researching the use of antenatal anti-D but the results are not yet conclusive.

Antenatal management

Blood grouping should be done at the first antenatal visit and all Rh-negative women tested for Rh antibodies. If antibodies are not present, the test should be repeated at 28, 32 and 36 weeks. If antibodies are found, the quantity of antibody should be measured frequently throughout the pregnancy, but an assessment of antibody levels alone does not accurately predict the severity of disease. Amniocentesis to assess the degree of staining of the liquor with bile pigment and the actual quantity of the antibody, undertaken between the 30th and 36th weeks of pregnancy, increases the accuracy.

As the disease often increases in severity in subsequent pregnancies, antibody levels must be interpreted in the light of previous experience. In the most severely affected cases, haemolysis causes such a fall in haemoglobin level that heart failure results. In such babies, ultrasound scans show fetal ascites or pleural effusions. In this situation, a transfusion of group O Rh-negative blood cross-matched against the mother's blood into the umbilical vein will often prevent fetal death in utero. This procedure is performed under direct vision at amnioscopy, but is only available at a few specialist centres. When such extreme measures are not needed, a judgement must be made when to deliver the baby, balancing the risks from increasing disease severity as the pregnancy progresses against the hazards of prematurity from early delivery. In general, intrauterine transfusions are preferable before 30 weeks' gestation whereas premature elective delivery with exchange transfusion after birth is the lesser-risk approach after that point.

Management at birth

The presence of maternal antibodies does not always imply an affected baby. For example, half the offspring of heterozygous fathers will be Rh negative and therefore unaffected, or antibodies may not be transferred across the placenta in sufficient quantity to affect the infant. To establish the diagnosis, specimens of cord blood must be taken to estimate the haemoglobin and serum bilirubin levels, to check the ABO and Rh blood groups and to perform the Coombs' (or anti-human globulin) test. In most centres this is recommended for all Rh-negative mothers regardless of whether antibodies were found antenatally. A positive Coombs' test on the cord blood means an affected infant; a negative one means that no sensitisation of the infant's red cells has taken place and that the infant will not develop the disease.

The treatment of Rhesus haemolytic disease depends on the severity of the condition. It is aimed at restoring a normal haemoglobin concentration and preventing the rise of bilirubin to a dangerous level. If the cord blood haemoglobin level is below 10 g/dL or the bilirubin concentration above 85 μmol/L (5 mg/dL), the disease is severe and immediate exchange transfusion is required. Otherwise, the rate of rise in the level of bilirubin should be monitored at intervals of not more than 8 hours, and an exchange transfusion is carried out if it exceeds 10 μmol/L (0.5 mg/dL) per hour.

These guidelines for treatment may have to be modified in favour of earlier exchange transfusion in a preterm baby of less than 36 weeks' gestation or where a previous infant has been severely affected. In exceptional circumstances, where there is a severe anaemia resulting in oedema and ascites at birth, resuscitation and urgent replacement of 20 mL of the baby's blood with a smaller volume of packed group O Rh-negative red cells will be needed. This must be followed by administration of a diuretic such as furosemide (frusemide) before proceeding with a limited exchange transfusion.

In less severely affected infants, the rate of rise of bilirubin can be reduced by giving phenobarbital to the mother for 2 weeks before the birth of the baby to stimulate the baby's liver enzymes into action. Continuous phototherapy (p. 195) from birth may also reduce the need for an exchange transfusion in some infants. The rise in serum bilirubin gradually slows as the liver becomes able to metabolise and excrete it and eventually the jaundice disappears. However, the haemolysis continues as long as there is some Rhesus antibody in the baby's circulation and this may result in a further fall of haemoglobin for which a top-up transfusion of blood is required.

Exchange transfusion

The aim of exchange transfusion is to reduce the level of circulating bilirubin, to restore the blood volume and the haemoglobin concentration to normal, and to remove as much as possible of the circulating maternal Rh antibody from the baby's blood in order to reduce the risk of further haemolysis.

The techniques for performing exchange transfusions vary and only a simplified outline is given here. They are normally carried out using catheters inserted into the umbilical artery and vein, continuously running the cross-matched blood into the venous catheter while slowly removing an equivalent amount from the arterial line. This is continued until about 200 mL/kg body weight of blood has been exchanged and will take between 1½ and 2 hours to complete. Monitoring of the ECG, heart rate and body temperature must be carried out throughout the procedure. Although in many cases one exchange is sufficient, in more severely affected infants further exchanges may be required.

Prognosis

With careful management, over 95% of infants born alive can be expected to survive intact (Stewart et al 1994), the deaths being those with severe hydrops fetalis and those of very low birth weight (Thompson et al 1993, Greenough 1999). About 40% of affected babies require no treatment. Later disability from kernicterus is now a rarity, though minor degrees of deafness have been found in prospective studies.

Haemolytic disease due to ABO incompatibility

In the other major type of haemolytic disease, known as ABO incompatibility, the anti-A or anti-B haemolysins develop in the blood of a group O mother and are transferred to the developing group A or B infant. In a small proportion of such cases, this results in haemolytic disease and jaundice. The incidence of significant disease in the baby is about one in 200 births and many of these are only mildly affected. There are also incompatibilities involving other rarer blood groups which occasionally cause similar trouble.

Diagnosis and management

Unlike Rhesus haemolytic disease, ABO haemolytic disease is as likely in the first-born child as it is in subsequent pregnancies. Prediction during pregnancy is much less precise than in Rh incompatibility and the severity does not relate to the level of antibody in the maternal serum. The Coombs' test on the baby's blood is usually negative and the cord bilirubin and haemoglobin levels do not have predictive value. The essential diagnostic observation is the development of clinically obvious jaundice within the first 24 hours – a situation which always requires laboratory investigation. Anaemia is rarely marked and is less of a feature than the rapidly rising level of bilirubin. Although exchange transfusion may be necessary when the jaundice is early and severe, in most cases of ABO haemolytic disease phototherapy effectively prevents a rise in bilirubin to dangerous levels (p. 190).

Inherited causes of haemolytic disease

Glucose-6-phosphate dehydrogenase deficiency

Deficiency of glucose-6-phosphate dehydrogenase, an enzyme which protects the haemoglobin molecules from oxidation, is inherited as an X-linked recessive disorder. It affects males severely and the carrier females less so. It occurs substantially more commonly in certain ethnic groups, notably those from the Mediterranean area, the Middle and Far East and some parts of Africa, where it is the commonest reason for exchange transfusion. The red cells of affected babies are highly susceptible to haemolysis when challenged by certain drugs such as antimalarials, sulphonamide-containing antibiotics, aspirin and paracetamol, or when the baby has an infection. Under these conditions, and sometimes without apparent provocation, neonatal haemolytic jaundice may occur. It should be remembered that certain drugs are excreted in the mother's milk and even these small quantities may cause haemolysis in the predisposed child. It is treated by phototherapy or exchange transfusion according to similar criteria to those described for Rhesus haemolytic disease.

Hereditary spherocytosis

In this condition, the red cells are spherical, in contrast to the usual biconcave disc shape, and are unusually susceptible to destruction by haemolysis. Anaemia with mild jaundice is often present in the newborn period but severe hyperbilirubinaemia is exceptional. It is usually inherited as an autosomal dominant condition, so the family history may give warning of the condition.

Jaundice in preterm infants

This is simply an exaggerated form of the jaundice commonly seen in term infants. It is due to a greater functional inadequacy of the liver enzyme system which normally conjugates bilirubin with glucuronic acid and enables it to be excreted. Arising on the second or third day, the jaundice reaches a peak usually between days 5 and 7. There is evidence that in some immature infants the passage of bilirubin to the brain, causing kernicterus, occurs at a relatively low blood level (p. 121).

Evaluation of the severity of jaundice

Clinical estimation of the depth of jaundice by simple observation of skin colour is notoriously inaccurate, particularly in preterm infants, because it depends on the type of lighting, reflection from surrounding objects and the state of the baby's skin capillary blood flow. This is even more so when there is dark racial pigmentation. Hand-held transcutaneous bilirubinometers which measure the depth of yellow coloration of the skin are reasonably accurate and are useful for those

babies discharged home early (Bertini et al 2001). Their measurements correlate moderately well with laboratory measurements. They cannot be used during phototherapy as the yellow pigment they measure is absent from the skin. They may even be suitable for dark-skinned babies (Rubaltelli et al 2001), though there is little evidence so far. Many units have ward-based apparatus which measures the bilirubin in the serum from centrifuged capillary blood. These are more accurate but the baby has to suffer one or two painful heelpricks regularly each day, sometimes more often in the preterm infant. Serial laboratory estimations of serum bilirubin are most accurate.

Treatment of haemolytic jaundice

Exchange transfusion is now rarely needed but phototherapy is often helpful in keeping the serum bilirubin concentration below danger levels. However, the photodegradation of retinoids as well as the bilirubin may, rarely, leave the infant deficient in vitamin A.

Phototherapy

Exposing much of the baby's skin to sunlight effectively reduces the bilirubin level in the baby's blood but is impractical for treatment in the UK. However, artificial blue light of wavelength 400–500 nm and in an intensity of 4–10 microwatts/cm^2 also has the effect of converting unconjugated, fat-soluble bilirubin in the superficial capillaries to harmless water-soluble metabolites which are then excreted in the urine and stools. Though it is not as effective as exchange transfusion in removing bilirubin rapidly from the blood, this treatment can often prevent the bilirubin from reaching dangerous levels if applied early and at the appropriate intensity to the whole body (Dicken et al 2000). It should be applied before the bilirubin level has reached a potentially harmful value (Bertini et al 2001).

Most phototherapy equipment uses either banks of fluorescent tubes which emit light of the correct wavelength or diffused light from a halogen bulb source.

Care of an infant receiving phototherapy (Edwards 1995) from an overhead unit includes:

- nursing the infant naked or covered with no more than a nappy
- nursing the baby in a suitably warmed environment such as an incubator or in a cot under a heat shield
- protecting the eyes with eyeshields or a tinted perspex hood – this is to reduce discomfort from the intense glare, though there is little evidence that it does permanent harm
- monitoring the baby's temperature – the phototherapy unit gives off some heat, as do the photochemical reactions taking place in the skin

- if necessary, giving the infant extra fluids to counteract the increased insensible water loss, of the order of 20–30 mL/kg/day
- explaining to the parents to relieve any anxieties; treatment may be interrupted for breast feeding.

A different form of phototherapy uses a matrix of fibre-optic strands bonded to a flexible backing sheet, which is applied directly to the baby's skin under his or her clothing. A cold light source illuminates the light filaments on the sheet through a connecting fibre-optic cable (Figs 12.3A&B). Thus, the infant can be cared for in an almost normal way while treatment is given and does not become overheated, though the skin may occasionally

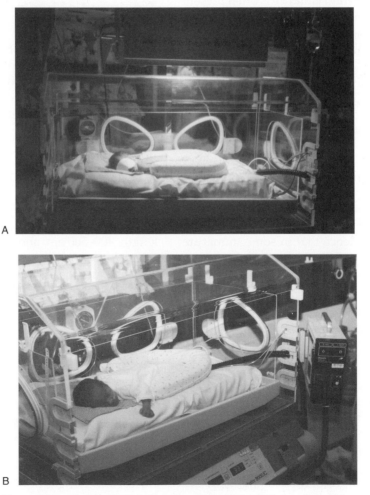

Figure 12.3 Phototherapy. A: In an incubator. B: Applied via a fibre-optic system.

become reddened where the sheet is applied. There is also no glare to the eyes. This system is most effective for the less severe forms of jaundice.

To judge whether or not a baby requires treatment, many maternity departments use charts on which the measured bilirubin levels are plotted against the baby's age at the time the sample was taken (Rose 2000). Action lines drawn on the charts indicate the bilirubin level at which phototherapy should be given, though the lines should be interpreted bearing in mind the underlying cause of the jaundice, whether the baby is well or sick and the infant's level of maturity. The more premature the baby, the lower the level at which treatment should be started (Fig. 12.4). Treatment usually continues for 2 or 3 days, with serial estimations of serum bilirubin once or twice a day to monitor its progress, and it is more effective in preventing a rise in serum bilirubin to a high level than in causing a significant fall once it has risen.

Although no serious sequelae have been shown to follow this form of therapy, fretfulness, fluid loss from overheating, rashes, looseness of the stools and vomiting have all been reported (Hart 1997). Clearly, the need for phototherapy must take into account the age of the baby, for the chances of a natural fall in the serum bilirubin after the fifth day are high.

In recent years, mothers and babies have been discharged home earlier from the maternity unit. One consequence of this is that there has been an increase in readmissions of babies for investigation of jaundice. In many cases, mild jaundice has been accentuated by a lack of milk intake and the treatment consists mainly in rehydrating the infant and improving the breast-feeding technique.

Other common causes of jaundice

Breast milk jaundice

Jaundice with serum bilirubin above 200 μmol/L (12 mg/dL) and continuing for more than 10 days is frequently associated with breast feeding.

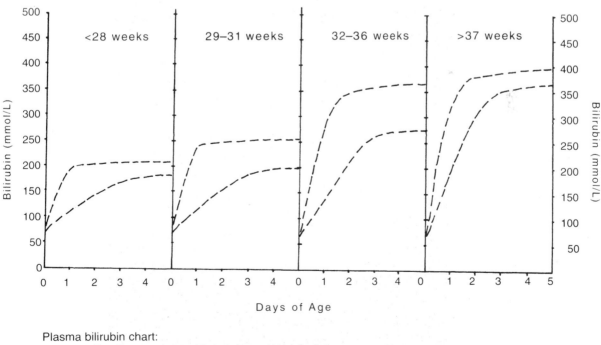

Plasma bilirubin chart:
    Top line   – consider exchange transfusion
    Bottom line – start phototherapy

Figure 12.4 Guidelines for the treatment of unconjugated neonatal jaundice.

Provided the baby is well and the other causes of prolonged jaundice have been excluded, the diagnosis of breast milk jaundice can be made with confidence even though there is no specific test for the condition (Hamosh 1990). Withdrawal of breast feeding temporarily, with replacement by artificial milk, results in a fall of bilirubin level but is rarely needed as a test since the slow decline in bilirubin value over the next week or two confirms the diagnosis. Although it may be that some factor in breast milk affects the conjugation and excretion of bilirubin, it may also result from interference with bilirubin metabolism in the gut which allows reabsorption of unconjugated bilirubin back into the circulation. Only rarely should discontinuation of breast feeding be recommended since the jaundice only occasionally reaches a level requiring treatment (Seidman et al 1995) and within 6–8 weeks it normally resolves without leaving any serious sequelae.

Jaundice due to sepsis

Apart from thrombophlebitis ascending from umbilical sepsis into the portal vein, which is extremely rare, jaundice may be a feature of any septicaemic illness in the first week of life. Unexplained jaundice, especially if associated with reluctance to feed, drowsiness or vomiting, should therefore always raise the suspicion of infection, particularly in the urinary tract (p. 172).

Congenital hypothyroidism

Unrecognised congenital hypothyroidism may cause abnormal prolongation of physiological jaundice beyond 2 weeks of age. However, the thyroid-stimulating hormone (TSH) screening test carried out on the seventh day of life should now identify these babies at an early stage (p. 77). The clinical signs are described on page 212.

Congenital galactosaemia

This rare error of metabolism is described on page 211 but is mentioned here since persistent jaundice is one of the early signs and because,

if the condition can be detected in the first few weeks of life, the treatment is rewarding and can minimise the mental retardation, permanent liver damage or death which may result from late diagnosis.

Congenital infection

Congenital infection by the rubella virus, cytomegalovirus, *Toxoplasma gondii* and *Treponema pallidum* (syphilis) may all present with jaundice as a prominent clinical feature. Initially of haemolytic type, the jaundice later has obstructive features and has to be differentiated from the many causes of neonatal hepatitis.

Obstructive jaundice

Jaundice may result from obstruction to the flow of bile either within the liver or from blocked extrahepatic bile ducts. In this situation, bilirubin is conjugated normally within the liver cells into its metabolites but, because they cannot pass through the bile ducts to the bowel, they are reabsorbed back into the blood. These water-soluble pigments circulate to the kidneys where they are excreted, colouring the urine a dark yellowish-brown. The stools remain pale as little or no bile flows into the gastrointestinal tract. Since the conjugated bilirubin is not fat soluble, it cannot cross the blood-brain barrier and there is no risk of kernicterus.

This uncommon clinical picture of a baby with persistent jaundice, conjugated hyperbilirubinaemia, pale stools and dark urine can result from both congenital atresia of the bile ducts and the many causes of neonatal hepatitis, and requires urgent investigation. The initial tests required in such a baby are given in Box 12.2, but extensive additional specific investigation is usually needed to reach a complete diagnosis. The most common conditions identified are biliary atresia and idiopathic neonatal hepatitis (Andres 1996). Alpha-1 antitrypsin deficiency is a relatively common cause in the UK though it is rarely seen in Australia and South Africa, where, respectively, cytomegalovirus infection and syphilis are more frequent causes.

Box 12.2 Initial investigation in conjugated hyperbilirubinaemia

- Standard liver function tests
- Prothrombin time
- Bacterial culture of blood and urine
- Viral culture of urine
- Reducing substances in urine
- Alpha-1 antitrypsin level and protease-inhibitor typing
- Serum and urine amino acids
- Hepatitis A, B and C antigens
- Serum thyroxine and thyroid-stimulating hormone levels
- Ultrasound examination of the liver and bile ducts

Congenital biliary atresia

Biliary atresia is a rare condition which may affect either the small intrahepatic ducts or the common bile duct or both. It is not a simple congenital malformation and may occur with metabolic causes of neonatal hepatitis such as alpha-1 antitrypsin deficiency. The condition appears to progress in the first few weeks of life. Jaundice may arise from birth or may be delayed until 2–3 weeks of age and the conjugated bilirubin level often fluctuates. The jaundice has a greenish tinge and the spleen may be enlarged. Liver function tests are not often helpful in diagnosis, though the transaminases are usually mildly elevated and the prothrombin time may be prolonged.

A progressive dilatation of the bile duct from partial or complete localised obstruction at the ampulla of Vater may cause a palpable choledochal cyst, which can be confirmed by ultrasound imaging.

Early surgery may relieve the obstruction provided the intrahepatic ducts are patent, and a portoenterostomy is usually recommended. In this operation, known as the Kasai procedure, a loop of small bowel is opened and anastamosed directly onto the surface of the liver to allow bile to drain straight into the gut lumen. If this is carried out before 8 weeks of age, the jaundice clears in nearly all infants, who then have up to 80% chance of long survival (Ishitani 2001). Surgery is less effective beyond this age and it is for this reason that the investigation of obstructive jaundice should be carried out urgently. If the operation is not successful, the only treatment which can prevent early death from cirrhosis is liver transplantation.

Neonatal hepatitis

Neonatal hepatitis is twice as common as biliary atresia and may be difficult to differentiate from it. The cause is not always established but in the UK about 20% of cases are associated with recessively inherited alpha-1 antitrypsin deficiency, in which circumstances cirrhosis of the liver is likely to follow and siblings have a high risk of being affected. The condition is diagnosed by protease-inhibitor (Pi) typing, which can also detect carriers and enable genetic evaluation of the risk of recurrence of the disease in other family members. Various intrauterine infections, including hepatitis A and C, rubella, toxoplasmosis, herpes simplex and those caused by cytomegalovirus or coxsackievirus, make up a further 10%, and maternal carriers of hepatitis B antigen can transmit the viral infection to the baby during labour (p. 180). Cystic fibrosis and a large number of very rare recessively inherited metabolic disorders, including galactosaemia and fructosaemia, can cause a similar clinical picture. In many cases, however, no cause is identified.

The course of the illness is very variable and in many cases the baby is not apparently unwell. Jaundice gradually appears over the first few weeks and there may sometimes be a low-grade pyrexia or reluctance to feed. When none of the serious causes mentioned above are identifiable, the chances of complete recovery are good. Among the rest, a few affected babies die in the early stages and about half of those who seem to be recovering develop later cirrhosis of the liver in addition to the other consequences of the underlying cause.

Diagnosis and management

Differentiation of biliary atresia and neonatal hepatitis is never easy and usually requires specialised experience. Moderately raised transaminases, high serum alpha-fetoprotein and low alpha-1 antitrypsin levels, though favouring hepatitis, may be found in either condition. Ultrasound examination of the liver may reveal a choledochal cyst, but rarely helps otherwise since the intrahepatic ducts are usually not dilated in biliary atresia. Metabolic and infective causes should be investigated. It is usually possible to distinguish the two disorders with a combination

of isotope excretion scans and histological examination of a liver biopsy (Lai et al 1994), though occasionally laparoscopy (Senyuz et al 2001) or laparotomy is needed to exclude extrahepatic biliary atresia. There is some evidence, however, that surgery may worsen the outlook for some babies who prove to have neonatal hepatitis.

REFERENCES

Andres J M 1996 Neonatal hepatobiliary disorders. Clinical Perinatology 23(2):321–352

Bertini G, Dani C, Pezzati M et al 2001 Prevention of bilirubin encephalopathy. Biology of the Neonate 79(3-4):219–223

Brown L, Arnold L, Allison D et al 1993 Incidence and pattern of jaundice in healthy breast fed infants during the first month of life. Nursing Research 42(2):106–110

Cao A, Galanello R, Rosatelli M C 1998 Prenatal diagnosis and screening of the haemoglobinopathies. Baillières Clinical Haematology 11(1):215–238

Dicken P, Grant L J, Jones S 2000 An evaluation of the characteristics and performance of neonatal phototherapy equipment. Physiological Measurement 21(4):493–503

Edwards S 1995 Phototherapy and the neonate: providing safe and effective care for jaundiced infants. Journal of Neonatal Nursing 1(5):9–12

Golding J, Birmingham K et al 1992 Intramuscular vitamin K and childhood cancer. British Medical Journal 305:341–346

Greenough A 1999 Rhesus disease: postnatal management and outcome. European Journal of Pediatrics 158(9):689–693

Hamosh M 1990 Breast milk jaundice. Journal of Pediatric Gastroenterology and Nutrition 11:145–149

Hart G 1997 Phototherapy for neonates. Journal of Neonatal Nursing 3(4):centre insert

Howard H L, Martlew V J, McFadyen I R et al 1997 Preventing Rhesus D haemolytic disease of the newborn by giving anti-D immunoglobulin: are the guidelines being adequately followed? British Journal of Obstetrics and Gynaecology 104(1):37–41

Hughes R G, Craig J I, Murphy W G et al 1994 Causes and clinical consequences of Rhesus (D) haemolytic disease in the newborn: a study of a Scottish population 1985-1990. British Journal of Obstetrics and Gynaecology 101(4):297–300

Ishitani M B 2001 Biliary atresia and the Kasai portoenterostome: never say never? Liver Transplantation 7(9):831–832

Kaplan C 2001 Immune thrombocytopenia in the foetus and the newborn: diagnosis and therapy. Transfusion and Clinical Biology 8(3):311–314

Lai M W, Chang M H, Hsu S C et al 1994 Differential diagnosis of extrahepatic biliary atresia from neonatal hepatitis: a prospective study. Journal of Pediatric Gastroenterology and Nutrition 18(2):121–127

McCormack K 1998 Neonatal blood transfusions: a case for guidelines. Journal of Neonatal Nursing 4(5):12–17

Roberts I A, Murray N A 2001 Neonatal thrombocytopenia: new insights into pathogenesis and implications for clinical management. Current Opinion in Pediatrics 13(1):16–21

Rose F M 2000 Monitoring bilirubin. Journal of Neonatal Nursing 6(5):centre insert

Rubaltelli F F, Gourley G R, Loskamp N et al 2001 Transcutaneous bilirubin measurement: a multicentre evaluation of a new device. Pediatrics 107(6):1264–1271

Seidman D S, Stevenson D K, Ergaz Z et al 1995 Hospital readmissions due to neonatal hyperbilirubinaemia. Pediatrics 96(4):727–729

Senyuz O F, Yesildag E, Emir H et al 2001 Diagnostic laparoscopy in prolonged jaundice. Journal of Pediatric Surgery 36(3):463–465

Stewart G, Day R E, Del Priore C et al 1994 Developmental outcome after intravascular intrauterine transfusion for rhesus haemolytic disease. Archives of Disease in Childhood Fetal and Neonatal Edition 70(1):F52–F53

Thompson P J, Greenough A, Brooker R et al 1993 Antenatal diagnosis and outcome in hydrops fetalis. Journal of Perinatal Medicine 21(1):63–67

Von Kries R 1999 Oral versus intramuscular phytomenadione: safety and efficacy compared. Drug Safety 21(1):1–6

Wariyar U, Hilton S, Pagan J et al 2000 Six years of experience of prophylactic oral vitamin K. Archives of Disease in Childhood Fetal and Neonatal Edition 82:F64–F68

Chapter 13

Congenital malformations and genetic disorders

CHAPTER CONTENTS

Introduction   202
Incidence of congenital anomalies   202
Aetiology, predisposing factors and causes   202
Prevention   203
   Prenatal identification of congenital
   malformations   203
   Deformities   203
   Life-threatening anomalies   203
Parental reactions to the birth of an abnormal
baby   204
Genetics and genetic disorders   204
   Dominant inheritance   205
   Recessive inheritance   206
   X-linked inheritance   207
Conditions associated with developmental delay   207
   Trisomies and other chromosome disorders   207
   The dysmorphic syndromes   209
Recessively inherited conditions   209
   Cystic fibrosis   210
   Inborn errors of metabolism   210

Structural congenital malformations   213
Alimentary tract   213
   Cleft lip and cleft palate   213
   Anomalies which cause intestinal obstruction   214
   Neonatal intestinal obstruction below the
   duodenum   217
   Disorders of development of the umbilicus   219
Respiratory tract   219
   Choanal atresia   219
   Lung malformations   220
The heart and great vessels   221
   Presentation of congenital heart disease   221
   Investigations   221
   Common heart malformations   223
Genitourinary tract   226
   Kidneys   226
   Obstruction in the urinary tract   227
   Ectopia vesicae   227
   External genitalia   228
   Ambiguous genitalia   228
Central nervous system   230
   Neural tube abnormalities   230

   Other abnormalities of head size and shape   232
Eyes   233
   Microphthalmia   233
   Macrophthalmia   233
   Congenital cataracts   233
Limbs and joints   233
   Congenital dislocation of the hip   233
   Talipes equinovarus and calcaneovalgus   235
   Scoliosis   236
Lymphatic system   236

INTRODUCTION

The identification of a physical malformation or a metabolic or genetic disorder in a baby before or after birth is very distressing for parents and the wider family, since such a defect may have an effect on the baby's health or threaten the baby's life or developmental progress in the future. In many cases, medical or surgical treatment can result in near normality; however, in others, intervention only corrects a physical feature while leaving the child permanently handicapped, or requiring prolonged medical or surgical attention, special education and social help. It is imperative that the parents are given as much information as possible about the suspected abnormality by informed and experienced staff so that they can make informed choices about the investigation and treatment of their baby. In some cases, the ethical or religious beliefs of the parents or family members may cause a difference of opinion between them and the professional advisors and this may be difficult to resolve.

INCIDENCE OF CONGENITAL ANOMALIES

Estimates of the total incidence of congenital abnormalities vary widely depending upon what is regarded as serious enough to include and up to what age the infants surveyed are followed. Some defects, such as those of the urinary tract, may not become apparent until middle or late childhood. The figures are also affected by how the information is collected. The incidence should include all live births and stillbirths as well as spontaneous and elective abortions, and those with multiple anomalies may be listed only under the major anomaly. On average, however, a congenital abnormality of significance occurs about once in every 30 live and stillbirths; in 25% of these babies there is more than one defect. Minor abnormalities occur in about another 3% of total births (Riley et al 1998).

AETIOLOGY, PREDISPOSING FACTORS AND CAUSES

Much has been learnt about the origin of congenital malformations from research in animals, but disappointingly little is known about the cause of many human anomalies, with a few notable exceptions.

Although many congenital anomalies have some genetic basis, a distinct pattern of inheritance is uncommon in structural abnormalities but is more common in the rarer inborn errors of metabolic or biochemical function. This subject is discussed in detail on p. 204.

In some conditions, there is a substantial difference in the occurrence rate of abnormalities in different racial groups. For instance, sickle cell disease is confined to those originating from Black Africa, thalassaemia is seen mainly in those of Mediterranean or Far Eastern origin, and glucose-6-phosphate dehydrogenase deficiency is commoner in many tropical and subtropical countries (p. 188).

Social class differences also occur, neural tube defects being more common where the father has an unskilled occupation whereas congenital dislocation of the hip is more prevalent in managerial and professional families.

Malnutrition, too, may play some part. Folic acid deficiency is a major factor in the origin of neural tube defects, for example, since there is a 75% reduction of recurrence of the condition if folic acid supplements are taken before conception and while the fetus is differentiating (p. 230).

Increasing maternal age is known to be a factor in the production of at least one major abnormality – Down syndrome – and probably in all trisomic chromosomal anomalies.

Birth order is of significance in anencephaly, spina bifida and congenital dislocation of the hip, which are all more common in first pregnancies.

The majority of malformations, however, are likely to be caused by factors adversely affecting the fetus in the early stages of its development. These include the following:

- Infections – the best-known example is rubella, with its effects on ears, eyes, heart and brain. These and the abnormalities caused by antenatal infection with *Toxoplasma gondii* and cytomegalovirus are described in Chapter 11. Infection with, for example, Coxsackie A and B or echoviruses may also cause anomalies, but associations with other viruses are less certain.

- Prescription drugs – the thalidomide tragedy in the 1960s had the beneficial side-effect of promoting caution in the use of all drugs in early pregnancy. Although many other substances have been suspected, few have been proven to be the sole cause of malformation. It seems likely that some drugs contribute to the production of a defect only in conjunction with other factors such as nutritional deficiency, hypoxia or a genetic predisposition. The excess of babies with cleft palate and congenital heart disease born to mothers taking sodium valproate or carbamazepine for epilepsy (Bertollini et al 1985) is a possible example of this. The effect of harmful drugs varies according to which organs are undergoing differentiation at the time of exposure.
  - Alcohol (p. 16).
  - Smoking (p. 16).
  - Drugs of addiction, e.g. cocaine (p. 18).
- Irradiation – although this is undoubtedly a danger to fetal development, proven ill-effects have occurred only after heavy exposure or following preconceptional irradiation of the parental gonads.
- Maternal disease (p. 53) – the incidence of congenital malformations is doubled in inadequately controlled diabetes in pregnancy.
- Multiple births – the risk of malformations is increased, though only one infant may be affected.
- Environmental factors – many other factors have come under suspicion of causing malformations. Toxic pollutants such as sulphur dioxide, carbon monoxide, solvents, lead, dioxins, pesticides and even electromagnetic radiation from overhead pylons have been considered, though there is little firm evidence to associate them with particular anomalies.

PREVENTION

Careful and comprehensive history-taking from the mother at the first antenatal visit, to identify familial inherited disorders, is of the utmost importance, but other opportunities for prevention are still often missed at this stage.

Publicity aimed at decreasing the proportion of women who reach antenatal clinics too late in pregnancy, and education about the importance of adequate nutrition before conception and during the early months of pregnancy might lead to some reduction in the incidence of genetic diseases.

Immunisation against infections to which the fetus is susceptible is, at present, only practicable in the case of rubella and to be effective and safe this has to be done before conception.

Prenatal identification of congenital malformations

Clinical findings which point to an increased chance of malformation in the current pregnancy and help in predicting the possibility include polyhydramnios, oligohydramnios and intrauterine growth retardation, all of which justify a careful ultrasound examination of the fetus. A newborn infant with a single umbilical artery is also at increased risk of renal tract anomalies.

Deformities

Deformities, as distinct from true developmental malformations, can undoubtedly be caused by abnormal mechanical stresses or pressures upon the developing fetus; examples of these are talipes and congenital scoliosis, although in both there may also be a hereditary predisposing factor. Amniotic bands can cause amputations of digits or even whole limbs.

Life-threatening anomalies

A small proportion of malformations can result in the death of the baby before or shortly after birth, though timely treatment can save life in many cases. In some cases where a truly lethal anomaly such as renal agenesis or anencephaly has been identified by ultrasound examination in early pregnancy, a termination may be recommended. Around 20% of life-threatening malformations are identified at postmortem examination of stillborn babies; about 50% cause death within the first month; in the remainder, death occurs during later infancy or childhood. The great majority affect the heart, central nervous system, gut or urinary systems, but many are associated with chromosomal abnormalities or are only one of several malformations in the same infant. Mortality rates from

Table 13.1 Examples of life-threatening congenital malformations

Central nervous system	Anencephaly
	Spina bifida
	—with hydrocephalus
	—encephalocele
	Spinal muscular atrophy
Cardiovascular system	Hypoplastic left heart syndrome
	Transposition of the great arteries
	Pulmonary atresia
	Cardiomyopathy
Gastrointestinal tract	Diaphragmatic hernia
	Exomphalos
	Gastroschisis
	Intestinal atresias
Urinary tract	Renal agenesis
	Dysplastic or cystic kidneys
Chromosomal disorders	Trisomy 18
	Trisomy 13
Multiple abnormalities	Recognisable 'syndromes'
Metabolic disorders	MCAD deficiency

MCAD = medium-chain acyl coenzyme-A dehydrogenase.

congenital malformations vary markedly between racial groups, the risk in the offspring of Asian-born mothers being more than twice as high as that in UK-born mothers. By contrast, the rate is low in Afro-Carribean mothers. Examples of these most serious defects are given in Table 13.1.

PARENTAL REACTIONS TO THE BIRTH OF AN ABNORMAL BABY

Parental responses to the birth of an unexpectedly malformed infant are complex but the interruption to the joy at the birth of the baby can have a lasting impact on the parents' relationship with the infant. It can be difficult for them to make appropriate decisions or give properly informed consent in such emotional turmoil, and great sensitivity and understanding is required by doctors, nurses and others in helping parents cope. These issues are discussed in Chapter 14 (p. 241).

GENETICS AND GENETIC DISORDERS

Genetics is the study of heredity and the transmission of characteristics from one generation to the next. As its techniques have rapidly developed in the last decade, the genetic basis of an increasing number of disorders has become apparent. Genetic screening can also identify apparently healthy carriers of inherited conditions and closely follow the gene patterns through the family. Although many congenital malformations have some genetic basis, a distinct pattern of inheritance is uncommon in structural abnormalities but is found frequently in the rarer inborn errors of metabolic or biochemical function.

In order to understand the implications of genetic inheritance, it is important to know something of the scientific basis of heredity, and the following section gives an introduction to the subject.

The normal baby has 22 identical pairs of chromosomes and two sex chromosomes, making 46 in all (23 pairs). These are located in the nucleus of all cells except the ova and sperm. One of each pair comes from the mother, the other from the father, and they carry the genetic material which determines the characteristics of the recipient baby. Chromosomes vary greatly in size and each carries a unique selection of genes which determine the characteristics of the baby, yet each gene is always found at the same location on its particular chromosome.

In the process of producing ova and sperm, each chromosome pair divides, so that each gamete will contain only half the genetic material of the parent. In the normal process of fertilisation, the chromosome material from the ovum and sperm matches with its equivalent partner, to form a full complement of 23 whole pairs in the zygote (fertilised ovum). The sex chromosomes, named X and Y, act differently. Each female has two X chromosomes and each male one X and one Y chromosome. Every ovum therefore has one X chromosome, but a sperm will have either an X or a Y chromosome. If the X chromosome from the father fertilises the ovum, the resulting baby will be XX – a girl. Conversely, his Y chromosome will produce an XY zygote – a boy.

Occasionally, errors occur in this process and the zygote receives either too many or, more rarely, too few chromosomes, or small parts of a chromosome may be deleted or duplicated. When this happens, it usually results in malformation of the baby.

Table 13.2 Some conditions diagnosed by DNA analysis and fluorescent in-situ hybridisation (FISH)

1. DNA analysis

Diagnosis	Mode of inheritance	Diagnostic findings
Cystic fibrosis	Autosomal recessive	Mutation of CFTR gene on chromosome 7 identified in 50–90% of cases
Werdnig–Hoffmann disease	Autosomal recessive	SMN and NAIP gene deletions found on chromosome 5 in over 95% of cases
Congentital adrenal hyperplasia	Autosomal recessive	Mutations of 21-hydroxlase gene on chromosome 6 in most cases
Myotonic dystrophy	Autosomal dominant	Trinucleotide repeat mutations of specific gene on chromosome 19 in almost all cases
X-linked hydrocephalus	X-linked	Mutation in L1CAM gene identified in most familial cases
Wiedemann–Beckwith syndrome		Visible deletion on chromosome 11 in 5%; uniparental disomy for 11p15 markers in 20%

2. FISH

Condition	Diagnostic findings
Prader–Willi syndrome	Deletions on short arm of 15 chromosome in 5%; maternal uniparental disomy for chromosome 15 in the rest
Williams syndrome	Deletion of elastin gene on chromosome 7 in 95% of cases
Velocardiofacial syndrome	Gene deletion on short arm of chromosome 22 in 90% of cases

The most common chromosomal abnormalities identified are trisomies, where the baby has three identical chromosomes of one type instead of just a pair. This can affect the number 13 or 18 chromosomes but most commonly the 21 chromosome, when it produces trisomy 21 – Down syndrome.

Genetecists have many techniques now to identify abnormalities of the chromosomes beyond simply finding abnormal numbers or missing fragments. These include conventional light microscopy, banding of the chromosomes with Giemsa staining and examination after culturing the chromosomes in special media, chromosome 'painting' and other more specialised techniques. The identification of 'fragile X chromosomes' (p. 209) in some children with mild learning difficulties is an example of the newer methods. In this case, culture of the chromosomes in a folate-poor medium results in the tip of one X chromosome breaking off from its body.

However, most genetic disorders are not associated with visible abnormalities of the chromosomes themselves but are related to errors in the genes on the chromosomes. Analysis of the genes themselves has become a reality since the introduction of highly specialised molecular genetic analysis of DNA, the complex chemical which forms the chromosomes. This can reveal abnormalities of the genes and identify an increasing number of inherited conditions even in early fetal life (Hanna et al 1994). It is now widely available in the UK. The number of conditions amenable to diagnosis in this way is growing ever larger and the technique is superseding other methods of diagnosis in many genetic disorders (Table 13.2).

Just as with the chromosomes themselves, each gene is one of a pair, one on each of the pair of chromosomes. Gene analysis is now able to identify a rapidly increasing number of individual genes and can in some cases accurately predict the gene abnormality responsible for a particular disease. It can also frequently identify healthy carriers of the abnormal genes for these conditions in other family members so that they can be advised with greater certainty of the risk of having an affected infant. The ability to identify the abnormal gene pattern enables many of these disorders to be identified in early fetal life and is the basis for the antenatal diagnosis of many genetic diseases.

There are three main ways in which genetic diseases may be transmitted. These are known as dominant, recessive and X-linked inheritance.

Dominant inheritance

In the dominant pattern of inheritance (Fig. 13.1A), the gene is present in one of the parents, who,

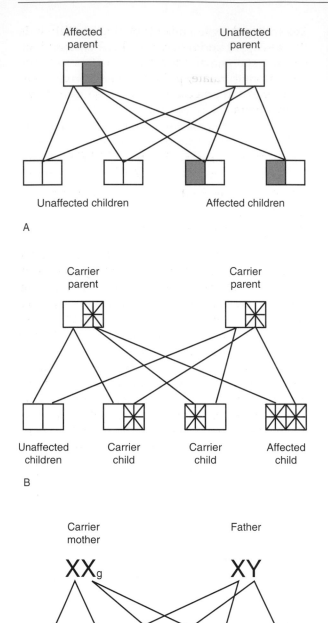

A

B

C

Figure 13.1 Patterns of inheritance of genetic disorders.
A: dominant; B: recessive; C: X-linked.

consequently, has the condition, and it is directly passed on to the baby, who inherits the same condition. The abnormal gene is located on only one of the pair of chromosomes and is dominant over the normal gene on the other. The offspring either inherit it or do not. In this situation, each baby has a 1 in 2 chance of having the condition and can pass it on to their offspring also. If they do not inherit the disorder, they cannot pass it on as they do not have the gene.

Examples of such conditions include:

- achondroplasia
- tuberous sclerosis
- Huntington's chorea
- neurofibromatosis.

Recessive inheritance

In recessively inherited conditions (Fig. 13.1B), both apparently healthy parents are carriers of an abnormal gene but it is dominated by the normal gene on the other chromosome in the pair. In this situation, both parents give either a normal or an abnormal gene to each baby. If either endows the baby with the normal gene, the baby will be healthy irrespective of whether he has inherited the normal or the abnormal gene from the other parent. If he inherits the abnormal gene from both parents, he does not have a normal gene and therefore expresses the abnormal gene, which results in the disease. Each child of such parents have a 1 in 4 chance of having the condition but 50% will be healthy carriers like the parents. The occurrence of such conditions is greater if the parents are blood relatives and are therefore more likely to share an abnormal gene. The increased incidence of malformations among Asian British families has been attributed to the higher rate of cousin marriage in some of these groups and to childbearing at an older age.

Conditions passed on in this way include:

- cystic fibrosis (p. 210)
- phenylketonuria (p. 211)
- galactosaemia (p. 211)
- congenital adrenal hyperplasia (p. 229)
- Friedreich's ataxia.

X-linked inheritance

In X-linked inheritance (Fig. 13.1C), an abnormal gene is located on the X chromosome and there is no equivalent balancing gene on the Y chromosome. In almost every case, the mother is healthy, as she has a normal gene on her other X chromosome. If she passes the abnormal gene to a male baby, the Y chromosome does not have the normal gene and the condition will be expressed. If the X chromosome with the normal gene is passed to her son, he will not have the disease. Female offspring of the carrier mother will have a 50% chance of receiving the abnormal gene and, therefore, being able to pass it on to their sons. In this situation, each pregnancy carries a 25% risk of producing an affected male and a 25% chance of a female carrier. All the female offspring of affected fathers will be carriers but his sons will be unaffected and unable to pass the condition on. Thus, the carrier females may pass on the gene to later generations without being aware of it, but the conditions are always expressed in carriers' sons.

Conditions inherited in this fashion include:

- fragile X syndrome (p. 209)
- Haemophilia (p. 187)
- Duchenne muscular dystrophy (p. 158).

More often there is a mixed aetiology, with heredity playing a less-well defined role. Conditions showing a sporadic pattern of inheritance include cleft palate, pyloric stenosis, congenital heart disease, most cases of Down syndrome and many others.

CONDITIONS ASSOCIATED WITH DEVELOPMENTAL DELAY

Trisomies and other chromosome disorders

Down syndrome (trisomy 21)

Occurring in total once in every 600 births, Down syndrome is recognisable at or shortly after birth in nearly every case. It is due to the possession of extra chromosome material, either as a separate additional 21 chromosome (Fig. 13.2) or as a translocation of extra chromosome 21 material onto another chromosome.

This abnormality usually follows non-disjunction of the parental chromosomes during one of the stages of cell division, and in this situation the risk of recurrence is closely related to advancing maternal age, though there is also an increased risk in teenage pregnancy. At 20 years

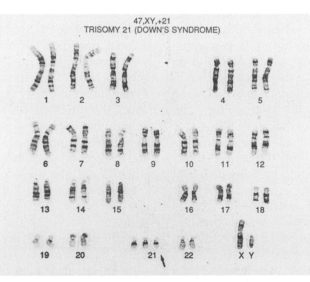

Figure 13.2 Chromosome pattern in Down syndrome, showing the extra 21 chromosome. (By kind permission of Prof. P Jacobs.)

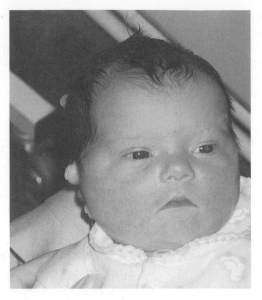

Figure 13.3 Down syndrome.

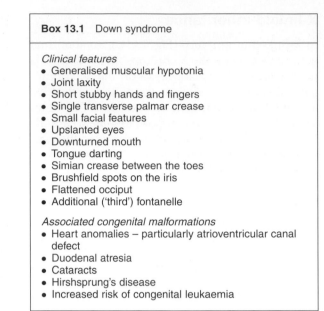

Box 13.1   Down syndrome

Clinical features
- Generalised muscular hypotonia
- Joint laxity
- Short stubby hands and fingers
- Single transverse palmar crease
- Small facial features
- Upslanted eyes
- Downturned mouth
- Tongue darting
- Simian crease between the toes
- Brushfield spots on the iris
- Flattened occiput
- Additional ('third') fontanelle

Associated congenital malformations
- Heart anomalies – particularly atrioventricular canal defect
- Duodenal atresia
- Cataracts
- Hirshsprung's disease
- Increased risk of congenital leukaemia

of age the chance of bearing an affected child is 1:1923; at 25 it is 1:1205; at 30, 1:835; at 40, 1:109; and at 45, 1:32. In spite of this, 70% of babies with Down syndrome are born to mothers under 35 years of age because childbirth is so much more frequent in the younger age group.

In the minority of cases, the abnormality is due to translocation of chromosome material. In about half of these cases, the balanced translocation can be identified in one or other parent, the risk of recurrence in this case being as high as 1 in 4. In the rest, it arises as new mutation. It is advisable for all parents of Down syndrome children to have chromosome studies to identify the small number with a translocational abnormality so that appropriate genetic counselling can be given. Amniocentesis or chorionic biopsy for chromosome analysis can then be offered in subsequent pregnancies, with the option of termination of pregnancy should the baby be found to be affected.

Recognition   Down's syndrome is usually recognised most easily from a general impression of the infant (Fig. 13.3) rather than by consciously taking note of the separate features (Box 13.1). Many abnormalities make up this clinical impression. The baby is often small. There is a general muscular hypotonia and laxity of joints.

The head is rounded and relatively short from front to back. An extra fontanelle may be present in the sagittal suture line just above the posterior fontanelle. The features of the face are grouped more closely than normal and are in themselves generally smaller. The eyes show an oblique slant of the palpebral fissure outwards and upwards. The mouth is often turned downward at the corners and the tongue frequently protrudes. The ears are small and simply formed. Small white flecks (Brushfield's spots) may be seen in a ring around the iris. The hands are short and wide with stubby fingers, an incurved little finger, and often a single transverse palmar crease. A congenital heart anomaly is present in nearly half of cases, though often it is not possible to recognise it on initial clinical examination. Cataracts, duodenal atresia and Hirschsprung's disease are also relatively common. One of the most constant features is the abnormal pattern of dermal ridge (fingerprint markings) on the palms, but they are not easy to see on the small hand of the newborn child.

Once the diagnosis has been made, the parents must be informed. This difficult task ought only to be undertaken by a doctor who fully understands the effect it may have, and who knows how to answer the many questions that will inevitably be asked about the future. This subject is discussed in more detail in Chapter 14 on Helping the Parents.

Trisomy 18

In trisomy 18, or Edward's syndrome, the multiple abnormalities include low-set ears, overlapping ulnar-deviated fingers, 'rocker' feet, and complex congenital heart anomalies which often result in the early death of these infants.

Trisomy 13

Trisomy 13 (Patau's syndrome) includes cleft palate, brain defects, microphthalmia, absent testes and renal abnormalities.

Both trisomy 18 and trisomy 13 are almost always incompatible with survival.

Turner's syndrome

In this anomaly, one X chromosome is missing (chromosomes are 45 XO) and is associated with absence of the ovaries which results in infertility in adult life. The abnormal chromosome pattern may be found incidentally during the pregnancy whilst screening the fetal cells for other anomalies such as Down syndrome. The disorder may be recognisable in the newborn by the presence of persistent oedema of the lower limbs or webbing of the neck, though most girls with the condition have no dysmorphic features and cannot be identified clinically on neonatal examination. Coarctation of the aorta is a common accompaniment. These girls often fail to thrive in infancy and grow slowly throughout childhood, ending up as short adults. The importance of early diagnosis rests in the hope of increased growth which may be achieved through giving low-dose oestrogen and growth hormone supplementation during childhood, but it is too early to know what increase in adult height can be achieved.

'Fragile X' chromosomes

Recently, the chromosomes of special-needs children with moderate learning difficulties have been examined and a small proportion found to have fragments which appear to break off the end of the X chromosomes during chromosome culture in a folate-deficient medium. This condition is not uncommon and is associated with a number of physical features such as a long face and prominent jaw, large ears and a normal head circumference. After puberty, the testes are often unusually large. It is inherited as an X-linked condition, thus often affecting other male members of the family, and some 30% of the carrier mothers have some degree of learning difficulty. The location of the gene on the X chromosome has been identified by DNA analysis and this can now be used to confirm the diagnosis in the fetus or in the child after birth.

Other syndromes associated with chromosome anomalies are comparatively rare.

The dysmorphic syndromes

Many infants with chromosome anomalies will be noticed initially because of unusual physical features. Others with dysmorphic characteristics have normal chromosomes but may, because of the recognisable association of clinical features, be given a diagnosis as a specific named syndrome, though in some cases no diagnosis can be reached (Fig. 13.4). All of them are rare but features which should suggest such a syndrome include:

- an odd facial appearance
- abnormalities of the limbs, particularly shortening
- malformations of the hands and digits
- abnormal genitalia
- unusual head shape
- abnormal position or structure of the eyes.

Since many of these babies will later become mentally handicapped and some are familial, the advice of a clinical geneticist should be sought if a syndrome cannot be easily diagnosed.

RECESSIVELY INHERITED CONDITIONS

Although very few recessively inherited conditions are common, in many cases they have a

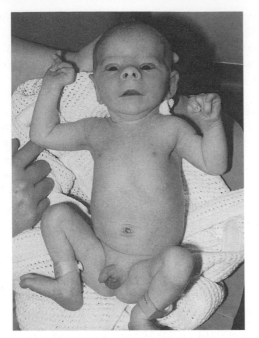

Figure 13.4 Dysmorphic facies, unusual posture of the fingers and bilateral undescended testes in a newborn baby. No diagnosis was reached in this case.

very serious impact on the life of the infant. A few examples of such conditions are given here.

Cystic fibrosis

Cystic fibrosis is one of the commoner recessively inherited conditions. Although its underlying biochemical abnormality is not known, it is a condition which affects the mucus-secreting glands throughout the body. Pancreatic enzyme secretion is limited, producing very sticky meconium which may block the lumen of the intestine before birth (a condition known as meconium ileus), causing either perforation of the gut and meconium peritonitis or acute intestinal obstruction at birth. X-ray of the abdomen reveals a characteristic finely mottled appearance due to the small air bubbles trapped in the meconium. The condition often requires surgery to relieve the obstruction.

After birth, the paucity of pancreatic enzymes causes maldigestion and malabsorption leading to failure to thrive during the first year of life.

The sticky mucus in the lungs leaves the infant vulnerable to repeated staphylococcal chest infections which often come to dominate the child's life during the school years.

Cystic fibrosis only occasionally presents in the newborn period, but the diagnosis should be sought at an early stage if a sibling has the condition. The diagnosis can only be confirmed by the finding of raised sodium and chloride levels in the sweat – test which is difficult to perform accurately in the first few weeks of life. The identification of one of the many known gene mutations associated with the condition may in time improve the early diagnosis of this disorder. Should the diagnosis be made in the neonatal period, treatment should begin with pancreatic enzyme replacement to ensure adequate digestion and absorption of the milk. The baby must then be followed up closely in a specialised cystic fibrosis clinic.

Routine screening for the condition in all newborn babies at 7 days of age by dried blood spot testing for raised levels of immunoreactive trypsin is performed in certain parts of Britain and the USA and is widely used in Australia, though there is insufficient evidence to prove unequivocally that the prognosis is improved by such early screening (Merelle et al 2000, Scotet et al 2000, Doull et al 2001).

Inborn errors of metabolism

Biochemical techniques have brought to light a large number of different metabolic errors which are associated with impaired mental and physical development in childhood. Most result from the lack of activity of an enzyme or defects in the transport of proteins and other metabolites. Some are recognisable by means of biochemical screening tests in the neonatal period, comprising analysis of dried blood spots taken at 7 days of age (Dezatuex 1998). In a small number of such conditions, treatment from the beginning with dietary restriction or replacement therapy has been proved to prevent disability or handicap. An early diagnosis is therefore essential if the damaging effect of the disease is to be prevented (Leonard & Morris 2000) (p. 211). Others present in a variety

---

> **Box 13.2** Modes of presentation of inborn errors of metabolism
>
> - Neurological symptoms, e.g. lethargy, poor feeding, vomiting, irritability
> - Severe neurological disease, e.g. coma, seizures
> - Severe biochemical disturbance, e.g. non-ketotic hyperglycinaemia, hyperammonaemia, ketonuria (neonates do not normally produce ketones)
> - Unexplained metabolic acidosis
> - Repeated episodes of hypoglycaemia
> - Heart failure
> - Liver disease
> - Dysmorphic features
> - Developmental delay

---

of ways (Box 13.2), ranging from delayed development to episodes of hypoglycaemia serious and life-threatening metabolic disturbance with acidosis and acute encephalopthy (Chakrapani et al 2001). They are almost all inherited as autosomal recessive conditions. All are complex but the development of gene therapy may provide a means of treatment for those for which no effective therapy is currently available.

Galactosaemia

Galactosaemia is one condition in which early treatment can be effective. Lack of an enzyme (galactose-l-phosphate uridyl-transferase) results in a failure of conversion of galactose to glucose, leading to an accumulation of galactose which in turn results in damage to the liver and brain. Since the disease is inherited as a recessive condition, the parents are themselves unaffected clinically but the risk to each subsequent child is 1 in 4. Though its incidence is only about 1 in 60 000, the condition should be suspected in any newborn infant who vomits, refuses feeds, fails to thrive and becomes jaundiced in the first week without any cause. Cataracts may be seen at an early stage. The diagnosis can be suspected if a reducing substance is identified in the urine using the Clinitest tablet method. A further test with Clinistix strips (which identify only glucose by the glucose oxidase method) confirms that the substance is not glucose and specific laboratory testing identifies it as galactose. The diagnosis is confirmed by direct measurement of the red cell

transferase enzyme content, which is greatly reduced. Since galactose forms half of the disaccharide lactose, which is the sugar found in breast and most formula milks, these must be withdrawn completely and replaced by a special low-lactose milk preparation. Symptoms will usually resolve quickly and the dietary restrictions must continue for life. Despite these measures, long-term effects will become apparent in many cases, including damage to the ovaries (in 80% of girls), speech delay and learning difficulties. In some parts of the USA, a blood spot test for the condition is included in neonatal screening programmes.

Phenylketonuria

Although occurring only once in 10 000–15 000 births, early recognition and treatment of the condition are essential to prevent severe learning difficulties from developing. It is inherited as a recessive characteristic, both parents are heterozygous carriers of the gene, and each subsequent child has a 1 in 4 risk of having the disorder.

Congenital deficiency of the liver enzyme phenylalanine hydroxylase prevents the conversion of the amino acid phenylalanine to tyrosine. Increased amounts of phenylalanine accumulate in the blood and tissues, while phenylpyruvic acid appears in the urine. The persistent high blood levels of phenylalanine are responsible for the progressive cerebral dysfunction and irreversible severe learning difficulties which will inevitably develop in untreated cases.

The diagnosis cannot be made clinically and is only identified by the routine screening heel-prick blood test on the seventh day of life. This measures the blood phenylalanine level by the Guthrie bacterial inhibition test or amino acid chromatography. A high value must be urgently confirmed by more detailed biochemical investigation. Significantly elevated phenylalanine levels (above 725 μmol/L or 12 mg/100 mL) confirm the diagnosis.

Treatment   As phenylalanine is an amino acid found in all animal and human protein and many vegetable proteins, breast and formula feeding must cease immediately and dietary treatment must then start using one of the low-phenylalanine milk substitutes with the necessary vitamin and mineral supplements. Regular blood phenylalanine checks are essential and the diet is subsequently regulated to maintain the level near the minimum required for normal growth and metabolism (120–240 μmol/L or 2–4 mg/100 mL) by means of calculated protein additions. Normal intellectual development can usually be achieved and no major deterioration results from relaxing the dietary restriction after 8–12 years of age. A woman with this disorder who wishes to become pregnant must, however, revert to a strict low-phenylalanine diet before conception in order to reduce the risk of severe damage to the developing brain of her fetus (p. 28) (Koch et al 2000).

Congenital hypothyroidism

In about one baby in 3000, the thyroid gland fails to develop or is ectopic and produces inadequate amounts of thyroxine. The clinical signs of established hypothyroidism are only exceptionally recognisable in the newborn and usually only become apparent in the second or third month, by which time some degree of brain damage is already established in a third of cases and this cannot be reversed by treatment. There is clear evidence from clinical trials that the incidence of learning difficulties associated with the condition is substantially reduced by early treatment of those babies identified by the screening programmes, though more minor neurological deficiencies may remain (Rovet 1999). Not all babies so ascertained will have permanently reduced thyroid function and a review of all those with positive tests should be carried out at a year of age to find those who need to continue treatment. Most authorities favour estimation of thyroid-stimulating hormone (TSH) on dried blood spots for routine screening although it fails to detect the exceptional case of secondary hypothyroidism (incidence about 1:100 000). Neonatal TSH screening is now universal in Britain.

Without screening tests, hypothyroidism may be recognised in at least 50% of cases in the first 2 weeks, though at this stage the signs are often subtle. These are sluggish movements, slowness to cry, dryness of the skin, subnormal temperature and unexplained persistent mild physiological jaundice. If X-ray of the long bones of the leg shows absence of the lower femoral epiphysis and the infant is not preterm, the diagnosis may be strongly suspected. Primary hypothyroidism may then be confirmed by finding a low serum thyroxine level with a high value of TSH.

Treatment should start immediately the diagnosis is confirmed, with thyroxine 0.025 mg daily, subsequently increasing the dose as the child grows.

Hypothyroidism associated with congenital goitre is more easily recognisable at this age but is very rare. Endemic hypothyroidism from iodine deficiency is not a problem in Britain but families in which goitrous hypothyroidism occurs are described. More commonly, goitre in the newborn infant is due to drugs used in therapy for maternal thyrotoxicosis in pregnancy or to the administration of iodine. The signs of hypothyroidism do not always accompany the goitre, which gradually diminishes in size, but occasionally thyroxine administration is necessary in the first few weeks.

Other inborn errors of metabolism

There are many other recessively inherited metabolic conditions caused by a specific enzyme deficiency whose gene locations have been identified very recently, thus offering the chance of early prenatal diagnosis of the condition in an at-risk fetus by DNA analysis. In the majority of such conditions, there are no distinguishing features in the neonatal period to point to such a diagnosis. However, a very small number, including, for example, medium-chain acyl coenzyme-A dehydrogenase (MCAD) deficiency, may present in the early weeks of life with a serious metabolic disturbance including acidosis, cerebral symptoms, or even sudden unexpected death. It is clearly important to identify accurately which disorder is causing the problem as early as possible since it is only feasible to test for it in a subsequent pregnancy if the enzyme defect has been characterised. In most cases, an examination of the urine for amino acids and organic acids will identify the offending disease but more extensive discussion of the subject is beyond the scope of this book.

Haemoglobinopathies such as thalassaemia and sickle cell disease are also recessively inherited from carrier parents. In both cases the parents have a mild form of the disease and often know they are carriers. Both conditions can be identified by haemoglobin electrophoresis on neonatal blood spot samples. Screening programmes for both conditions have been introduced into certain parts of the USA where a sizeable proportion of the population is from ethnic black or other predisposed races.

STRUCTURAL CONGENITAL MALFORMATIONS

Sometimes, a congenital abnormality will have been identified before birth by ultrasound examination, e.g. hydrocephalus, spina bifida, hydronephrosis, severe congenital heart disease and many others (p. 21). Most are either obvious at birth or are identified in the first few days or weeks (e.g. gut atresias), but some are only revealed by a deliberate search (e.g. congenital dislocation of hips, phenylketonuria).

In the following descriptions, stress is laid mainly upon those malformations in which early recognition is important so that appropriate management or advice can be given; most of the rarer anomalies are omitted unless some specific form of early treatment is essential.

ALIMENTARY TRACT
Cleft lip and cleft palate

This type of deformity occurs in between 1 in 300 and 1 in 600 births. The lip is involved in 60% of these, the remainder involving the palate alone. Both genetic inheritance and environmental factors are involved in its causation. If either parent has the condition, the occurrence in their offspring is up to 1 in 20, and 1 in 25 siblings of an index case will be affected. For an isolated midline cleft palate, which is a genetically distinct condition comprising about a quarter of the total,

the risk is about half this figure. Ten per cent of clefts are associated with other congenital malformations, particularly trisomies and other chromosome anomalies. Maternal anticonvulsants taken in pregnancy increase the risk and small 'epidemics' of cleft lip and palate have been reported in association with outbreaks of Coxsackie B4 virus infections.

The cleft lip may be single (Plate 11) or double (Plate 18A); if double, the central portion (globular process) between the clefts may protrude forward.

Management

Though the parents are often shocked by their baby's appearance, the main problem for the child in the neonatal period is difficulty with feeding. The method of feeding depends upon the extent of the deformity. In many cases of cleft lip alone, or small clefts of the soft palate, breast feeding is possible and should be recommended. For those infants who from choice or because breast feeding is unsuccessful are to be bottle fed, feeding can often be managed remarkably well using an ordinary bottle and a big soft teat, with an enlarged hole in it if necessary, even when the cleft is quite severe. Specially designed flanged teats are available to try and close the gap during suction, but they are seldom helpful. A fitted solid palatal prosthesis may help in some cases. If this fails, spoon or cup feeding is always possible and should be practised at some time before the operation in order that mother and child will be accustomed to it when it is used temporarily after repair of the lip. Great parental anxiety is natural at first and a full explanation of the management, including discussing the likely outcome of the operation and showing the parents photographs of the final result in other children (Plates 18A & B), is time well spent.

Respiratory difficulty occurs only in a rare group, known as the Pierre Robin syndrome, in which a midline cleft of the soft palate is associated with micrognathia (short mandible); the tongue tends to protrude upwards and backwards through the cleft, obstructing the respiratory passages. Although the resulting cyanotic attacks can potentially endanger life, they may almost always be prevented by nursing the infant in the prone position, which sometimes requires a special arrangement for supporting the head face-downward whilst keeping the airway clear.

Surgical treatment

Repair of the lip is usually carried out at around 3 months of age, palatal closure being performed after 9 months. Around 80% of babies treated at this age will have normal or near normal speech (Sell et al 2001, Timmons et al 2001), the rate being substantially lower if palatal surgery is delayed until later in childhood. The growth of the maxilla is unaffected by early surgery.

Middle ear infections are not rare even after closure of the palate and some degree of hearing impairment is common. Regular hearing tests should minimise this. Frequently, grommets will be inserted by an ENT surgeon in the tympanic membranes to prevent hearing loss associated with chronic serous otitis media. Continuing orthodontic care is required to ensure a good cosmetic appearance of the teeth and speech therapy may be required later to improve speech. Teamwork is essential, each playing complementary roles to achieve good long-term results. Some cosmetic surgery is often needed through childhood to achieve acceptable appearances.

Anomalies which cause intestinal obstruction

There are many malformations which cause obstruction to the passage of food through the gut, from oesophageal atresia to anal atresia. Each presents with a characteristic combination of symptoms and is a surgical emergency requiring referral to a unit specialising in neonatal surgery to restore the patency of the gut. Symptoms relate to the distance from the mouth to the point of the blockage, but all present within a few hours of birth.

Oesophageal atresia

In this anomaly, the upper part of the oesophagus is present only to the level of the second to fourth thoracic vertebrae (about a third of its length), where it ends blindly. In most cases there is also a fistula between the trachea and the lower section of the oesophagus, which leads to the stomach. In about 8% there is a blind oesophagus without a tracheo-oesophageal fistula, and the remainder consists of other variations. The anomaly occurs about once in 3000 live births.

Diagnosis   A large amount of amniotic fluid is normally swallowed by the fetus each day; however, this is impossible when the oesophagus is blocked, and polyhydramnios results. About 1 in 30 cases of polyhydramnios is associated with upper intestinal obstruction or diaphragmatic hernia. It should therefore be routine practice to pass a nasogastric tube to exclude oesophageal atresia soon after delivery in all cases of polyhydramnios. The abnormality should also be suspected in any newborn infant who accumulates excessive saliva and mucus secretions in the mouth and pharynx, particularly when this secretion is frothy and the baby has periodic attacks of choking with obstruction to breathing and perhaps cyanosis.

It is vital to make the diagnosis before the first feed is given, to avoid choking and aspiration of feed into the lungs. The midwife should, without delay, attempt to pass a firm polythene nasogastric tube through the mouth and down the oesophagus. If atresia is present, the tube is held up by an obstruction 7–10 cm down the oesophagus, though if the tube is not fairly rigid it may curl up in the oesophageal pouch (Fig. 13.5). The absence of acid in the fluid aspirated from the tube also supports the diagnosis. Instillation of a radio-opaque medium is contraindicated since the inevitable aspiration into the lungs adds to the problem already present. Gas in the intestine on X-ray indicates the presence of a tracheo-oesophageal fistula as well as atresia (Fig. 13.5), but absence of gas does not exclude it.

Management   The mouth, pharynx and blind oesophagus must be aspirated frequently to remove accumulating secretions. This is best performed using a double lumen replogle tube attached to a low pressure continuous suction pump. A search should be made for additional congenital malformations. Prompt transfer of the

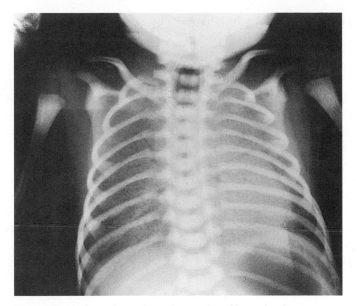

Figure 13.5 Oesophageal atresia – a chest X-ray showing a large-bore nasogastric tube coiled up in the upper oesophagus. (By kind permission of Dr Jo Fairhurst.)

infant to a paediatric surgical team for urgent operative repair is essential. The two ends of the oesophagus are anastomosed through a thoracic approach. Sometimes a temporary gastrostomy to allow enteral feeding is needed if primary anastamosis is not possible, but this is combined with an oesophagostomy opening to the outside at the root of the neck. This allows the infant to retain the art of sucking and swallowing until the oesophagus is joined to the stomach at later surgery. The main risk to the infant is from pneumonia following aspiration of the oesophageal contents into the lungs, from any accompanying anomalies or from prematurity.

Congenital oesophageal hiatus hernia

In congenital oesophageal hiatus hernia, the cardiac portion of the stomach protrudes through the oesophageal hiatus in the diaphragm. Often it remains undiagnosed until later infancy. Sometimes it can be intermittent, a condition known as a sliding hernia. There is free reflux of gastric contents up the oesophagus due to interference with the valvular mechanism at the cardia and acid-induced ulceration may occur at the junction of oesophageal and gastric mucosa, followed occasionally by stricture formation. The condition is not uncommon and it may become symptomless after mixed feeding begins at about 4 or 5 months.

Vomiting usually occurs from birth but it is not always profuse or consistent; later, the vomit may contain small amounts of blood due to oesophagitis, and, very occasionally, anaemia from persistent occult bleeding is the presenting feature. Confirmation of the diagnosis can only be made by X-ray screening during a barium feed, which demonstrates the pouch of stomach above the diaphragm. Reflux of gastric contents into the oesophagus is not in itself enough to make the diagnosis since it occurs in some normal infants. Medical treatment, consisting of the use of thickened feeds and maintaining the semi-upright position throughout the day and night for several months, successfully tides over most cases until they become symptomless towards the end of the first year. Persistent acid oesophagitis, which may be suspected when there is continued altered blood in the vomit and confirmed by oesophagoscopy, may respond to supression of acid production by H2 antagonists such as ranitidine. Surgery is rarely required except for stricture formation.

Congenital hypertrophic pyloric stenosis

In this condition, the muscle at the pylorus of the stomach hypertrophies over the first few weeks of life, causing an increasing obstruction to the passage of milk feeds. It is doubtful whether this relatively common disorder should be classed as congenital or as a malformation even though it presents so early in life. Heredity plays a part in its causation, for the normal incidence of about 2 per 1000 births is much increased where either parent or a previous child has suffered from it, and it is five times as common in boys as in girls. The risk of occurrence of the condition in the children of women who have had pyloric stenosis is 1 in 5 for sons and 1 in 15 for daughters. In the case of an affected father, the risks are 1 in 20 for sons and 1 in 40 for daughters.

Clinical features and management Whether or not there is some pyloric hypertrophy present at birth, the obstruction rarely begins until after the second week. Vomiting, which is the major presenting feature, sometimes starts in the first week but more often it is delayed until the third to fifth weeks or even occasionally as long as 2 months. It starts as small possets but gradually becomes projectile and occurs immediately after feeding, the vomit containing no bile; weight is lost, but, unless dehydration or electrolyte disturbances become severe enough to cause apathy, the infant will continue to take the feeds hungrily. Stools may become infrequent and small.

Visible gastric peristalsis in the left upper quadrant of the abdomen after a feed is characteristic but not diagnostic and only palpation of the thickened pylorus during a feed, which requires patience and some experience, is conclusive clinical evidence. Occasionally, an ultrasound examination or barium meal (Fig. 13.6) will confirm the diagnosis in a case where the tumour cannot be felt.

Surgical treatment by means of Ramstedt's pyloromyotomy, in which the hypertrophied muscle is split along its length to widen the pyloric canal, relieves the problem rapidly and

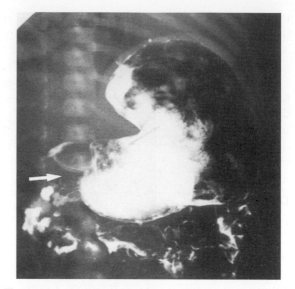

Figure 13.6 Barium meal in congenital hypertrophic pyloric stenosis showing the pyloric canal (arrowed) narrowed to a fine line by the hypertrophied surrounding muscle.

effectively. It is never a surgical emergency and significant fluid and electrolyte imbalance should be fully corrected intravenously before the operation.

Duodenal atresia

In this condition, the site of obstruction is usually in the third part of the duodenum, below the opening of the common bile duct. Maternal polyhydramnios is a common accompanying sign and the infant frequently has evidence of intrauterine growth retardation. There is a substantially increased incidence in babies with Down syndrome. If a congenital abnormality ultrasound scan has been carried out in the early stages of pregnancy, this anomaly is identifiable, since the stomach and duodenum are shown distended with fluid in contrast to the rest of the gut which is empty.

After birth, the condition presents as repeated vomiting of bile starting within the first 24 hours of life without noticeable distension of the abdomen. Meconium may be passed normally at first. The yellowish staining of vomit caused by pigment in swallowed colostrum is to be distinguished clearly from the greener colour of bile. Also it must be remembered that, on the rare occasions where the atresia is above the bile-duct opening, no bile will be present in the vomit. Straight X-ray of the abdomen in the erect posture is diagnostic, the double gas shadows of the dilated stomach and duodenum only being visible, usually with fluid levels. The operation of duodenojejunostomy must be carried out urgently and usually relieves the condition.

Duodenal stenosis

This is more difficult to diagnose. Vomiting is usually present from birth and is often bile stained. Since the obstruction is only a partial one, meconium and normal 'changing' stools are passed.

Straight X-ray of the abdomen is not likely to be conclusive; screening after a small feed containing contrast medium may safely be used for diagnosis if there is no evidence of lower intestinal obstruction from straight X-ray films.

Neonatal intestinal obstruction below the duodenum

Obstruction below the duodenum gives rise to a recognisable clinical picture, for which there are several different causes. The onset of vomiting of bile-stained or brownish material and an increasingly distended abdomen and, sometimes, visible peristalsis within the first few days of life are the characteristic features. A straight X-ray of the abdomen in the erect posture will confirm the diagnosis by showing the characteristic dilated loops of bowel and fluid levels in the gut.

Differential diagnosis of the site and cause of the obstruction can often be made from the clinical signs and X-ray appearance, and the principal types are described here with their main characteristic features.

Atresia of the jejunum or ileum

Abdominal distension is early in onset and erect straight X-ray shows the large gas shadows of dilated small intestine – usually with fluid levels

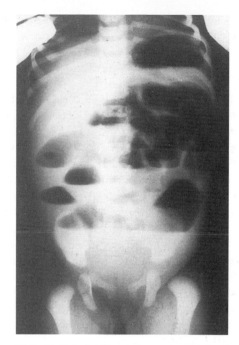

Figure 13.7 Multiple fluid levels in an erect abdominal X-ray in ilieal atresia.

but with no gas in the colon (Fig. 13.7). Occasionally the X-ray appearance of slight generalised dilatation of the gut with occasional fluid levels may be caused simply by swallowing a lot of air, but in atresia of the small gut the distended loops of intestine terminate abruptly at the point of obstruction. Early operation is usually successful, but it is often necessary to resect a portion of the very dilated gut before anastomosis.

Malrotation of the midgut

Malrotation of the midgut, though often remaining undetected and symptomless until later childhood, may also cause obstruction in the neonatal period. There may be either duodenal obstruction from compression by the abnormal mesentery or a volvulus involving the ileum and jejunum.

Meckel's diverticulum

Meckel's diverticulum causes an obstruction that gives rise to a similar picture. There is nothing diagnostic about the clinical features except the timing of onset, which is generally after the first 2 days of life.

Hirschsprung's disease

Hirschsprung's disease may present in the neonatal period as abdominal distension with gas and severe retention of faeces amounting sometimes to obstruction. It is almost entirely a disease of males, with an incidence of 1 in 5000 births and, like duodenal atresia, is relatively more common in children with Down syndrome. The hold-up in the passage of faeces through the lower part of the colon is caused by a length of large gut which lacks parasympathetic ganglion cells (the 'aganglionic segment') and fails to pass on the peristaltic wave. This segment may be a short one extending from the rectum into the last few inches of sigmoid colon, or less commonly it may extend upward for a variable distance in the colon. Persistent dilatation of the normal gut behind it results in the so-called megacolon.

Usually no meconium is passed at all in the first few days, but sometimes there are infrequent loose offensive stools thereafter. The outstanding feature of Hirschsprung's disease is in the abdominal distension from retained gas. On rectal examination it is possible sometimes to produce a temporary dilatation of the aganglionic segment with relief of symptoms by a rush of gas and faeces. A barium enema may reveal the characteristic narrowed segment of colon but a rectal biopsy showing the absence of ganglion cells is necessary for diagnosis; however, even these can be difficult to interpret.

The use of repeated saline washouts may help postpone surgery during the neonatal period. If a laparotomy is required to exclude other causes for the obstruction, it is usual to fashion a colostomy and take a biopsy of the rectal mucosa for histological diagnosis. The colostomy may have to remain for several weeks or months before the operation of rectosigmoidectomy is performed, consisting of resection of the aganglionic segment and most of the rectum followed by anastomosis of the proximal colon to the remaining rectal stump. In subsequent pregnancies there is a risk of about 1 in 5 for any male child developing the same condition.

Incarcerated inguinal hernia

Incarcerated inguinal hernia is another occasional cause of obstruction, usually occurring in the preterm male baby (p. 122).

Imperforate or ectopic anus

There is a great variety of different anomalies in this region (Plate 19). In the female, the commonest type is displacement forward of the anal opening so that it opens immediately behind the vulva, inside the vulva or, rarely, inside the vagina. In the male there may be no sign of an anus at all, a bulging membrane or triangular portion of skin at the anal site, or a narrow subcutaneous channel leading forward from the true anus to a fistulous opening anteriorly (the 'covered anus'). Rectourethral fistulae also occur rarely in males.

Even when there is simple anterior displacement of the anal opening, it is usually a narrow one which allows some temporary passage of meconium but generally leads to partial obstruction sooner or later. It can be treated initially simply by dilatation, though often further surgery is needed later.

The extent of the anomaly and the type of operation which is required should be determined by a paediatric surgeon. In many cases, a simple cutting-back operation to enlarge the displaced opening is all that is necessary and does not interfere with sphincter control, but the more serious forms of the condition require operation via the abdomen in order to define the abormal anatomy. A colostomy may be necessary until the definitive surgery is carried out. Provided that use can be made of the puborectalis muscle sling, good results with faecal continence can be obtained in most cases.

Meconium plug

Temporary obstruction from the presence of a meconium plug (not in association with meconium ileus) is relatively common. The plug occupies the lower colon and rectum, and its leading end consists of white mucoid jelly which may sometimes be removed by gentle rectal examination. Occasionally, a small repeated saline washout may be necessary to achieve this.

Meconium peritonitis

Meconium peritonitis may be a complication of meconium ileus or necrotising enterocolitis, or may be due to congenital defects in the intestinal wall. X-ray of the abdomen shows gas in the peritoneal cavity and, sometimes, calcification outside the bowel. Exploratory laparotomy is essential to detect the site of the perforation and to repair it.

Disorders of development of the umbilicus

Exomphalos

This anomaly (Plate 20A) occurs once in every 5000 births. In this type of abdominal hernia, the protrusion occurs into the umbilical stalk itself, so that the cord is inserted into part of the hernial sac, consisting of amniotic membranes and peritoneum. Occasionally this may rupture during delivery, allowing the abdominal contents to spill out. Association with other congenital malformations, particularly of the alimentary tract, is common and exomphalos is one of the features of Beckwith's syndrome (p. 56).

Gastroschisis

In this condition (Plate 20B), the herniation occurs through a large defect in the abdominal wall adjacent to the umbilicus, so there is no covering sac. The protruding gut is usually inflamed from irritation by amniotic fluid and the baby often has peritonitis at birth. The bowel is oedematous, thickened and often appears blue due to interference with its blood supply.

Both exophalos and gastroschisis cause a rise in maternal alpha-fetoprotein levels in early pregnancy but they can be distinguished from the more usual cause – an open spina bifida – by antenatal ultrasound scanning (p. 23).

Treatment

Immediate treatment of both exomphalos and gastroschisis is directed towards preventing drying out and infection of the protruding gut until the baby can be brought to neonatal paediatric surgery. One effective means of doing this is to wrap the whole abdomen, including the herniated intestine, loosely in clingfilm to prevent loss of fluid and dress the baby with warm clothing to maintain his temperature.

Fluid and electrolyte losses from an exposed hernial sac or the protruding gut can be severe and an intravenous infusion of human albumin is essential if the baby is to be transferred to a distant hospital for surgery. Parenteral nutrition is often required postoperatively until the gut recovers its function.

The difficulty in surgical treatment is proportional to the amount and size of the viscera which have to be replaced. It is sometimes impossible to return all the abdominal contents and still close the abdominal muscles over them without compromising the baby's breathing, so in some cases a temporary cover with skin or a Dacron sheet is made and full repair attempted later.

RESPIRATORY TRACT
Choanal atresia

Obstruction to the upper airway should be excluded whenever a baby seems to be in respiratory difficulty immediately after birth. Choanal atresia is a congenital abnormality in which there is bony or cartilaginous obstruction in the posterior nasal passages. Since a newborn baby has the greatest difficulty breathing through the mouth when the nasal airway is obstructed, repeated vigorous inspiratory efforts are made before a small intake of air passes the tongue, momentarily relieving the shortage of oxygen which may be severe enough to cause cyanosis. When seen immediately after birth, this struggle for effective respiration can be mistakenly attributed to a disorder of lung function until it becomes clear that no air is passing the nose. Thick stringy mucus usually occupies the nasal space. The diagnosis is likely if a nasogastric tube cannot be passed beyond the posterior part of the nose, and confirmed by the absence of airflow past a wisp of cotton wool held under the nostril. Feeding from the breast or bottle is impossible for any length of time and orogastric tube feeding is necessary until the condition can be relieved surgically.

Treatment

Breathing may be eased temporarily by pulling the tongue forward to allow air to pass through the mouth into the pharynx and nursing the baby in the prone position. A small oral airway strapped into position can be very effective as a temporary measure. The next step involves surgical treatment in a specialised unit, and the methods of relieving the obstruction vary. Good results have been obtained by using a trochar and cannula to make a new opening through the solid occlusion in the posterior nasal passages, followed by the insertion of polythene tubing as an airway to keep the passage from closing until epithelium has formed.

Unilateral atresia can go unnoticed until later in childhood as many such infants can breathe adequately through the one open side. The condition is occasionally associated with other congenital malformations and nerve deafness in a rare syndrome known as the CHARGE association. Early assessment of the baby's hearing is essential to enable hearing aids to be provided and language training to be introduced from an early age.

Lung malformations

Congenital lung cysts

These rare malformations usually present at birth with respiratory difficulty, though they occasionally remain symptomless until later childhood. They are often identifiable on examination of the fetal lungs on prenatal ultrasound; after birth, the chest X-ray may resemble a diaphragmatic hernia but the condition can be distinguished from it by passing a nasogastric tube into a normally positioned stomach. The abnormal part of the lung should be removed surgically to prevent recurrent infection.

Sequestration of the lung

In this condition, the bronchi fail to communicate properly with a portion of lung tissue which remains unaerated after birth. It is often symptomless, but if it is identified on an X-ray, surgical removal is indicated.

Diaphragmatic hernia

Around once in 2000 births part of the diaphragm fails to develop, allowing the abdominal organs to occupy the left side of the chest, and displacing the heart and mediastinum to the right. Polyhydramnios often accompanies the malformation and ultrasound scanning can often demonstrate the abnormality before birth. If it is identified antenatally, it is important that the infant is resuscitated by endotracheal intubation at birth and that positive pressure by mask is avoided since it may cause distension of the stomach which will further embarrass respiration. When large amounts of the abdominal contents are located in the chest, severe respiratory distress and cyanosis are present from birth, and, if not diagnosed antenatally, the condition may be suspected when the maximum area of intensity of the heart sounds is over the right side of the chest and the abdomen is noticeably hollowed.

A chest X-ray (Fig. 3.5b) shows the loops of bowel in the chest and often displacement of the heart to the opposite side. Symptomatic diaphragmatic hernia is a surgical emergency, for early operation may be life saving. Sometimes the lungs are hypoplastic and are unable to sustain adequate oxygenation despite maximal endotracheal ventilation, and the respiratory failure may be compounded by persistence of fetal pulmonary hypertension. The resulting hypoxia accounts for the high mortality of the condition, particularly in the preterm infant.

Hypoplasia

Hypoplasia of the lungs with diminished lung function and pulmonary hypertension may complicate several conditions including diaphragmatic hernia, idiopathic oligohydramnios and the very rare bony abnormalities which restrict the growth of the chest wall. So long as the underlying problem is remediable, the lungs will usually develop improved function as the child grows.

THE HEART AND GREAT VESSELS

The true incidence of congenital malformations of the heart is uncertain because many, including some of the more serious lesions, are not detectable at birth by present methods of routine examination and some – for instance, the smaller ventricular septal defects – resolve completely without treatment. The documented incidence is about 8 per 1000 births and around half of these will require medical and surgical treatment in the neonatal period. In a quarter of cases, the cardiac malformation is only one of several congenital anomalies or is one feature of a syndrome associated with a chromosomal abnormality, such as Down syndrome.

Surgical techniques have developed so rapidly that the number of completely inoperable abnormalities is now small. An increasing number of corrective procedures can now be undertaken in the newborn period and techniques to relieve cyanosis can reduce the morbidity of others considerably. It follows that early recognition of serious congenital heart disease is of great importance and it is this, rather than detailed differential diagnosis of the numerous types of abnormality, that will be described here. About 25% of congenital heart lesions can be diagnosed before birth by ultrasound examination (Garne et al 2001) but to date there is little evidence that the outlook is improved by prenatal diagnosis.

For those who look after newborn babies, what matters is the ability to identify the infants whose problems are attributable to heart disease, to know how to select the ones who require early surgical treatment, and to have the means of maintaining the infant in the best condition to enable a safe transfer to a paediatric cardiology centre at the optimal time.

Presentation of congenital heart disease

In the neonatal period, congenital heart disease presents itself in one or more of the following ways:

- Cardiac failure (p. 226) – tachypnoea, costal recession, tachycardia, enlargement of the liver and, occasionally, oedema are the main features. It can be difficult to be certain whether respiratory distress is due to pulmonary or cardiac disease.
- Central cyanosis, affecting the whole body and the mucous membranes of the mouth and conjunctiva, which is persistent and not confined to the extremities, in the absence of a pulmonary cause.
- A cardiac murmur – it must be remembered that moderately loud transient systolic murmurs may sometimes be heard in some normal babies in the first few days. Conversely, the murmurs of certain types of congenital heart disease do not become audible for several days or weeks, and not all types of congenital heart disease cause a murmur.
- An arrhythmia (e.g. bradycardia with heart block, ectopic beats, supraventricular tachycardia).
- Lethargy, inactivity, poor feeding and, later, failure to thrive.

Investigations

The purpose of investigation of suspected congenital heart disease is to identify the type of defect present, to aid in the assessment of risk to the infant's immediate health and to monitor the need for, and the effects of, treatment. The investigations usually performed are:

- chest X-ray
- electrocardiogram (ECG)
- echocardiography
- blood gases
- pulse oximetry
- oxygen saturation test.

A chest X-ray shows the heart size, outline and position, and the vascularity of the lungs. Apparent cardiac enlargement may be due to a large thymic shadow. Sometimes, enlargement of the whole heart or a specific chamber or vessel can be seen, but the rapid circulatory changes at this time and the variations of the normal chest X-ray make interpretation difficult at this age.

The ECG

At birth, the ECG pattern reflects the hypertrophy of the right side of the heart which has ensured the effectiveness of the fetal circulation. As the baby rapidly adapts to independent existence, alterations occur in the ECG within the first 24 hours. Thereafter the pattern becomes fairly stable, although certain characteristics differ from those in later infancy. The electrical axis of the normal neonatal heart is between +110° and +180° (as shown by a dominant S wave in lead I and R wave in lead III), caused by the dominant right ventricle, which is represented as prominent R waves in V4R and V1 chest leads and S waves in V5 and V6. Notching of the R wave in V1 is a common variation of normal. The T waves in the right chest leads are usually upright for the first 24 hours but become inverted by the fourth day.

Disorders of conduction and rhythm, particularly atrial premature beats, are present in about 1% of newborn infants, though rarely do they cause clinical disturbance and usually they disappear by 3 months of age. They may also be seen on fetal heart recordings in labour.

Neonatal ECGs are difficult to interpret because large changes in the dynamics of the circulation are occurring. However, findings that should alert suspicion include a superior axis, left axis deviation, left ventricular hypertrophy (tall R waves in V6 and deep S waves in V2), marked right ventricular hypertrophy (upright T wave after the fourth day, together with a tall R wave in chest lead VI), or conduction abnormalities.

Blood pressure

It is very difficult to measure the blood pressure by auscultation or even by palpation. The most accurate measurements are made by placing a Doppler ultrasound probe over the brachial or tibial artery below the cuff. Automated electronic apparatus using a pressure-sensitive transducer can make repeated measurements in even the smallest infant and is now a standard part of intensive neonatal care, particularly of the sick baby with respiratory distress syndrome. A blood pressure recording may also help in the diagnosis of aortic coarctation, where the pressure in the legs is significantly lower than in the arms.

The normal range of blood pressure is wide and varies with gestational age. In a term baby, the systolic pressure in the arm rises from about 70 mmHg on the first day to around 85 mmHg by the second week and 95 mmHg at 6 weeks. Variation in the size of the cuff causes big differences in the readings, too small a cuff giving too high a value. The inflatable section should cover over half the length of the upper arm and more than two-thirds of its circumference. For the term newborn infant, a width of 5 cm and a length of 7–10 cm is ideal, with relatively narrower cuffs for smaller babies.

Other investigations

Echocardiography provides a non-invasive means of demonstrating the anatomical structure of the chambers, valves and vessels of the heart and the connections between them, together with measurement of pressure gradients across the valves if Doppler equipment is available. Colour flow mapping can also demonstrate abnormal pattern of blood flow in septal defects or in more complex anomalies. In some conditions it provides enough information to plan surgical treatment, though cardiac catheterisation is still required in a proportion of cases.

In a baby with significant cyanotic heart disease, transcutaneous pulse oximetry will demonstrate the degree of arterial oxygen desaturation. The oxygen saturation test can be used to distinguish cardiac from pulmonary cyanosis. An infant with cyanotic heart disease breathing 100% oxygen will fail to raise the arterial pO_2 above 13 kPa, whereas the pO_2 will rise significantly above this value in lung conditions. Blood gases are particularly important in the cyanosed infant and will show whether the baby is becoming acidotic as a result of hypoxia. If much time is likely to elapse before the baby's arrival at the cardiac centre, the control of acidosis is crucial to the outlook for either survival or minimisation of the risk of later neurological handicap. In some conditions an infusion of prostaglandins is needed to keep the ductus arteriosus open during transfer (p. 225).

Common heart malformations

There are many different types of cardiac malformation. Those producing symptoms in the neonatal period are often complex or multiple. Those that most commonly occur will be described, classifying them according to their mode of presentation.

Malformations presenting mainly with cyanosis

Cyanotic congenital heart disease is usually complex and the physical signs vary greatly in the same basic condition from one infant to another; distinguishing the conditions clinically is often impossible and an accurate anatomical diagnosis can only be made with echocardiography or more complex investigations. All babies suspected of having a cyanotic heart malformation require urgent investigation and most require surgical intervention to improve the oxygenation of the blood.

Transposition of the great arteries In transposition of the great arteries, the aorta arises from the right ventricle and the pulmonary artery from the left (Fig. 13.8). Thus, unless a septal defect or open ductus arteriosus is also present, the two circulations are completely separated. Cyanosis from birth is usual, and typically the baby seems otherwise well in the first day or two until the ductus arteriosus begins to close. Thereafter the progress depends upon how much oxygenated blood flows across any associated septal defect between the pulmonary and systemic sides of the circulation. Cyanosis and respiratory difficulty usually become progressively worse within the first week. Murmurs and other signs, even the X-ray and ECG findings, are so variable at different stages that they prove to be of little diagnostic help. Echocardiography can demonstate the pulmonary artery arising from the left ventricle,

and the aorta in an abnormally posterior position coming off the right ventricle (Fig. 13.8).

The development of balloon septostomy (Rashkind's procedure), which creates a large interatrial communication by the use of a balloon catheter alone and relieves cyanosis rapidly by allowing mixing of the saturated and unsaturated blood, means that early transfer to a cardiac centre on suspicion of the diagnosis is essential. Later, a surgical procedure to create a cross-over of the circulations can be achieved by an arterial switch procedure (Brown et al 2001) or, less commonly, by a Mustard procedure in the atria. These have a high success rate and a relatively low operative mortality.

Pulmonary atresia and critical pulmonary stenosis In these conditions, the pulmonary artery, pulmonary valve and the right ventricle are all hypoplastic, and often cyanosis is the only abnormality on clinical examination. On the ECG there is usually left axis deviation, because of the diminished forces from the hypoplastic right ventricle, and the tall peaked P waves of right atrial hypertrophy. The X-ray shows gross cardiac enlargement with pulmonary arterial oligaemia but often obvious bronchial artery shadows. Immediate referral to a cardiac centre is essential since some cases may be helped by urgent pulmonary valvotomy or balloon valvuloplasty, or an arterial shunt operation, but the prognosis is often poor.

Tricuspid atresia Atresia of the tricuspid valve is always accompanied by hypoplasia of the right ventricle (Fig. 13.9). A large ventricular septal defect is usually present, allowing enough pulmonary blood flow to maintain adequate oxygenation of the blood. Treatment can often be deferred until much later in childhood. It is often associated with the presence of marked left-sided dominance on the ECG.

Total anomalous pulmonary venous drainage This condition, in which the pulmonary veins enter the right atrium instead of the left, is usually associated with cyanosis and the early onset of cardiac failure. Murmurs may be absent. The lung fields on X-ray appear hazy due to pulmonary vascular congestion and the ECG shows right ventricular hypertrophy.

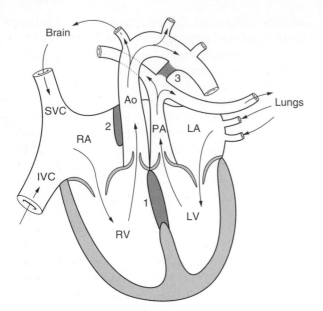

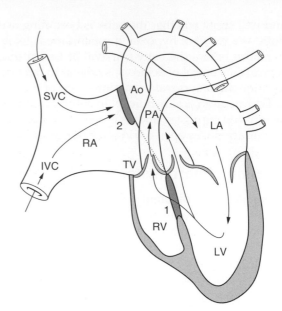

Figure 13.8 Transposition of the great arteries. The aorta (Ao) arises from the right ventricle (RV) and the pulmonary artery (PA) from the left ventricle (LV). The pulmonary and systemic circuits have no connection unless a defect in the ventricular (1) or atrial (2) septum coexists or the ductus arteriosus (3) remains open. SVC = superior vena cava; IVC = inferior vena cava; RA = right atrium; LA = left atrium.

Figure 13.9 Tricuspid atresia. With an absent tricuspid valve (TV) and a hypoplastic right ventricle (RV), the returning venous blood crosses the foramen ovale (2). Pulmonary and systemic blood mix in the left atrium (LA) and venticle (LV). Some crosses a ventricular septal defect (1) to reach the pulmonary artery (PA). SVC = superior vena cava; IVC = inferior vena cava; RA = right atrium; Ao = aorta.

Persistent truncus arteriosus Persistent truncus arteriosus consists of a single artery leaving the heart which supplies both the aorta and pulmonary vessels. A systolic murmur and mild cyanosis are usually present, with breathlessness from increased pulmonary blood flow. Echocardiography shows the single arterial trunk emerging from the ventricles. A proportion of babies with this or other conotruncal abnormalities have a gene deletion on chromosome 22 (p. 205).

Single ventricle A single ventricle, with or without other anomalies, is also likely to present with cyanosis.

Fallot's tetralogy Pulmonary stenosis associated with right ventricular hypertrophy and an aorta which overrides a ventricular septal defect is known as Fallot's tetralogy. Initially there is a murmur at the left sternal edge from the stenotic pulmonary valve, but cyanosis develops as hypertrophy of the infundibular muscle of the right ventricle obstructs pulmonary blood flow. A chest X-ray shows reduced pulmonary

vascularity and the heart is usually of normal size. Echocardiography shows the abnormal anatomy well and surgical correction of the ventricular septal defect and the pulmonary stenosis is often very successful.

Poor pulmonary perfusion Occasionally, cyanosis can result from poor pulmonary perfusion associated either with polycythaemia or with persistence of fetal pulmonary hypertension without a cardiac malformation. This latter problem requires treatment with oxygen and pulmonary vasodilator drugs, e.g. tolazoline, and sometimes the condition is sufficiently severe to need mechanical ventilation. It is often only diagnosed after full cardiac investigation has excluded any anatomical abnormality.

Management of the severely cyanosed infant

In transposition and pulmonary atresia in particular, the baby's survival may depend on the small amount of oxygenated blood flowing through an open ductus arteriosus. Closure, which may occur at any time, results in the rapid onset of acidosis and severe hypoxia which can cause brain damage. In these infants, an intravenous infusion of dinoprostone at a rate of 0.01–0.05 µg/kg per minute may improve mixing of the circulations for long enough to enable the safe transfer of the infant to the cardiac centre (Penny et al 2001).

Malformations presenting mainly with heart failure and respiratory distress

Hypoplastic left heart syndrome This condition, consisting of aortic atresia and severe under-development of the left ventricle, is the commonest fatal cardiac malformation in the newborn period. The only treatment available is heart transplantation, though results are currently very disappointing. Heart failure, which does not respond to medical treatment, appears within the first few days of life together with poor peripheral pulses and some degree of cyanosis. Occasionally, a murmur may be present. The ECG usually shows gross right ventricular dominance and the diagnosis is readily confirmed on echocardiography. Death usually occurs within a week or two of birth.

Coarctation of the aorta Coarctation of the aorta (Fig. 13.10) is a localised narrowing of a small segment of the aortic arch which partially obstructs aortic blood flow. It is often associated with other anomalies, such as persistent ductus arteriosus or ventricular septal defect, and only presents in the newborn period if it is severe. The femoral pulses are either not palpable or diminished and delayed, and the blood pressure is higher in the arms than in the legs. Cardiac failure usually occurs within the first 2 weeks. A murmur is often heard most easily between the scapulae. Unexpectedly, the ECG usually shows right dominance, probably because the ductus remains open. Urgent corrective surgery in the neonatal period is needed if the baby is in heart failure, and is successful in most cases. Restenosis with the development of hypertension occurs in a minority of babies later in childhood.

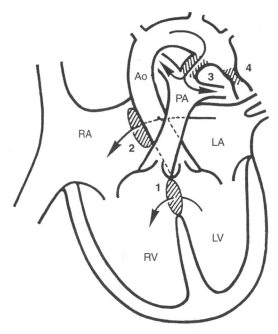

Abbreviations:

RA – Right atrium
LA – Left atrium
RV – Right ventricle
LV – Left ventricle
PA – Pulmonary artery
Ao – Aorta

Heart abnormalities illustrated:

1 – Ventricular septal defect
2 – Atrial septal defect
3 – Patent ductus arteriosus
4 – Coarctation of the aorta

Figure 13.10 Diagram to show the position and direction of blood flow in the main acyanotic congenital heart lesions.

Less severe coarctation without additional malformations, which is more common, can only be diagnosed at this age by the finding of absent or delayed femoral pulses and raised blood pressure in the arms.

Ventricular septal defect, persistent ductus arteriosus and atrial septal defect In most cases of isolated ventricular septal defect or persistent ductus arteriosus (Figs 13.10 and 9.10) the baby remains well and the heart clinically normal in the newborn period. A murmur usually appears 2 to 6 weeks after birth. If the defects are large or are associated with other cardiac anomalies, heart failure may ensue during the first week. In ventricular septal defect, a short systolic murmur appears in the first 2–3 weeks and only becomes pansystolic after about 6 weeks of age, as the pressures in the right side of the heart fall naturally below the left, allowing blood to flow from left to right across the defect. The classical continuous or machinery murmur of the ductus arteriosus is not usually audible at this age for the same reason. Secundum atrial septal defects (Fig. 13.10) rarely present in the first few weeks of life, though infants with the more complex primum defects, which are often associated with defects of the mitral and tricuspid valves, often develop heart failure in the first few days of life.

Heart failure   Heart failure due either to congenital heart disease or to an arrhythmia frequently shows itself first as laboured breathing or tachypnoea. The diagnosis and investigation are described on page 221 but the clinical features which should give rise to suspicion are:

- rapid respiration with marked indrawing of the lower ribs on inspiration
- tachycardia
- enlargement of the liver
- cyanosis
- oedema with unexpected weight gain
- heart murmurs (not always present at this stage).

Paroxysmal supraventricular tachycardia   In this condition, which is caused by an abnormality of the conducting tissues within the heart and is not uncommon, the rate of the heart suddenly rises, often reaching rates of well over 200 per minute. Although the infant can often tolerate these rates and remain largely asymptomatic for many hours, eventually heart failure ensues. The diagnosis is made on the ECG, which shows the very rapid rate (Fig. 13.11). The treatment consists of trying to reduce the rate to normal as quickly as possible. This can be achieved in an emergency by inducing a very strong vagal reflex by dipping the baby's face into ice-cold water momentarily, or by giving an intravenous injection of adenosine 0.1–0.2 mg/kg, but in any case it is advisable to treat only in consultation with an experienced paediatric cardiologist. An ECG after the tachycardia has resolved

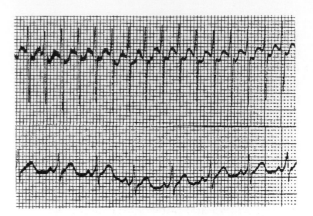

Figure 13.11   ECG traces showing supraventricular tachycardia above, and, below, the short PR interval and slurred upstroke of the R wave in the baby's underlying Wolff–Parkinson–White syndrome.

often shows the Wolff–Parkinson–White anomaly (Fig. 13.11). The condition recurs in infancy in most, but not all, cases, and may require treatment with other antiarrhythmic drugs.

Other rarer causes of heart failure   Fibrosis of the inner lining of the ventricles of unknown origin, which is known as subendocardial fibroelastosis, and myocardial infarction from anomalous origin of the coronary arteries are also rare causes of early heart failure. Myocarditis, sometimes due to coxsackievirus infection, and mitochondrial disease can also rarely present in this way.

The medical management of heart failure

The infant is best nursed in a semi-erect posture and may be helped by raising the oxygen content of the inspired air to about 30%. Reduction of the venous pressure using a diuretic such as furosemide (frusemide), 1 mg/kg intravenously or intramuscularly, is essential. Maintaining the diuresis can be achieved using oral furosemide (frusemide) or bendrofluazide together with potassium supplements or spironolactone.

GENITOURINARY TRACT
Kidneys

Absence or severe dysgenesis of both kidneys gives rise to impaired fetal growth and oligohydramnios from lack of fetal urine production. Ultrasound examination of the fetus can confirm the absence of the kidneys, and at birth there is a diagnostic frog-like appearance of the face (Potter's facies) with wide-set eyes, low-set ears and a parrot-beaked nose.

Absence of one kidney may be suspected at routine neonatal examination if this is done carefully, since the lower poles of both are normally palpable in the newborn. Ultrasonography or isotope renography helps to confirm the diagnosis. A large mass in one or both renal regions is an occasional finding on prenatal ultrasound examination or at birth, and the differential diagnosis lies between Wilms' tumour (nephroblastoma), polycystic kidneys (usually bilateral) and severe hydronephrosis. Differentiation of the causes of the mass can be achieved using ultrasound, computerised tomography (CT) scanning or intravenous pyelography. If obstruction to the urinary tract or a tumour is suspected, early referral to a paediatric surgeon is essential to relieve the obstruction or remove the tumour.

Polycystic disease of the kidneys

Polycystic disease of the kidneys is usually classified into two main types. The 'infantile' variety is inherited as an autosomal recessive characteristic and the parents would therefore be expected to have normal kidneys. It presents as bilateral abdominal masses which can cause a marked abdominal distension, and is often accompanied by cystic disease of the liver. It has a relatively poor prognosis owing to the deterioration of renal function or the development of hypertension which ensues, often within the first year. The 'adult' type is transmitted as a dominant condition from one or other parent and renal function is not usually impaired until adult life.

'Prune belly' syndrome

Congenital absence of part of the abdominal musculature in association with renal abnormalities, usually hydronephrosis, and undescended testes constitutes a rare condition known as the 'prune belly' syndrome.

Obstruction in the urinary tract

Congenital abnormalities resulting in obstruction to the flow of urine occur at the level of the pelviureteric junction, the lower ends of the ureters or at the outlet of the bladder; many are identifiable on prenatal ultrasound examination of the fetal abdomen since they all result in dilatation of the renal tract. Since many cases of obstruction show no symptoms or abnormal physical signs in the neonatal period, but present later with pain, urinary tract infection or diminished renal function, the introduction of ultrasound screening has improved the outlook for these infants by allowing surgical correction, where necessary, before complications arise (Aviram et al 2000).

The most likely anomaly to present with symptoms in the newborn period is congenital valvular obstruction of the male posterior urethra. It may be possible to diagnose this condition in the first week if a poor stream of urine or infrequent micturition is recognised. Delay in first passing urine beyond 24 hours is common but seldom has any serious significance, the apparent delay being caused by the fact that urine has passed unnoticed during delivery. Significant urethral obstruction is accompanied by a hypertrophied bladder which is often palpable after micturition. Where such an obstruction is suspected, it is possible to confirm the presence of valves by radiography after introduction of radio-opaque material into the bladder. Surprisingly, little or no resistance to the passage of the catheter is encountered.

In female infants, an ectopic ureter, usually arising from one portion of a duplex kidney, may open into the vagina and cause continual dribbling of urine from birth.

Ectopia vesicae

This defect of the bladder and abdominal wall results in an everted bladder (and sometimes urethra), the ureteric orifices being visible on the surface. The symphysis pubis is often lacking and the pubic rami are widely separated. Although the condition is compatible with a long lifespan, the disability of complete incontinence is such that surgical treatment is always worthwhile.

The type of procedure and the timing of it depends on the detail of the anatomy, but reconstruction operations are seldom done before 6 months of age. Until then, the exposed mucous membrane of the bladder is covered with non-adherent dressings and padding to collect the urine until it becomes covered with thicker epithelium. The surrounding skin should be protected by a water-repellent ointment. Ureteric transplants into an isolated jejunal loop may be best if reconstitution of the bladder is impractical.

External genitalia

Hypospadias

In this malformation, the urethra fails to extend the whole length of the penis and opens at some point on its ventral surface or even onto the perineum. The further down the shaft it opens, the more severe the deformity and the more difficult is the surgical correction. In coronal hypospadias (Fig. 13.12), the urethral opening is situated at the junction of the glans and the shaft of the penis, and the prepuce covers only the dorsal surface of the glans. Anchoring of the ventral surface of the penis by a fibrous structure (chordee), which results in a curvature of the penis on erection may

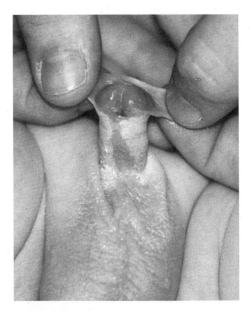

Figure 13.12 Coronal hypospadias.

necessitate surgical correction, but otherwise treatment is not essential since the condition is compatible with normal micturition and sexual function. Where the urethral opening is placed further down the shaft or on the perineum, immediate surgery is only necessary if the urinary stream is poor or narrow, which suggests that there is some obstruction to the flow of urine. Otherwise, surgery to move the urethral meatus as near the tip of the penis as is possible is undertaken much later, usually between the age of 3 and 5 years. In the most severe forms of the condition, especially where there is a bifid scrotum, the various causes of ambiguous genitalia must be borne in mind (p. 228).

Epispadias

Epispadias is much rarer than hypospadias, the urethral opening being on the dorsal surface of the penis.

Imperforate hymen

Imperforate hymen may be identifiable in the newborn, presenting as a cystic swelling between the labia minora. Accumulation of mucus in the vagina may occasionally result in a swelling palpable in the lower abdomen. A cyst of Gaertner's duct may also produce a mucus-containing swelling in the vagina.

Adhesion of the labia minora

Adhesion of the labia minora is rarely seen at birth but is a fairly common disorder in the first 3 years; it is normally acquired rather than congenital. Separation can often be achieved after application of an oestrogen cream, and surgical separation is seldom necessary.

Ambiguous genitalia

The presence of external genitalia whose appearance is neither definitely male nor unequivocally female is distressing both for the parents and for the professionals involved. It results from a hormonal imbalance in early embryonic development preventing the differentiation of the genitalia. The strong temptation instantly to declare the child male or female should be resisted for it is very important to establish the underlying cause from appropriate investigations so that the best ultimate decision about the sex of rearing can be made.

The investigations required include chromosome evaluation, ultrasound examination of the pelvic organs to demonstrate the presence of a uterus, endocrine studies of the several metabolic abnormalities known to cause this picture, and even surgical exploration to identify the gonads. The main anomalies encountered are described in greatly simplified terms below.

Female pseudohermaphroditism

In this condition, the gonads are ovaries and ultrasound examination confirms the presence of a uterus in the pelvis. The external genitalia give the impression of being male, with a hypertrophied clitoris, which resembles a penis, and sometimes wrinkling of the skin of the labia majora, which simulates that of an empty scrotum.

Smears from the buccal mucosa show that cell nuclei contain the chromatin body which indicates that there are two X chromosomes and analysis of the chromosome complement in the white blood cells confirms the normal female pattern of 46XX. The great majority of these children have congenital adrenal hyperplasia, the clitoral hypertrophy resulting from overproduction of androgens. Occasionally, a similar picture but of rather lesser degree may result from administration of progesterone preparations to the mother in pregnancy. Even more rarely, the condition is found to have no hormonal basis and is of genetic origin.

Congenital adrenal hyperplasia

Congenital adrenal hyperplasia (Plate 21A) is inherited as an autosomal recessive condition, so each baby of the outwardly normal carrier parents has a 1 in 4 risk of being affected. The gene mutation responsible for the condition is on chromosome 6 and can be identified in many cases by DNA analysis. The condition results from the

absence of an enzyme (most commonly 21-hydroxylase) concerned in the synthesis of cortisol by the adrenal gland. The lack of cortisol causes increased adrenocorticotrophic hormone (ACTH) production by the normal 'feedback' mechanism to the pituitary gland, which results in an overstimulation of androgen production. The condition can be diagnosed by finding a high level of 17-hydroxyprogesterone in the blood. In nearly half the cases, a salt-losing adrenal crisis develops in the second or third week as a result of a lack of mineralocorticoid hormone secretion. The infant refuses feeds, fails to gain weight and vomits repeatedly, with resultant dehydration, electrolyte imbalance, hypotension and circulatory impairment. There is an elevation of the serum potassium level and usually a lowering of serum sodium. This requires immediate attention, though it can be prevented if the diagnosis is suspected and the salt-losing state anticipated.

Intravenous normal saline and dextrose together with administration of fludrocortisone (0.05–0.1 mg daily) will correct the fluid and electrolyte disturbance initially. Life-long hydrocortisone replacement treatment is started, which will also suppress ACTH production, reduce virilisation and enable normal growth. The dosage is about 2.5 mg twice daily, though greater amounts will be required temporarily during intercurrent illnesses. Surgery may be needed to correct the appearance of the external genitalia.

Male pseudohermaphroditism

In male pseudohermaphroditism (Plate 21B), the gonads are testes and the chromosome complement is 46XY, confirming that the child is genetically male. The external genitalia are feminised to a variable extent. The penis is hypoplastic and may resemble a clitoris, being bound down ventrally by a chordee. It usually results from either an inherited lack of sensitivity of the genitalia to the male hormone testosterone or the lack of an enzyme responsible for its production. Some of these conditions are inherited in an autosomal recessive or X-linked fashion.

Full investigation of all male pseudohermaphrodite babies is essential in the first few days of life in order to establish a precise diagnosis, and therefore the prognosis. A decision must also be made as to whether surgery can help to create genitalia that are recognisably and functionally male. If not, it may be necessary to bring the child up as a girl.

True hermaphroditism

True hermaphroditism is extremely rare. Both testicular and ovarian tissue are present in the gonads and the external genitalia are variable in appearance, usually resembling one form of male pseudohermaphrodite as described above.

CENTRAL NERVOUS SYSTEM
Neural tube abnormalities

Anencephaly and spina bifida (p. 23) are examples of neural tube abnormalities. In the first weeks after fertilisation, some cells form a groove along the length of the developing embryo; these then roll into a tube-like structure which eventually forms the fetal brain and spinal cord and its surrounding spine. A failure of complete closure of this tube is responsible for this group of disorders.

The incidence of this group of serious abnormalities has fallen substantially in Britain, from approximately 4 per 1000 births in the 1970s to less than 0.3 per 1000 now. Both genetic and environmental factors are involved in their aetiology, the risk of malformation being greatly increased when a previous child has been affected and being significantly greater in some parts of the country than in others. The incidence of liveborn affected infants has fallen, partly as a result of the introduction of alpha-fetoprotein screening, ultrasound diagnosis and termination of affected fetuses. More significantly, the supplementation of certain foodstuffs with folic acid (Ali & Economides 2000, Oleary et al 2001) has reduced the natural occurrence rate, and the provision of preconceptional vitamin supplements with folic acid 0.4 mg daily for mothers who have had one affected baby has reduced the recurrence rate in a subsequent pregnancy from 3.5% to 1.0%. In some countries, a daily folic acid dose of 4–5 mg is recommended for women at high risk. Such doses are not known to have any harmful effects in healthy pregnant women, though they may counteract the anticonvulsant activity of some drugs used in epilepsy. A surviving affected girl who herself becomes pregnant has a 1 in 30 chance of bearing a child with a neural tube abnormality.

Anencephaly

This fatal malformation, in which the forebrain is largely absent and the overlying skull and its coverings are missing, is usually identified at routine ultrasound screening. The pregnancy is normally terminated, but if not, the infant will be stillborn or will live only a few hours. Maternal polyhydramnios often accompanies the condition.

Encephalocele

Encephalocele, in which there is a large midline protrusion of brain substance through a skull defect either at the occiput or above the nose, is a severely disabling or lethal condition which is only rarely susceptible to successful surgical treatment.

Spina bifida with myelomeningocele or meningocele

A myelomeningocele (Fig. 2.3, p. 23) most commonly occurs in the lumbar region where there is a midline defect in the spine, with or without a swelling, covered only by a thin membrane of neuroepithelium and abnormal blood vessels; it contains either spinal cord or spinal nerve roots and almost always the surface oozes moisture, giving the appearance of a large ulcer. Less commonly, it may be covered by true skin. Hydrocephalus of varying degree due to a malformation of the cerebellum in the region of the foramen magnum (Arnold–Chiari malformation) is almost always present, though it may not always be severe enough to need immediate treatment.

The degree of disability which the child may be expected to suffer as he gets older depends upon the level and extent of the lesion, and the severity of the hydrocephalus. In the majority of cases where the lumbar spine is involved, there is marked weakness or complete paralysis of the lower limbs, often with talipes and congenital dislocation of the hips. With a small sacral lesion there may be no loss of mobility, though, because the nerve supply to the bladder and anal sphincter mechanism is impaired, urinary and faecal incontinence results. The bladder dysfunction frequently leads to secondary disorders of the upper urinary tract, often with hydronephrosis and chronic urinary infection. In about 80% of cases, the hydrocephalus is associated with sufficiently raised intracranial pressure to require insertion of a ventriculoatrial or ventriculoperitoneal shunt to reduce the pressure and minimise the potential brain damage.

Follow-up studies of children with severe myelomeningocele treated surgically in the neonatal period have shown that many become severely physically handicapped and have major learning disabilities, though early treatment limits this to a small degree. Features that have a particularly poor prognosis include established hydrocephalus at birth, multiple spinal defects and extensive paralysis of the legs. The implications of this for the child and family require a thorough discussion with both parents by an experienced paediatrician. Even without treatment most babies will survive and closure of the back is usually recommended. Thereafter, if hydrocephalus is present, its extent is monitored by repeated ultrasound measurements of the size of the ventricles. Treatment of increasing hydrocephalus is by insertion of a shunt, using one of the variations of the Spitz–Holter valve and catheter which drains the cerebrospinal fluid from one lateral ventricle to the right atrium or into the peritoneum.

The long-term treatment of these children must be a matter of well-organised teamwork by those with special experience in different fields, including neurosurgery for the hydrocephalus, orthopaedics for the hip and foot deformities, and urological surgery for the management of the bladder problems. Physiotherapists can encourage and facilitate the child's development, particularly his mobility, and advise about appropriate aids for walking or wheelchairs if needed. The Social Services will provide support for the family, and advice from the education authorities about special education will normally be needed.

Occasionally, spina bifida is accompanied by a meningocele only, the sac containing no spinal cord structures and being covered by skin. Hydrocephalus is much less common in these children and there are often no neurological complications, so the outlook for normal mobility and cerebral function after operation is good.

Spinal dysraphism

In spinal dysraphism, the cord in the lumbar region is divided by a cartilaginous spur which gives rise to dysfunction of the nerves to the bladder and lower limbs in later childhood. It should be suspected whenever there is a small midline defect of skin or a sinus above the sacrococcygeal region, especially when associated with a tuft of fine hair.

Congenital hydrocephalus

The great majority of cases of congenital hydrocephalus are associated with spina bifida and myelomeningocele.

Isolated hydrocephalus is most commonly due to obstruction of the cerebrospinal fluid pathways by adhesions somewhere in the subarachnoid space. More rarely it is due to a malformation of the ventricular system such as aqueduct stenosis – in which a stenosed channel between the third and fourth ventricles obstructs the flow of cerebrospinal fluid – or an intracranial cyst. Intracranial haemorrhage, particularly in preterm infants, is another important cause and intra-uterine infection with toxoplasmosis accounts for a few cases. In a small number of cases, it is familial and is inherited as an X-linked disorder (p. 207).

Undiagnosed isolated hydrocephalus is now a rare cause of disproportion giving rise to difficulties in labour. Increasingly early detection by antenatal ultrasound may lead to termination of pregnancy in severe cases, so the incidence in liveborn infants is falling. If it develops after birth, hydrocephalus rarely causes immediate clinical disturbance in the baby, though exceptionally some drowsiness or vomiting may occur. Usually, an enlarging head draws attention to the diagnosis, which is confirmed by serial measurements of head circumference. An increase of more than 2.5 cm in the first 2 weeks justifies further investigation by ultrasound examination.

Clinical examination shows a wide and often tense anterior fontanelle with separation of the cranial sutures. As the pressure rises, the eyes become down-turned, so that only the upper halves of the cornea can be seen (the 'setting sun' sign), and the scalp veins are dilated. The amount of neurological disturbance that results depends upon the cause of the hydrocephalus and the degree and duration of the raised intracranial pressure. Cerebral function is often surprisingly normal. Treatment of advanced hydrocephalus can be compatible with normal intelligence. However, if ventricular dilatation is identified in utero or occurs as a consequence of intraventricular haemorrhage, the prognosis is usually poor, with severe developmental delay.

About 40% of cases of isolated hydrocephalus progress for a time and then arrest spontaneously. Full investigation by ultrasound (Fig. 13.13) or CT scanning is necessary if early arrest does not take place, and surgical treatment with some form of bypass valve of the Spitz–Holter type is nearly always possible (p. 231).

Hydranencephaly

In hydranencephaly, the skull is intact and often of normal shape and size, but there is absence of most of the cerebral hemispheres, the space being filled by cerebrospinal fluid. Initially, the condition may be hard to diagnose, because the baby sucks without difficulty and abnormal neurological signs are not at first obvious. Transillumination of the head using a very bright light in a dark room is a simple and useful means of investigation for this at the bedside, but scanning by ultrasound is replacing it as it is now becoming a ward procedure.

Other abnormalities of head size and shape

Congenital microcephaly

In this condition, the skull, particularly the frontal region, is small and the rest of the facial development relatively normal, producing a characteristic appearance. The outcome is severe learning difficulties. One form of the disorder is inherited as an autosomal recessive characteristic occurring only in homozygotes (p. 206), but there

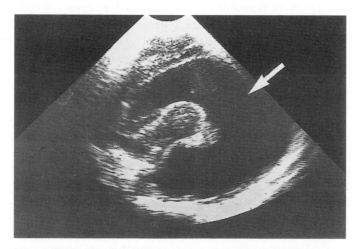

Figure 13.13 Cerebral ultrasound scan showing greatly dilated lateral ventricles (arrowed) in congenital hydrocephalus.

are other causes, including intrauterine cytomegalovirus infection.

Craniosynostosis

Microcephaly must be distinguished clearly from the various forms of craniosynostosis in which early union of the cranial sutures forms a skull of reduced capacity and of deformed shape. For example, in turricephaly, a tall narrow head results from early fusion of the coronal sutures, and in scaphocephaly, a boat-shaped head with a prominent occiput is caused by premature closure of the saggital suture. In both of these situations, the restriction of space interferes with brain growth and may cause increasing intracranial pressure, resulting in fits, learning difficulties and reduced sight from optic atrophy. Microcephaly and craniosynostosis can be differentiated usually on clinical findings, but X-rays of the skull are necessary for confirmation. If craniosynostosis is confirmed, early surgical excision of the fused sutures is required to allow more normal skull and brain growth.

EYES

In the course of the neonatal examination, the size and position of the eyes, as well as other ocular abnormalities, should be noted (p. 65).

Microphthalmia

The abnormally small eye (microphthalmia) – apart from being a feature of congenital toxoplasmosis, the rubella syndrome and cytomegalovirus infection – may occur as an isolated congenital defect or associated with colobomata and possibly with cerebral agenesis. No treatment is available and sight in the affected eye is usually very limited.

Macrophthalmia

More important from the point of view of early diagnosis is the abnormally large eye which may be due to congenital glaucoma (buphthalmos). This causes cloudiness of the cornea over the first few months of life as the pressure of the fluid in the anterior chamber of the eye rises. The condition should be referred urgently to an ophthalmologist since the only hope of preserving vision lies in early surgical reduction of intraocular pressure.

Congenital cataracts

These are best seen when the eyes are examined with a light shining obliquely across them. Though usually the sole abnormality and often hereditary, they may also point to the diagnosis of other disorders. These include the rubella syndrome, congenital toxoplasmosis, Down syndrome, Lowe's oculorenal syndrome, congenital ectodermal dysplasia, and punctate epiphyseal dysplasia. They may develop later in congenital galactosaemia and neonatal hypocalcaemia.

Treatment is never urgent but early detection and referral to the ophthalmologist is advisable since early surgery, often involving lens aspiration and insertion of plastic lenses (Cassidy et al 2001) can restore vision and improve acuity and prevent a permanent amblyopia from developing.

LIMBS AND JOINTS
Congenital dislocation of the hip

Because early recognition and treatment of this condition from the newborn period is largely effective in preventing future disability from established dislocation, it is given special attention in the routine clinical examination. The manoeuvres for its detection are fully described on page 71.

Genetic factors must play a part in its causation since it is commoner in girls than boys and in close relatives of affected children. Environmental factors are also involved since it is more common where the baby is of above average birth weight or, curiously, has suffered fetal growth retardation, and where there has been oligohydramnios, breech presentation or delivery by caesarean section. However, in 40% of cases, no predisposing factors are found. The incidence varies in different parts of the world (Riley et al 1998), but in Britain it is approximately 1–1.5 per 1000 births. Many more than this are found to have an unstable, but not actually dislocated, hip when examined within the first 2 days of life, the number varying from 3 to 20 per 1000 births depending on the way in which the routine examination is carried out and interpreted. The shape of the acetabulum and the degree of instability of the joint can easily be demonstrated by ultrasound imaging (Fig. 13.14) and this should always be performed if instability is suspected. Among these unstable hips are some that would become firmly dislocated if not treated, however, some of them stabilise spontaneously, leaving a normal hip joint, without treatment within a week or so. There is therefore some difference of opinion about the correct approach to treatment by abduction splintage.

The unstable hip which can be easily relocated by gentle abduction should be kept in at least partial abduction and flexion by an abduction splint until it has stabilised. The hip which is in place at rest but can be displaced by testing may be treated in the same way, but it is equally reasonable to wait and review the hip with ultrasound

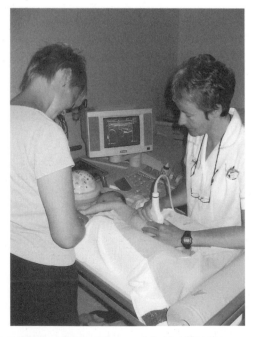

Figure 13.14 Ultrasound accurately identifies the structure and stability of the neonatal hip.

evaluation to see whether it becomes stable within a few weeks.

If on first testing the hip shows limitation of abduction, suggesting that the joint is actually dislocated, no force should be used and abduction splinting should not be undertaken in view of the risk of damage to the femoral head. Treatment should be in the hands of an orthopaedic surgeon with neonatal experience, because early open surgical reduction or adductor tenotomy may in some cases be necessary.

Splintage

There are several accepted ways of keeping the hip joints in the flexed and abducted position until the hip joint is stable. The von Rosen or Malmo splint is commonly used. It consists of a padded frame, the malleable metal arms of which bend to the position required for fixing the hips in relation to the trunk. It has the disadvantage of sometimes causing discomfort at first, which is reflected also in the baby's mother, who may feel that it impairs normal closeness and her confidence in handling the infant.

The 'Aberdeen' splint is simply a rigid cover for the napkin, the padded edges of which keep the thighs apart when it is strapped in place. It is less disturbing for both infant and mother but its weakness lies in the fact that it has to be taken off and reapplied each time the nappy is changed, which requires some practice to ensure that it is effective. The Pavlik harness (Morino et al 1998) (Fig. 13.15) is a more complicated device but has the advantage of allowing the baby a little more freedom to move.

Whatever method is used, the apparatus must be put on very gently by someone experienced in its use, and the baby's progress followed carefully until he is walking satisfactorily. X-rays in the first month give limited information since the femoral head only becomes visible at around 4–6 months of age, but are most helpful thereafter.

Ultrasound

Ultrasound examination of the hip joint shows its structure accurately in the first few weeks of life

(Fig. 13.16) and can be used to follow its maturation for 6 months or more in babies with clinically unstable hips to identify those hips which are likely to dislocate later or benefit from early surgery. Although it is used as a means of screening for the condition in some parts of Europe, it has not yet replaced the clinical identification of the unstable hip in most areas of Britain.

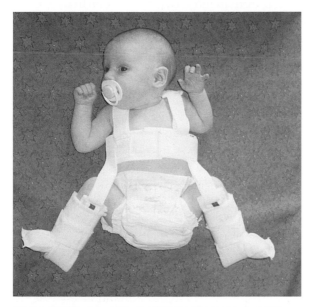

Figure 13.15 Infant fitted with a Pavlik harness to treat her unstable hips.

Talipes equinovarus and calcaneovalgus

These deformities are partly genetic in origin and partly the result of malposition or abnormal pressures in utero. The baby can usually be 'folded' easily into the abnormal position that he occupied within the uterus, and reduction of the amount of amniotic fluid is commonly associated. The condition can be diagnosed before birth in some cases by ultrasound scanning, which shows the abnormal posture of the feet (Fig. 2.2B, p. 21).

Talipes equinovarus

The deformity (Fig. 13.17) consists of plantar flexion at the ankle with varus deformity at the subtaloid joint and adduction of the forefoot. There is some degree of rigidity of the foot in this position and the deformity cannot be immediately corrected passively, thus distinguishing it from the temporary exaggerated postural inversion of the feet which is so common and which corrects itself.

Treatment should be started if possible in the first few days of life. The deformity is partially corrected by stretching and then is held in position either by the use of felt and adhesive strapping or by a splint. Frequent repetition of the stretching and strapping is necessary until overcorrection is achieved, and the treatment must be followed up carefully until growth of the feet is complete.

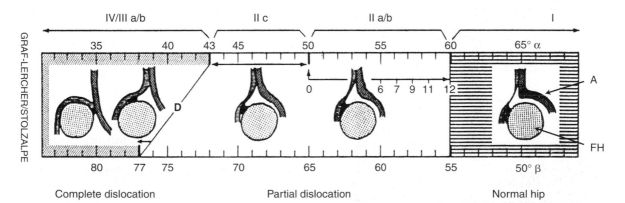

Figure 13.16 Ultrasound appearances in congenital dislocation of the hip. The diagram illustrates the progressive displacement of the femoral head in different degrees of dislocation. Graf type I is normal, showing good covering of the head (FH) by the acetabulum (A) in the iliac bone. As the head is increasingly displaced laterally, the acetabulum becomes more shallow, until it is barely identifiable in complete dislocation (type IV). (With kind permission of Dr R Graf.)

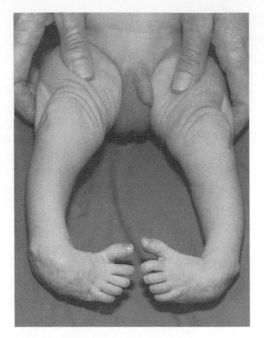

Figure 13.17 Bilateral talipes equinovarus.

Occasionally, an early operation to release the tight medial foot ligaments may be required, with later lengthening of the Achilles tendon in severe cases. Night splints should be worn to maintain a good foot posture until the child is about 3 years old and good foot function is usually obtained.

Talipes calcaneovalgus

Talipes calcaneovalgus is the opposite deformity, with the foot in extreme dorsiflexion and metatarsus valgus, so that the fifth toe approximates towards the outer border of the lower leg. There are all degrees of this deformity. In most cases, the foot can easily be replaced passively into the normal position and no treatment is necessary. Cases with the more severe valgus deformity require manipulation of the foot towards the normal position and splints or strapping to maintain the foot posture. The incidence of congenital dislocation of the hip is significantly greater with this type of talipes.

Scoliosis

This is infrequently recognised at birth unless it is due to structural abnormalities of the vertebrae, which may produce a relatively sharp angulation of the spine. Infantile idiopathic scoliosis may, however, have its origin in intrauterine malposition and if a lateral curve or an asymmetrical 'incurvation response' is noted at routine examination, the baby should certainly be examined again later. Most straighten spontaneously as the baby grows, but there may be a case for early postural treatment in selected instances.

Many other skeletal deformities, types of chondrodystrophy and soft tissue malformation are clearly recognisable in the newborn period. Major paediatric or orthopaedic textbooks describe them in full and they are not included here because of their individual rarity, and because early recognition is not important for effective treatment.

LYMPHATIC SYSTEM

Lymphangiomas most commonly occur as cystic hygromas – soft multilocular cysts in the region of the neck or axilla. They are less common in other sites but may be associated with haemangiomas. The feasibility of surgical excision depends upon the extent and site of the lesion.

REFERENCES

Ali S A, Economides D L 2000 Folic acid supplementation. Current Opinion in Obstetrics and Gynecology 12(6):507–512

Aviram R, Pomeran A, Sharony R et al 2000 The increase of renal pelvis dilatation in the fetus and its significance. Ultrasound in Obstetrics and Gynecology 16(1):60–62

Bertollini R, Mastroiacova P, Segni G 1985 Maternal epilepsy and birth defects: a case-control study in the Italian Multicentric Registry of Birth Defects (IPIMC). European Journal of Epidemiology 1(1):67–72

Brown J W, Park H J, Turrentine M W 2001 Arterial switch operation: factors impacting survival in the current era. Annals of Thoracic Surgery 71(6):1978–1984

Cassidy L, Rahi J, Nischal K et al 2001 Outcome of lens aspiration and intraocular lens implantation in children aged 5 years and under. British Journal of Ophthalmology 85(5):540–542

Chakrapani A, Cleary M A, Wraith J E 2001 Detection of inborn errors of metabolism. Archives of Disease in Childhood Fetal and Neonatal Edition 84(3):F205–F210

Dezatuex C 1998 Evaluating newborn screening programmes based on dried blood spots: future challenges. British Medical Bulletin 54(4):877–890

Doull I J, Ryley H C, Weller P et al 2001 Cystic fibrosis-related deaths in infancy and the effect of newborn screening. Pediatric Pulmonology 31(5):363–366

Garne E, Stoll C, Clementi M 2001 Evaluation of prenatal diagnosis of congenital heart disease by ultrasound: experience from 20 European registries. Ultrasound in Obstetrics and Gynecology 17(5):386–391

Hanna E J, Nevin N C et al 1994 Genetic study of congenital heart defects in Northern Ireland 1974–8. Journal of Medical Genetics 31:858–863

Koch R, Hanley W, Levy H et al 2000 Maternal phenylketonuria: an international study. Molecular Genetics and Metabolism 71(1–2):233–239

Leonard J V, Morris A A, 2000 Inborn errors of metabolism around the time of birth. Lancet 356:583–587

Merelle M E, Lees C M, Nagelkerte A F et al 2000 Newborn screening for cystic fibrosis. Cochrane Database of Systematic Reviews 2:CD001402

Morino T, Miyake Y, Matsushita T et al 1998 Pavlik harness applications for congenital dislocation of the hip. How short can they be made? Archives of Orthopaedic and Trauma Surgery 117(1–2):89–91

Oleary M, Donnell R M, Johnson H 2001 Folic acid and prevention of neural tube defects in 2000: improved awareness – low periconceptional uptake. Irish Medical Journal 94(6):180–181

Penny D J, Shekerdemian L S 2001 Management of the neonate with symptomatic congenital heart disease. Archives of Disease in Childhood Fetal and Neonatal Edition 84:F141–F145

Riley M M, Halliday J L, Lumley J M 1998 Congenital malformations in Victoria, Australia, 1983–1995: an overview of infant characteristics. Journal of Pediatrics and Child Health 34(3):233–240

Rovet J F 1999 Congenital hypothyroidism: long-term outcome. Thyroid 9(7):741–748

Scotet V, de Braeckeleer M, Roussey M et al 2000 Neonatal screening for cystic fibrosis in Brittany, France: assessment of 10 years' experience and impact on prenatal diagnosis. Lancet 356(9232):789–794

Sell D, Grunwell P, Mildinhall S et al 2001 Cleft lip and palate care in the United Kingdom – the Clinical Standards Advisory Group (CSAG) study. Part 3: Speech outcomes. Cleft Palate and Craniofacial Journal 38(1):30–37

Timmons M J, Wyatt R A, Murphy T 2001 Speech after repair of isolated cleft palate and cleft lip and palate. British Journal of Plastic Surgery 54(5):377–384

USEFUL WEBSITES

www.ncbi.nlm.nih.gov/Omim/ – On-line Mendelian Inheritance in Man (Omim)

www.rarediseases.org – National Organisation for Rare Diseases (NORD)

Chapter 14

Helping the parents

CHAPTER CONTENTS

Preparation for the birth of the baby   240
The ill or abnormal infant   241
   Parental reaction to the birth of a sick or
   malformed infant   241
   Breaking the bad news   242
   Counselling the distraught parent   243
The dying baby   244
   Helping parents after a perinatal death   245
   Postmortem examination of the baby   246
   Stillbirth   246
   Continuing care for the parents   247
Useful addresses   247

The birth of a healthy and contented infant who feeds and sleeps well is a fulfilling experience for both parents, especially if this has been achieved with the minimum of professional assistance. 'Preparation for parenthood' classes are a most valuable training for the birth and care of the infant, but the reality of having a real baby to nurture is not always as smooth as anticipated. The emotions of the delivery, the commonly experienced 'blues' in the first few days and the frequent demands from the infant all affect the parents' confidence. If they have had little prior experience of baby care, they have to learn quickly how to understand, anticipate and respond to the baby's needs. No two babies are alike, yet, fortunately, the majority of newborns slip easily into a regular pattern of activity, feeding and sleep and present few problems to new parents. However, if the baby does not conform to the expected pattern of behaviour, anxiety easily arises. Successful breast feeding, for instance, is not necessarily natural to a new mother nor easily achieved. The baby may have an irregular sleep pattern or simply be unsettled and such features can result in one or both parents becoming very tired. In such instances, understanding and informed nursing support is invaluable.

As many as one baby in 12 will require medical attention for a problem of some sort in the first few weeks. In such cases, the added anxiety will greatly affect the parents' confidence in the future and this will need considerable understanding from all medical and nursing staff concerned. It is essential that, as well as having knowledge of the conditions affecting the newborn infant, those caring for the family must be aware of their likely emotional reactions when faced with caring for a sick, handicapped or malformed child and know how best to support them. They should also know about the services available to assist in providing care and support to the family on their return home.

PREPARATION FOR THE BIRTH OF THE BABY

During the pregnancy, the information given in the 'education for parenthood' classes will concentrate largely on the care of the healthy baby. This should cover such information as listed in Box 14.1. The programme of care in the community for healthy infants from the midwife, health visitor and family doctor should also be described, together with the schedule of immunisations against infectious diseases in infancy which the baby should receive.

The best medical support that can be given to parents during a pregnancy is to assure them that

---

Box 14.1 Information provided at 'preparation for parenthood' classes

Antenatal period
- Diet
- Exercise
- Fetal movements
- Aspects of normal pregnancy
- Birth plans for parents, highlighting choices for labour and delivery, e.g. no analgesics for pain relief, delivery in the squatting position, deliver to music, water birth

The birth
- Signs of the onset of labour
- Pain-relief choices
- Equipment used during labour
- Modes of delivery
- Maternal positions for delivery
- Tour of maternity hospital

Postnatal period
- Breast and bottle feeding
- Parenting skills
- Basic baby care, e.g. bathing, nappy area care
- Car seat information
- Different sleep and feeding patterns of healthy babies
- Normal weight gain
- Normal developmental patterns of baby

---

all is well with mother and fetus. However, it is also important to identify any increased risk to the infant before birth so that plans for the future can be made. Mothers with high-risk pregnancies, for example those with a medical condition such as diabetes, are usually advised to deliver in a main obstetric unit and they need to be aware of these recommendations. A past history of many miscarriages, a stillbirth or neonatal death, a malformed infant or a family history suggesting a genetic disorder may increase the parents' anxieties about their anticipated infant and it is wise to notify the paediatric team of such situations so that they can be prepared for it. In some areas, a special programme of support is introduced in the antenatal period to parents who have previously lost a baby from the sudden infant death syndrome. This provides a package of care for the baby after birth involving frequent assessment of his progress by the health visitor. She will plot the infant's weight gain weekly on a special chart designed to identify those babies whose weight gain is suboptimal, and ensure accelerated access to medical or paediatric examination when needed. Provision of an apnoea alarm or weighing scales for use at home may be advised to monitor the baby's progress even more closely. After the baby's birth, the parents are also taught how to resuscitate him should he be found to be seriously ill. When there has been a previous neonatal death or stillbirth, some hospitals place an identification mark on the mother's notes to remind all professionals of the fact so that they can be more aware of the parents' feelings and avoid careless and upsetting remarks.

If a congenital abnormality is found on prenatal examination (p. 21) of the baby, it is often appropriate to involve a paediatric specialist to discuss its significance and to describe any treatment which may be available. Since about 8% of all infants born have some condition needing paediatric attention and may need admission to the neonatal unit, a case can be made for discussing this possibility with the parents during the antenatal period. However, those advising the parents must also take into account how much anxiety this might create for them and judge accordingly what to tell them and when. It must be remembered that, because of religious or cultural beliefs, prenatal intervention may not be acceptable to some parents and such views must colour the discussion about the management of the baby's condition. On the whole, it is best to tell the couple something of the range of possibilities since they are then less likely to be shocked if mother and baby do have to be separated at birth.

The antenatal period also affords the opportunity to identify any social problems or disadvantages which might affect the mother's ability to cope with the baby after delivery. These may include lone parenthood, housing problems, social isolation, unemployment, drug and alcohol misuse, and poverty. Where the first language of the mother is not English, interpreters may be necessary, or leaflets in the appropriate language may need to be supplied to ensure the information provided is understood. Parental physical or psychiatric illness or the presence in the family of other children with illness or disability may affect parenting ability. In a small number of cases there may be more serious social concern, such as another child in the family whose name is on the Child Protection Register for child abuse or a person in the home who has a conviction for offences against children. In such circumstances, Social Services or, occasionally, legal action may be required during the pregnancy to protect the baby after birth. Support from the social worker may be needed in such cases and this will become more important if the baby is found to have medical problems after birth.

There may also be cultural matters about which those caring for the mother and baby should know. Such things as dietary taboos, religious customs, mothers who find it unacceptable to be examined by a male doctor, and which family member will make the decisions about the care of the baby may be of great importance, particularly for a family from a minority group in society. Religious circumcision requirements may also need to be considered. Blood transfusion may be unacceptable to some groups. Each of these should be discussed, and an acceptable way found of accommodating the parents' requirements.

THE ILL OR ABNORMAL INFANT

It is when a sick, malformed or immature infant is born that the greatest understanding of the emotional and psychological needs of the parents is required. They will experience emotions which have features in common with the grief reaction following bereavement, and each parent will react individually, influenced by their beliefs, their past experiences and how responsible they feel for what has happened.

Parental reaction to the birth of a sick or malformed infant

The parents' initial reaction on realising or being told that their baby is malformed, handicapped or ill is one of shock, emotional disorganisation and confusion. Soon afterwards these feelings may turn into a period of denial in which the parents cannot believe the facts they have heard and they may even become hostile to the midwife, paediatrician or other professional who gave them the news. Feelings of rejection and even malice towards the child may follow, sometimes subsequently being replaced by feelings of guilt at having had such thoughts. Each parent may react in different ways at different times and in varying order and they may become bewildered in their attempts to support each other.

Such questions as 'why did it happen?', 'why did it happen to our baby?', 'did we do something wrong?', or 'did we fail to do something we should have?', 'could it have been caused by ...?' are all common and indicate that the parents are experiencing a feeling of guilt that they are in some way at fault for having a baby who is not perfect. This may be particularly poignant in cultures which believe malformations to be an act of God. 'There is nothing like this on my side of the family' is another frequent statement in which a parent tries to absolve himself or herself from responsibility for the baby's condition. This fear of 'blame' becomes particularly acute when the baby's condition has a genetic origin. When it is X linked, the fact that the condition is passed to a male child by an asymptomatic mother who carries the abnormal gene can cause particularly acute tension (p. 207).

Gradually, as the condition of the infant becomes clearer or the diagnosis is confirmed, the parents' reactions may become less acute and other, more considered reactions emerge. These too vary enormously, ranging from complete acceptance of the situation, through resignation to their plight or denial that anything is wrong, to outright rejection of the child. For most conditions there are now organisations set up by parents to provide information and help to other parents facing the situation for the first time. Many parents find great solace and help from joining such groups, which often fundraise for research into the disorder and to provide help for those parents who need support. Much useful medical information has come from such groups, which could not have been gained without them, and other professionals too learn from them about the condition so that they can themselves counsel families using the experience gained. It is important to inform parents about such groups so that they can make an informed choice as to whether to join or not. There are even support groups for twins and multiple births, not just for medical or genetic conditions. Contact addresses for a few of these organisations are listed at the end of the chapter. Health professionals should be aware of these groups and where the addresses, telephone numbers, websites and other information are kept. Such groups are now catalogued and their details are available in most paediatric departments. The internet also acts as an excellent source of information about such groups.

Breaking the bad news

The way in which the parents are first told that their baby has a serious abnormality has an important bearing upon how they come to terms with it. It is essential that they should be given every possible help to accept the child, and that trust in those responsible for the medical care should be firmly established from the beginning.

The timing must depend on circumstances but, if the abnormality is obvious at birth, the first explanation of what the parents can expect is best given as soon as the condition has been clinically assessed. Even when a full diagnosis cannot be made without further investigation, a preliminary discussion at the earliest possible time is necessary. If the birth is in hospital, all staff should be aware of who is to take on this responsibility and should themselves avoid impulsive, well-intentioned, but often misleading, advice or reassurance based upon their own feeling rather than on sound knowledge of all the circumstances. The parents may have to take difficult decisions about their child and it is important that whoever gives them guidance must be thoroughly informed about the family so that they can feel comfortable about those decisions.

The explanation should in general be given by a senior paediatrician, preferably by the one who will be responsible for the baby's ongoing care, and certainly one who understands the background culture of the family. If the first language of the clinician is not that of the parents, a skilled interpreter with some understanding of the medical problems and insight into the religious, cultural and family issues is invaluable. It is wise to arrange to see both parents together to hear the news so that they can provide support for each other. It is also helpful for a familiar nurse or midwife who has been involved in looking after the baby to be present when the doctor talks to the parents. If the parents find it difficult to take in what they are told about the baby, the nurse can be aware of what has been said and can repeat it to parents later. She will also be able to explain the situation further after the parents have had time to digest what has been said. If one of the parents can hold the baby during the discussion, this helps them to recognise the reality of the situation and often enhances the bond between parents and baby. Disbelief and denial, which are common reactions at this stage, are diminished by this approach. The other siblings should be cared for by another member of staff so that the parents can spend sufficient time to recover from their reaction to the news without having to cope with their other children too. They may also feel more able to express their emotions without the other children being present. Other family members, especially grandparents, may also require support and their needs should be considered.

Occasionally, where there is real doubt about the diagnosis, it may be thought best just to sow the seeds of doubt in the parents' minds, but there is seldom justification for withholding information so far as it is known. Parents are very perceptive and frequently deduce from the actions and manner of the caregivers that they have concerns about the infant. It is not helpful simply to restrict the explanation to answering questions from the parents – for the most important ones are usually not asked. The parents often recognise that there is a problem with the baby when, for example, the infant has Down syndrome, and in these circumstances it is best to confirm their suspicions and begin to explain the significance of the abnormality at once. It is often helpful to offer both parents a bed to stay on in the unit at such times, to enable them to be near their infant and supportive to each other. Rarely is it advisable for the mother and baby to be separated at this time unless there is an overriding medical reason to do so.

If the concern about the infant is that she will have significant learning difficulties as a result of a serious cerebral insult or a complication occurring during intensive care in a preterm infant, the same principles apply. Giving both parents together an honest appraisal of the situation, including its uncertainties, is almost always the best policy in the long term. Great patience, an unhurried approach and a real concern for the family are some of the qualities that help to establish trust, and opportunities must be found at agreed dates for further interviews to expand upon aspects which may not previously have been dealt with. Often the parents will take in only a small amount of what is said and they are frequently confused about the significance of the abnormality. It may be necessary to repeat almost everything at subsequent interviews. There should also be close liaison with those asked to give support, including the family doctor and health visitor, and some agreement should be reached about who should be the person to whom the family turns first for advice when they are uncertain about the infant's care. The parents should be informed of the support they will receive from the multidisciplinary team of doctors, nurses, therapists and social workers in the community for children with special needs, so they are aware of what help is available when they take the infant home.

Bringing up a child with a handicap, whatever its nature, is a difficult task and it can be most helpful for parents to meet at an early stage the therapists and social workers available to treat the child and support the family. These personnel can then introduce the parents to the local and national voluntary organisations from which they can obtain additional help. Although the best place for any baby is at home with the natural parents, there are occasions when they cannot provide the necessary care for the child, in which case the paediatric social worker will help in advising about the financial benefits available and assist the family in discussing the available alternatives to care at home should this become necessary.

Counselling the distraught parent

Although doctors, nurses and midwives have their own skills in understanding and counselling people in distress, there are some attitudes which are known to be helpful and others which can be destructive. The empathic person is one who can feel for the parents and get alongside them in their distress and it is this type of caregiver who will be most supportive to them. Such a person will respect the parents' feelings and help them to understand that their emotions are natural and acceptable, however uncomfortable for others. They will share in the parents' sorrow and encourage them to know that they will grow through the experience, that they do have the strength to cope and will have the support they need to enable them to do so. They will also allow the parents the space and time they need, and respect those times when they need privacy. By contrast, additional burdens can be placed on the parents by a person who fails to get alongside them, being obviously in a hurry, offering quick and slick solutions rather than listening to what they are really saying, or, worst of all, implying disapproval and giving the impression that the parents are behaving unreasonably. It is not an easy task to help distressed parents and even quite experienced professionals sometimes feel out of their depth. Courses exist to train nursing and medical staff in counselling following bereavement and after the birth of a disabled baby, and it is very profitable for nurses and doctors to attend one. Although all staff need to be aware of the principles involved in caring for such families, not everyone will feel comfortable with it and careful selection of the right nurse to support the family is vital.

THE DYING BABY

Approximately eight babies in every 1000 are stillborn or die in the first month of life in the UK despite the best available attention; in places where experienced antenatal and neonatal care is not well developed, the rate is much higher. Thus, the death of a newborn infant is not an uncommon event and every midwife, neonatal nurse and doctor caring for newborn infants should know how to care well for the dying baby and help the parents. It should be remembered that the staff themselves will be affected by the death and they too may need some support from other staff members.

The types of condition which result in the death of a newborn baby nowadays are discussed in Chapter 1. Many of them relate to incomplete antenatal care, premature birth, birth asphyxia, maternal illness associated with the pregnancy, or unexpected malformation of the baby. In some cases, such as stillbirth or overwhelming sepsis, death may be sudden and unexpected, but in the rest it is possible to anticipate, at least briefly, that the baby's life is ending, though there is often little time for the parents to prepare themselves for the event. Whatever the cause, it must be remembered that, however small and immature, every dying baby deserves all the dignity and respect which is afforded to an older child or adult. Many dying neonates will be undergoing some form of intensive care with all its associated equipment, but this should not blind the care-givers to the human needs of both the baby and

the parents. It is often possible to involve the parents in their baby's physical care however intensive it is, and if it is clear that the baby is dying, their contribution can be increased if they so wish. They should also be encouraged to express their wishes about the care to be given and the religious or cultural customs they wish to be observed, and those caring for the baby should adapt the treatment to accommodate them appropriately. It can be helpful to parents if some of the doctors and nurses are involved in such ceremonies, to demonstrate that they too share in the family's feelings (McHaffie et al 2001a). Flowers may be placed on top of incubators after religious ceremonial customs as a mark of respect and as an indication to other staff that this ceremony has taken place, to avoid any unnecessary words.

Although it is entirely proper to strive to maintain the life of an infant, a time may come when it is more important for the parents to have and hold their baby without the apparatus and accompaniments of intensive care, so that her last moments may be peaceful and dignified and the parents' later recollections more personal. If this can occur in a private place away from clinical activity, it gives a greater opportunity for the parents' grief to be expressed more naturally. Sometimes the presence of medical, nursing or other staff is helpful in this process, but all carers should be sensitive to the wishes and feelings of the family and, as far as possible, the family should be allowed to choose those they wish to support them at that time (Chiswick 2001).

The parents often value a photograph of themselves with the baby, even one taken after the infant has died. A lock of hair and footprints and handprints from the baby may be placed in a special card to be presented to the family at an appropriate time. The parents will often also value the baby's namebands and cot card as keepsakes with which they will remember the baby's brief life (Fig. 14.1). Any photographs taken of the baby should also be offered to the parents. It is not unusual for parents to display these at home for a long time after the baby has died, such is the impact of his life on the family. Some cannot cope with such items and in those cases the mementos

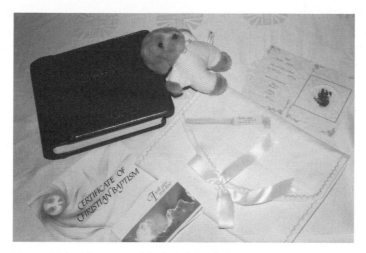

Figure 14.1 Mementos of the baby's brief life help the parents to grieve the loss of their infant.

should be kept in the baby's notes in case the family asks for them at a later date.

Helping parents after a perinatal death

The support of parents after the death of their newborn baby is complex and requires particular understanding and empathy. They will require comfort in their initial sorrow, advice about arranging the funeral, and information on how to register both the birth and the death of their infant. All available information relating to the cause of the death must be sought and collated by the medical and nursing staff so that later on the family can be given the opportunity to discuss it with the paediatrician to help them understand more fully what happened and why.

Whatever the cause of death, the parents will be deeply affected by their loss after the great hopes and expectation raised during the pregnancy. The grief of such a loss affects people in different ways and at different rates. Sometimes this can confuse a couple who are at different stages of the process and lead to additional tension between them. Simply explaining to such parents that this is a natural and normal situation can often be very supportive. The emotional reactions experienced during the initial grieving include bitterness, anger, helplessness,

fear, disbelief and sometimes a guilt that they may have contributed to the death of the baby. If the parents' anger is turned towards one or more of the carers, perhaps focussed on a decision made or a perceived delay in an action being taken, it can be hurtful to the person concerned but it is not helpful to the family to discuss the substance of the complaint at this stage. It is also out of place to offer casual words of sympathy to the parents or a hollow reassurance that they will be able to have a replacement for the dead infant. The opportunity must be found for an unhurried listening to the parents' natural desire to unburden their sorrow and their concerns about the circumstances of the death.

In most cases the parents are present when the baby dies, but if not they can be gently encouraged to see and hold their dead infant as this can help them overcome their sense of disbelief. Even when there is a severe congenital malformation, ways can usually be found to present the baby with much of the affected area covered, thus highlighting the good and positive features of the baby, and to draw the attention away from the malformation. This should enable the parents to see and hold the infant without causing undue shock, if this is what they wish. For others, it is important that they see the abnormalities for themselves to help them understand what has happened and why the baby has died. The caring staff themselves often feel deeply for the family and sharing their grief can provide comfort to them.

Most maternity departments have a checklist of all those professional carers who need to be informed of a baby's death so that they can continue to provide appropriate advice and help. Giving the parents the contact numbers for appropriate support groups which offer excellent support, advice and counselling, is often of great value to the parents.

In the UK it is the parents' responsibility to register the birth and death of the infant, a task which can accentuate the confused emotions of the situation. If the death was expected and its cause beyond doubt, the doctor caring for the baby will complete and sign a death certificate which the registrar will need in order to complete the necessary registrations. After this, the baby's body can be released for the funeral. If the parents express a wish for the staff to attend the funeral, every effort should be made for one or more of the nurses who were involved with the infant and parents to do so, as a mark of respect and continued support. The parents may need advice on how to arrange the funeral and will want to do it themselves, though many hospitals will make the arrangements for them if they so wish. Occasionally, the death may be of uncertain cause or unexpected. In these situations, the local coroner should be consulted. He will often require a postmortem examination to be carried out to establish the cause of death before he allows the death to be registered and the body released for the funeral.

Postmortem examination of the baby

Confirmation of the clinical diagnosis by postmortem examination has traditionally been thought to help the clinician without providing the parents with much useful information. Developments in autopsy techniques have now added cytogenetic analysis and X-rays of the bones to the traditional direct inspection of the internal organs, microscopical analysis of relevant tissues and microbiological culture of fluids and organ surfaces. Recent research into the value of such extended postmortem examination on

stillbirths and neonatal deaths has shown that, where there was uncertainty about why the baby died, either the cause of death or important information of relevance in future pregnancies was found at autopsy in about a quarter of cases. Unexpected congenital abnormalities, cytogenetic abnormalities and infections were particularly frequently found. Clinicians have been reticent about suggesting such examinations in the past, but as their value is now clear, an autopsy should be offered to parents in most cases. Because of recent controversy concerning the retention of tissues and organs of children following postmortem examinations, the doctor should explain sufficient details of the procedure, allowing time for parents to express any concerns and fears. It is good practice to ensure that the parents know fully what to expect and give adequately informed consent to the examination (McHaffie et al 2001b). It takes sensitivity and time, but the benefits are worth the effort.

Some groups, such as Muslims, will not normally allow postmortem examination for religious reasons, except where the law requires one to be done (Gatrad & Sheikh 2001). Other people may refuse permission for cultural or emotional reasons and this should usually be respected. Some will allow very limited examination, such as an organ biopsy, blood sampling or X-ray imaging, and these can provide valuable information in some cases.

Although there is a need to inform the parents at the time of death of what is known about its cause, detailed discussions, including the result of the autopsy and any subsequent tests, are best left until the initial shock has receded. This explanation should wait until both parents can be present and must be given by a senior paediatrician who is well informed of all the facts and understands the implications for the parents' decisions about having further children.

Stillbirth

Until a few years ago, there was a tendency to treat the misfortune of a stillbirth somewhat differently from that of a neonatal death, but it is now better understood that the needs of these parents are much the same and their expressions of grief very similar. Counselling as described for neonatal death is equally appropriate and the parents should be offered the benefit of a post-mortem examination of the baby. A dignified disposal of the baby's body should be arranged according to the parents' wishes and customs. It may assist the parents' grieving to realise that they can give the baby a personal name.

Whether the baby was stillborn or died in the first few days, some parents find comfort from having a tangible reminder of the infant, such as a photograph, a handprint or footprint, or a lock of hair, and these should be offered if they so wish (Fig. 14.1). Parents should be allowed to spend time with their baby as if it were a neonatal death, to enable them to hold their stillborn child if they so wish. Ideally this should be in a room away from the sound of crying babies but still close to staff for support. It is important to remember to remove the cot from the mother's room on the ward, and that the section of the postnatal notes relating to the baby be taken out, thus minimising unnecessary reminders and stress. It is equally important, however, not to forget that the mother has just given birth to a baby.

Continuing care for the parents

Grieving will continue long after the parents return home and will involve the other members of the family, so it is important that those providing care in the community should have all possible information to enable them to help the family through the process of adjustment. Other children in the family will also grieve for the lost baby and their understanding of what has happened which will vary according to their ages. Their needs should also be taken into account as part of the support given to the family.

The continuing flow of lochia and secretion of milk serve as frequent reminders of the bereavement and may accentuate the depression that often ensues as part of the normal grieving process.

To assist parents to grieve the loss of their baby, many hospitals provide a Book of Remembrance in which parents may record a personal memory and the name of their infant. Some hospitals hold an annual memorial service for any bereaved families in a local church and these are often greatly valued, especially if some of the staff are also able to attend and take part in the service. Personal letters of invitation are sent to families and notices are distributed to doctors' surgeries and health visitor clinics to try and ensure all affected families are aware of the service. Other hospitals send out a card to the parents on the anniversary of the death to show parents that the child is not forgotten. Some families may wish to turn their tragedy into a positive contribution and can be advised about relevant charitable organisations and self-help groups which they may join. For others, the sense of loss may be so great that more formal treatment may be needed, but fortunately only a small number are affected to this extent.

If the baby's death was due to a congenital abnormality, referral to a clinical geneticist is advisable since it is being increasingly recognised that genetic factors are involved in the origin of many such abnormalities and information gained may be important in the management of subsequent pregnancies.

USEFUL ADDRESSES

Most neonatal anomalies have their own support group. Below are listed some of the broader associations. Almost all support groups have a website address, and information may be found on line.

CLEFT LIP AND PALATE ASSOCIATION (CLAPA)
235–237 Fichley Road
London
NW3 6LS
Tel: 020 7431 0033
Website: www.clapa.cwc.net/
Email: clapa@mcmail.com

DOWN'S SYNDROME ASSOCIATION
155 Mitcham Road
London
SW17 9PG
Tel: 020 8682 4001
Website: www.dsa-uk.com/
Email: info@downs-syndrome.org.uk

NATIONAL CHILDBIRTH TRUST
Alexandra House
Oldham Terrace
London

W3 6NH
Tel: 020 8540 4577
Website: www.nct-online.org/
Email: nctconnect@aol.com

SCOPE (Cerebral Palsy Support Group)
6 Market Road
London
N7 9PW
Tel: 020 7619 7100
Website: www.scope.org.uk
Email: cphelpline@scope.org.uk

STILLBIRTH AND NEONATAL DEATH SOCIETY (SANDS)
28 Portland Place
London
W1N 4DE
Tel: 020 7436 5881 (Helpline)
    020 7436 7940 (Office)
Website: www.uk.sands.org/
Email: support@uk-sands.org/

THE CHILD BEREAVEMENT TRUST
Aston House
West Wycombe
High Wycombe
Buckinghamshire
HP14 3AG
Tel: 01494 446648
Website: www.childbereavement.org.uk/
Email: enquiries@childbereavement.org.uk

THE FOUNDATION FOR THE STUDY OF INFANT DEATHS
Artillery House
11–19 Artillery Row

London
SW1P 1RT
Tel: 020 7222 8001
Website: www.sids.org.uk/fsid/
Email: info@sids.org.uk

TOFS (Tracheo-oesophageal Fistula & Oesophageal Atresia)
St George's Centre
91 Victoria Road
Netherfield
Nottingham
NG4 2NN
Tel: 0115 961 3092
Website: www.tofs.org.uk/
Email: info@tofs.org.uk

TWINS AND MULTIPLE BIRTH ASSOCIATION (TAMBA)
Harnott House
309 Chester Road
Little Sutton
Ellesmere Port
CH66 1QQ
Tel: 0870 121 4000
Website: www.tamba.org.uk
Email: enquiries@tambahq.org.uk

UNICEF
UNICEF Baby Friendly Initiative
Africa House
64–78 Kingsway
London
WC2B 6NB
Tel: 020 7312 7652
Website: www.babyfriendly.org.uk

REFERENCES

Chiswick M 2001 Parents and end of life decisions in neonatal practice. Archives of Disease in Childhood Fetal and Neonatal Edition 84:F1–F3

Gatrad A R, Sheikh A 2001 Muslim birth customs. Archives of Disease in Childhood Fetal and Neonatal Edition 84:F6–F8

McHaffie H E, Laing I A, Lloyd D J 2001a Follow up care of bereaved parents after withdrawal of treatment from newborns. Archives of Disease in Childhood Fetal and Neonatal Edition 84:F125–F128

McHaffie H E, Fowlie P W, Hume R et al 2001b Consent for autopsies for neonates. Archives of Disease in Childhood Fetal and Neonatal Edition 84:F4–F7

Chapter 15
Neonatal pharmacopoeia

Prescribing drugs for the newborn infant is more complex than for the older child. Drug doses are almost all related to the weight of the infant, which can at times mean greatly different doses of the same drug for two babies in the same unit. The rate at which the infant metabolises or excretes drugs is often slower, so doses must be given at less frequent intervals to prevent side-effects from accumulation of the substance. Drugs excreted primarily by the renal route can accumulate rapidly because of the limited capacity of the immature kidneys to excrete such substances quickly. In such circumstances, measurement of blood levels and adjustment of the frequency or dose of the drug can prevent harmful blood levels arising. This is particularly relevant for certain antibiotics which, while highly effective, need to be given in doses very close to their toxic dose. Aminoglycoside antibiotics – for example gentamicin, tobramicin and netilmicin – are highly nephrotoxic and ototoxic when only slightly over the maximum recommended doses. For these drugs, the measurement of levels is mandatory. As nerve deafness can result from both meningitis (p. 171) and its treatment, it is particularly important to prevent iatrogenic hearing loss (p. 175).

The relatively lower blood albumin level found in the neonate may mean that less of the drug is able to be bound and more is available in a free, active state in the circulation. Some compete for albumin binding sites and others may displace bilirubin from them, e.g. sulphonamide-containing drugs, and thus increase the risk of bilirubin encephalopathy. It is for these reasons that the drugs recommended for use in the newborn baby are limited and why it is unwise to use others until sufficient experience has been obtained and the results of such trials published. Some drugs interact with others and alter their effectiveness or increase the risk of toxicity. It is advisable to avoid using such drugs together. Information about such interactions in adults is listed in comprehensive prescribing manuals or the British National Formulary and it is always good policy to consult these before giving unfamiliar combinations of drugs.

Great care must be taken in the prescribing and administration of drugs at this time of life, and the doses given in this pharmacopoeia (Tables 15.1 & 15.2) are a guide to the amount a baby requires rather than a firmly fixed dose. Published doses of drugs for use in the newborn baby vary considerably from one text to another. In many cases, drugs have not had the benefit of widespread clinical trials in the newborn as the ethics of doing such research are so complex. In this section, therefore, the doses given correspond closely to those most commonly encountered in other recent books and journals. As experience accumulates, the recomended doses may vary from those given here. It is important to consult a specialist neonatal formulary when prescribing for pre-term infants.

Certain drugs such as morphine and other opiates, whose effective dose also causes respiratory depression, should be used with great caution. The infant may need respiratory support because the dose required to obtain adequate analgesia seriously depresses the baby's respiratory drive.

Though rarely needed, insulin often causes a serious drop in blood glucose. As neonates are particularly susceptible to hypoglycaemia, the blood glucose should be followed very closely.

Such drugs should not be neglected for fear of side-effects, but all persons involved in the care of the infant need to be aware of the potential side-effects and how to prevent or identify them.

Table 15.1 gives details of drugs commonly used in the neonatal period. Antibiotics have been listed separately in Table 15.2. Certain information has been given to prevent serious problems arising from the administration of many of the drugs, but it is always wise to consult more complete texts before giving an unfamiliar drug. Examples of such texts and other sources are cited below.

Special attention must be paid to the units in which the drugs are given. In many cases, microgram (μg) doses are listed. Drugs are made mostly to suit adult doses and it may appear that the dose is very small compared with the amount in an ampoule. It is good practice for all doses to be checked before giving the drug to the baby. Where it is feasible, doses on the prescription chart and doses prepared for administration should be checked by two experienced nurses. Errors in prescribing and administration should be minimised by this practice.

REFERENCES

Royal College of Paediatrics and Child Health 1999 Medicines for children. RCPCH, London
Speidel B, Fleming P, Henderson J, Leaf A, Marlow N, Dunn P 1998 A neonatal vade mecum. Edward Arnold, London

The Northern Neonatal Network 2000 Neonatal formulary. BMJ Publishing Group, London

FURTHER READING

British National Formulary – current edition. British Medical Association and Royal Pharmaceutical Association of Great Britain, London

USEFUL WEBSITE

www.bnf.org – British National Formulary

www.neonatalformulary.com

Table 15.1 Drugs used in the newborn baby (excluding antibiotics)

Drug	Route	Single dose	Frequency[a]	Comments
Adenosine	i.v.	0.1–0.2 mg/kg	Single	Dilute to concentration of 1 mg/mL with 0.9% saline. Flush in with 1 mL of 0.9% saline. Use only with ECG monitoring
Adrenaline (epinephrine) 1 : 10 000	i.v. via ETT	0.1–0.3 mL/kg 1 mL/kg		See section on neonatal resuscitation (p. 39)
Aminophylline	i.v. i.v. Rectal	5 mg/kg 2.5 mg/kg 2.5–5 mg/kg	1 2 4	Loading dose – infuse slowly Infuse over 30 minutes Blood level monitoring needed
Caffeine citrate	Oral i.v. Oral	20 mg/kg 5 mg/kg	1 1	Loading dose – infuse slowly Daily maintenance
Calciferol (Vit D2)	Oral	10 μg	1	Daily requirements
Calcium chloride	Oral	33 mg/kg	4	With milk feeds
Calcium gluconate	i.v.	0.07 mmol/kg (0.3 mL/kg of 10% solution)	1	Slow infusion in 0.9% sodium chloride solution under ECG monitoring
Chloral hydrate	Oral	30 mg/kg 45 mg/kg	Up to 4 1	Single hypnotic dose
Chlorothiazide	Oral	10 mg/kg	1–2	Give spironolactone 1 mg/kg twice daily also, to counteract potassium loss
Chlorpromazine	Oral	500 μg/kg	4	Reduce only slowly in babies of drug-addicted mothers
Clonazepam	i.v.	100–200 μg/kg		Short infusion only
Dexamethasone	i.v./oral	100–500 μg/kg	1	Infuse over 5 minutes. Dose for bronchopulmonary dysplasia (p. 143)
Diamorphine	s.c. i.v.	50 μg/kg 10–15 μg/kg	6 Up to hourly	Respiratory depression can be reversed by nalorphine
Diazepam	i.v. Rectal	0.3 mg/kg 0.3 mg/kg	1–3	Bolus injection over 3 minutes Repeat after 10 minutes if fitting persists
Digoxin	i.v. Oral	10 μg/kg 5–10 μg/kg	1–3 1	Loading dose Daily maintenance
Dinoprostone	i.v.	0.01–0.05 μg/ kg/min	Continuous infusion	
Dobutamine	i.v.	5 μg/kg/min	Continuous infusion	Monitor heart rate and blood pressure closely and adjust infusion rate according to response
Dopamine	i.v.	2–5 μg/kg/min	Continuous infusion	Monitor heart rate and blood pressure closely and adjust infusion rate according to response
Edrophonium	i.v.	100–200 μg/kg	1	Diagnostic test dose in myasthenia gravis
Epoprostenol	i.v.	10 ng/kg/min	Continuous infusion	
Erythropoietin	s.c.	250 units/kg		3 times per week for 4–6 weeks
Folic acid	Oral	100 μg	Daily	
Furosemide (frusemide)	Oral	1 mg/kg	1	Monitor electrolytes. Potassium supplements may be required
	i.v.	0.5–1.0 mg/kg	Single	
Gaviscon	Oral	1/2 sachet	At each feed	Dose per 50 mL of feed
Heparin	i.v.	2 units/hour	Continuous infusion	Infuse as a solution of 2 units per mL
Hepatitis B vaccine vaccine	i.m.	0.01 mg (0.5 mL)	Single dose	Single dose; repeat at 6 and 12 months of age
Hepatitis B immunoglobulin	i.m.	200 IU	Single dose	Give with hepatitis B vaccine

Table 15.1 (cont'd)

Drug	Route	Single dose	Frequency[a]	Comments
Indomethacin	i.v./oral	0.1–0.3 mg/kg	1	Give for up to 6 days as bolus injections over 10 minutes
Insulin	i.v.	0.1 units/kg	Continuous infusion	Dose adjusted according to response
Magnesium sulphate 50%	i.m.	0.2 mL/kg	1–2	Maximum of 3 doses
Mannitol 20% solution	i.v.	0.5–1.0 g/kg	1	Infuse over 30 minutes
Midazolam	i.v.	150 μg/kg	1	For sedation for painful procedures. Effect may be reversed by flumazenil 20 mg/kg i.v.
Morphine	i.v.	50 μg/kg	1	Loading dose for preterm infants
	i.v.	5 μg/kg/hour	Continuous infusion	Preterm infant dose. May be increased up to 30 μg/kg if needed
	i.v.	50–100 μg/kg	1	Loading dose for term infants
	i.v.	10–20 μg/kg/hour	Continuous infusion	Term infant dose
Naloxone	i.v./i.m.	10–30 μg/kg	1	For immediate reversal of opiate effect
	i.m.	70 μg/kg	1	For continued effect over 24 hours
Pancuronium	i.v.	50–80 μg/kg	Up to hourly	Repeat every 1–4 hours as needed
Paracetamol	Oral/rectal	10–15 mg/kg	Up to 4	For pain relief
Paraldehyde	i.m.	0.1 mL/kg	Up to 6	Inject deep into muscles
Pethidine	i.m./i.v.	0.5–2.0 mg/kg	4	Lower doses by the i.v. route
Phenobarbital	i.v./i.m.	20 mg/kg	1	Loading dose
	Oral	2.5 mg/kg	1–2	Maintenance dose
Phenytoin	i.v.	20 mg/kg	1	No faster than 1 mg/kg/min; may be repeated after 1 hour
	Oral	5 mg/kg	2	Blood level monitoring essential for maintenance therapy. Keep blood level in target range 40–80 μmol/L
Phosphate	Oral	1 mmol/kg	1	Prevention of rickets of prematurity. Dose given for Phosphate Sandoz
Potassium chloride	Oral/i.v.	0.5–1.0 mmol/kg		As a supplement to prevent hypokalaemia. Maximum concentration for i.v. use 40 mmol K$^+$ per litre, given at a rate not greater than 0.2 mmol/kg/hour
Ranitidine	Oral	1 mg/kg	3	
Sodium bicarbonate 4.2%	i.v.	2–4 mL/kg	1	See sections on neonatal resuscitation (p. 39) and intensive care (p. 134)
Sodium chloride	Oral/i.v.	2–5 mmol/kg/day		Daily requirements during parenteral nutrition regimen
Sodium valproate	i.v.	10 mg/kg	1	Loading dose; infuse over 5 minutes
	Oral	10 mg/kg	1–3	Maintenance dose
Spironolactone	Oral	0.5–1.5 mg/kg	2	Potassium-sparing drug for use with diuretics
Theophylline	Oral	5 mg/kg	1	Loading dose
	Oral	2–3 mg/kg	4	Maintenance dose
Tolazoline	i.v.	1.0 mg/kg	1	Infuse over 10 minutes
	i.v.	0.1–1.0 mg/kg	Hourly	Maintenance infusion
Vitamin E	i.m.	25 mg/kg		3 daily doses
	Oral	10 mg		Daily requirement
Vitamin K	i.m./oral	1 mg		Single i.m. dose to correct deficiency or for prophylaxis. Repeat doses required for routine prophylaxis in breast-fed infants (p. 186)

[a] Number of doses per day, or as stated.
i.m. = intramuscular; i.v. = intravenous.

Table 15.2   Antibiotics commonly used in the newborn baby

Antibiotic	Route of administration	Single dose per kg body weight	Number of doses per day[a]	Comments
Amikacin	i.v.	7.5 mg/kg	2	
Ampicillin or amoxycillin	i.v./i.m./oral	30–50 mg/kg	2–3	
Azlocillin	i.v.	100 mg/kg	2	Dose should be halved in preterm infants
Cefotaxime	i.v./i.m.	50 mg/kg	2–3	Dose may be increased up to 150 mg/kg in severe infections
Ceftazidime	i.v./i.m.	30 mg/kg	2–3	
Cefuroxime	i.v./i.m.	30 mg/kg	2–3	Dose may be increased up to 100 mg/kg in severe infections
Chloramphenicol	i.v./oral	12.5 mg/kg	2	Dose may be doubled after 2 weeks of age; blood levels should be monitored
Cloxacillin or flucloxacillin	i.v./oral	25–40 mg/kg	4	Dose may be increased up to 100 mg/kg in severe infections
Erythromycin	Oral/i.v.	12.5 mg/kg	4	i.v. by slow infusion
Gentamicin	i.v./i.m.	3.0 mg/kg	2–3	Monitor blood levels; keep peak level 8–10 mg/L and trough level <2 mg/L
Isoniazid	Oral	5 mg/kg	2	Pyridoxine supplement required
Metronidazole	i.v./oral	7.5 mg/kg	3	Infuse over 1 hour
Netilmicin	i.v./i.m.	3.0 mg/kg	2–3	Monitor blood levels; keep peak level 8–10 mg/L and trough level <2 mg/L
Penicillin	i.v./i.m.	15–30 mg/kg	2–3	Dose may be increased to 50 mg/kg in severe infections
Tobramycin	i.v.	2.0 mg/kg	2–3	Monitor blood levels as for gentamicin
Vancomycin	i.v.	10–15 mg/kg	2–3	Infuse over 60 minutes
Antifungal agents				
Amphoterocin	Oral	100 000 U	4	Give after feeds;
	i.v.	0.25–1.0 mg/kg	1	infuse over 6 hours; use higher dose in severe infections
5-Fluocytosine	Oral	50 mg/kg	4	
Miconazole	i.v.	10 mg/kg	2	Infuse over 1 hour
Nystatin	Oral	100 000 U	4	Give after feeds
Antiviral agents				
Acyclovir	i.v.	10 mg/kg	3	Infuse over 1 hour

[a] The lower dose frequency should be used in the first 7 days in term infants and for 10–14 days in preterm infants.
i.m. = intramuscular; i.v. = intravenous.
For further details, consult the current *British National Formulary*, either in its regular book publication or on-line, or the *Neonatal Vade Mecum*.

Index

Numbers in bold refer to figures and tables.

A

Abdomen, examination, 68–69
Abdominal distension, 68, 105, 121, 217, 218
Abdominal X-ray
  ileal atresia, **217**
  necrotising enterocolitis, **140**
Aberdeen splint, 234
ABO incompatibility, 192, 194
Abortion
  drug addicted mothers, 18
  mid-trimester, 3
Abscess
  breast, 99, 166
  lung, 172
Absorption of food, 92
Accessory auricles, 65
Accessory digits, 70
Achondroplasia, 70, 206
Acidosis
  in asphyxia, 33, 34
  in congenital heart disease, 41
  persistent metabolic, 43
  preterm infants, 112
  in respiratory distress syndrome, 134
Acquired immune deficiency syndrome (AIDS), 29, 96, 178, 179–180
Acupuncture in pregnancy, 27
Acute illness in pregnancy, 19, 20
Acute renal tubular necrosis, 128
Acyclovir, **252**
Adaptation to independent life, 31–33
Adenosine, **250**
Admission to neonatal unit, selection of infants, 60–61
Adrenal hyperplasia, congenital, 69, **205**, 206, 229
Adrenaline (epinephrine) in resuscitation, **39**
Age, maternal, 14
  and congenital anomalies, 202
  and Down syndrome, 22, 202, 207
  and perinatal mortality, 6, **15**
Air leaks in RDS, 139
Albumin infusions, 128, 134, 174
Alcohol, effect on fetus, 16
Alimentary tract
  function, 86
    preterm infants, 112
    unusual bowel actions and stools, 105
  infections, 167
  structural congenital malformations, 213–219
Allergens
  in breast milk, 95
  in cow's milk protein, 94

Allopurinol, 155
Alpha-1 antitrypsin deficiency, 198, 199
Alpha-fetoprotein
  in Down syndrome, 22
  in gastroschisis, 219
  in neural tube defects, 23
Ambiguous genitalia, 69, 228–230
Amethocaine local anaesthetic gel, 144
Amikacin, **252**
Amino acid chromatography, 211
Aminophylline, 120, **250**
Amitriptyline in pregnancy, 25
Ammoniacal dermatitis, 87–88
Amniocentesis, 22
  in rhesus haemolytic disease, 193
Amnioscopy, 23
Amniotic bands, 203
Amniotic fluid, 86
  meconium staining, 33, 40
  swallowed, 105
Amoxycillin, 171, 173, **252**
Amphoterocin, **252**
Ampicillin, 167, 169, 171, **252**
Anaemia
  at birth, 183, 184
  haemolytic, 119, 122, 192
  haemorrhagic disease of the newborn, 186
  hiatus hernia, 215
  malaria, 182
  in pregnancy, 15
  preterm infants, 119, 122
  twins, 56
Anaesthetics in labour, effect on neonate, 26
Analgesics
  in labour
    effect on neonate, 26
    in preterm labour, 113
  neonates
    before endotracheal intubation, 136, 144
    in intensive care, 144
Anencephaly, 202, 203, 230
Angiotensin-converting enzyme inhibitors, effect on fetus, 24
Anniversaries of death, 247
Antenatal care
  availability, 5
  identifying inherited disorders, 203
  infant feeding education, 97
  'preparation for parenthood' classes, 97, 239, **240**
Antenatal diagnosis, 8, 9, 203
  cytogenetic and DNA analysis, 22–23
  fetal blood sampling, 23
  fetal cardiac monitoring, 23
  maternal blood tests, 22, 23
  ultrasound, 20, 21, 23
Antepartum haemorrhage, 5

Anterior fontanelle, 63
  imaging through, 152
  tense, 48, 152, 232
Anti-D globulin, 22, 192
Antibiotic resistance, prevention, 175
Antibiotics
  in newborn, 130, 174–175, **252**
    dosage, 175
    eye infections, 166
    meningitis, 171
    osteomyelitis, 174
    pneumonia, 172
    septic arthritis, 174
    septicaemia, 169
    skin infections, 165, 166
    upper respiratory tract infections, 167
    urinary tract infections, 173
  in pregnancy, 24, **25**
Antibodies, 163
  maternal, 85, 112, 163
  rhesus
    clinical impact of, 192
    development of, 22, 191, 192
  see also Immunoglobulins
Anticoagulants in pregnancy, 24–25, 27
Anticonvulsants
  in neonates, 154, 157, 193, 251
  in pregnancy, 24, **25**, 203, 213
Antidepressants in pregnancy, 25
Antiseptic solutions, preterm infants, 115, 130
Anus
  examination, 69
  imperforate, 218
Aorta, coarctation, 68, 209, 225
Apgar score, 36, 151
Apnoea, 33, 41, 67
  light for dates infants, 52
  preterm infants, 112, 120
Aqueduct stenosis, 231
Arms
  examination, 70
  posture, 72, 73
Arnold-Chiari malformation, 230
Aromatherapy in pregnancy, 27
Arrhythmias, 18, 23, 221, 226
  see also Bradycardia; Tachycardia
Arterial switch procedure, 223
Artificial tears, 138
Asphyxia, 5, 16, 43, 50
  assessment at birth, 36
  Doppler blood flow studies, 21
  intracranial haemorrhage, 150
  morphine and pethidine effects, 26
  predisposing factors, 33, 151
  prognosis, 155
  recognition, fetal distress, 33–34
  resuscitation, 36–40
Aspiration
  meconium, 40, 43, 133
  pneumonia, 172
Aspirin, effects on fetus, 26
Asthma, 94

Asymmetric tonic neck reflex, 74, 152
Atelectasis, 42
Atenolol, effect on fetus, 19
Athetosis, 123
Atresia
    biliary, 198, 199, 200
    choanal, 65, 219–220
    duodenal, 216–217
    ileal, 217
    intestinal, 144
    jejunal, 217
    oesophageal, 214–215
    pulmonary, 223
    tricuspid, 223, **224**
Atrial septal defect, 225, 226
Attachment, mother-child, 8–9, 95
    fostering process of, 83–84
Audit, perinatal, 2
Auditory brain-stem-evoked response
    tests, 76
Autopsy see Postmortem examination
Azlocillin, **252**

B

Back arching, 152
Bacterial infections, 165–167
    clinical signs, **167**, 168
    congenital pneumonia, 171–172
    eyes, 166
    gastroenteritis, 174
    meningitis, 167, 168, 169–171
    osteomyelitis, 174
    septic arthritis, 174
    septicaemia, 141, 167, 168, 169
    skin, 165–166
    syphilis, 29, 164, 167, 175, 181, 198
    tuberculosis, 164, 176, 178
    upper respiratory tract, 166–167
    urinary tract, 172–174
Bacteroides infections, 169
Bag and mask ventilation, 37–38
Ballard's method, gestational age
    assessment, 108, **109**
Barlow's test, 71
Barotrauma, 138, 143
Barrier creams, 87
Bathing, 87
    preterm infants, 87, 114–115
BCG immunisation, 178
Beckwith's syndrome, 56, 66, 219
Bed sharing, infants and parents, 88
Bedding, 82
Behaviour, normal, 72
Benign congential hypotonia, 159
Benign familial neonatal fits,
    syndrome of, 156
Benzodiazepines in pregnancy, 26
Benzylpenicillin, **252**
Beta-human chorionic gonadotrophin
    (bHCG), Down syndrome
    testing, 22

Bicarbonate infusions, 134
Bifidobacteria in milk formula, 102
Bile in vomit, 105
Biliary atresia, 198, 199
    diagnosis and management,
        199–200
Bilirubin
    critical serum levels, 191
        for phototherapy, 197
    encephalopathy, 190–191
    metabolism, 188–189
Bilirubinometers, transcutaneous,
    195
Biochemistry values, 77
Birth
    assessment at, 36
    circulatory changes, 31–32
    onset of respiration, 32–33
    procedure at normal, 79–80
Birth weight, 3, 45
    and maternal diet, 14, 15
    and maternal smoking, 15–16
    see also Low birth weight infants
Birthmarks, 62–63
Bladder, palpation, 68
    see also Ectopia vesicae
Blankets, 82, 85
Bleeding see Haemorrhage
Blood
    emergency group O-negative, 36
    preterm infants, 111
    vomited, 105
Blood cultures, 41, 168
Blood gases
    in hypoxic-ischaemic
        encephalopathy, 154
    in respiratory distress, 41, 133–134,
        138, 142
    in weaning from ventilator, 138, 139
Blood group, 193
    ABO incompatibility, 192, 194
    see also Rhesus haemolytic disease
Blood loss, signs, 40
Blood pressure, 222
    hypotension, 140, 141
    in hypoxic-ischaemic
        encephalopathy, 154
    persistent pulmonary hypertension
        of newborn (PPHN), 139–140
    preterm infant, 111
    in RDS, 140
Blood sampling
    in bleeding and clotting disorders,
        186
    fetal scalp, 34
    in total parenteral nutrition, 129
Blood tests
    antenatal diagnosis, 22, 23
    neonatal biochemistry, 77
Blood transfusion, 184–185
    preterm infants, 122
    in rhesus haemolytic disease, 193
    see also Exchange transfusion
Blood volume, 183, **184**

Bonding, 83–84, 95
Book of Remembrance, 247
Bottle feeding, 93, 101–104
    amount and frequency, 104
    cow's milk formulae, 94, 101, 102
    equipment sterilisation, 85
    giving feeds, 103–104
    infants' stools, 86
    preparing feeds, 102–103
Bottled water, 103
Brachial plexus injuries, 159–160
    see also Erb's palsy
Bradycardia
    fetal, 33, 34
    neonatal, 67
    preterm infants, 120, 128
Brain stem damage, 72, 152
Branchial cysts, 67
Breaking bad news, 242–243
Breast abscess, 99, 166
Breast care, 99
Breast engorgement, 95, 99–100
    preventing, 98
Breast feeding, 93–95
    antenatal education, 97
    benefits, **94**
    contraindications, 96, 179
    difficulties, 100–101
    drug addicted mothers, 18, 19
    immediately after birth, 84, 97
    infant's stools, 86, 94, 105
    jaundice, 197, 198
    light for dates infants, 51
    making more effective, 98–99
    positioning for, 97–98
    preterm infants, 94, 96, 118
    promoting, 8
    reasons for not, 95–97
    twins, 57
    urine output, 86
Breast milk
    comparison with formula milks,
        102
    composition, 92, 93, 94, 98
    control of gut organisms, 164
    donated, 117
    drugs secreted in, 18, 19, 96
    expressed, 117
    fortifiers, 117, 118
    inadequate supply, 95, 96
    physiology of secretion, 98
    storage, 117
    viral transmission, 165
Breast pads, 99
Breast surgery, cosmetic, 95
Breasts, neonatal
    examination, 67
    preterm infant, 109
Breath sounds, 67
Breathing movements, fetal, 32
Breech presentation, 56, 69, 70, 187
Bronchopulmonary dysplasia (BPD),
    143
Brown fat, 80, 92

Bruising, 187–188
  external genitalia, 69
  head, 149
  preterm infants, 111, 187
Bulbar reflexes, 75
Bullous impetigo, 165
Buphthalmos, 233
Bupivacaine in labour, effect on
  neonate, 26
Burst-suppression pattern, EEG, 153

C

C-reactive protein, 168
Caffeine, 120, 138, **250**
Calciferol, **250**
Calcium channel blockers, effect on
  fetus, 24
Calcium chloride, **250**
Calcium gluconate, 157, **250**
Calorie intake, 92, **93**
Campylobacter infection, 174
Candida infections, 141, 164, 167
  see also Thrush
Cannabis, 19
Captopril, effect on fetus, 24
Caput succedaneum, 61, 63
Carbamazepine, 203
Carbimazole in thyrotoxicosis, 28
Carbon dioxide levels, ventilated
  infants, 138
Cardiac massage, 39
Cardiotocography, 23, 33–34
Care, normal infants, 83–85
  alimentary tract function, 85
  minimising infection risk, 85–86
  procedure at birth, 79–80
  renal function, 86–87
  skin care, 87–88
  sleeping position, 88–89
  weighing baby, 89
Casein-based milks, 102
Cataracts, 66, 233
'Catch-up growth', 92
Categories of care, 125, **126**
Cefotaxime, 130, 166, 169, 171, 172,
  173, **252**
Ceftazidime, **252**
Ceftriaxone, 171
Cefuroxime, 169
Cellular immune systems, 164
Central venous catheters, insertion
  technique, 130
Cephalhaematoma, 63–64, 149, 185
Cerebral blood flow, 21, 151, 154
Cerebral injury, 150–155
  associated features, 75
  prognosis, 155
Cerebral irritation, 151, 152
Cerebral palsy, 2, 7, 151, 155
  periventricular leucomalacia (PVL),
  141, 142

preterm infants, 7–8
  primitive reflexes, 73
  triplets, 57
  twins, 56, 57
Cerebrospinal fluid (CSF)
  examination, 170, 171, 181
CHARGE association, 220
Chest, examination, 67
Chest 'shake' in HFOV, 137, 138
Chest X-ray, 67
  chronic lung disease (CLD), **143**
  congenital heart disease, 222
  diaphragmatic hernia, **42**
  meconium aspiration syndrome, 43
  oesophageal atresia, **215**
  respiratory distress syndrome, 41,
  132
  septicaemia, 168
  tension pneumothorax, **42**
Child abuse, 8, 9, 17, 83, 85, 241
Child Health and Development
  Record, 59
Child protection issues, 17, 18
Chlamydia trachomatis infection, 164,
  166
Chloral hydrate, **250**
Chloramphenicol, **252**
  in eye infections, 166
  in meningitis, 171
Chloroquine, 182
Chlorothiazide, 121, **250**
Chlorpromazine, **250**
  effect on fetus, 25
Choanal atresia, 65, 219–220
Choledochal cyst, 200
Chordee, 228
Chorionic villus sampling, 22, 23
Choroid plexus cysts, 21
Christmas disease, 187
Chromosomal disorders, 7, 22–23,
  204–210
  see also Down syndrome
Chromosomes, 204
Chronic illness in pregnancy, 19, 20
Chronic lung disease (CLD), 143
Chronic pulmonary insufficiency of
  prematurity (CPIP), 143
Circulation
  assessment, 67–68
  changes at birth, 31–32
  preterm infants, 111, 131
  problems in RDS, 139–140
Cirrhosis of liver, 199
Clavicle fracture, 70, 160
Cleansing skin, 87
  preterm infants, 114, 115
Cleft lip/palate, 16, 27, 66, 100, 203,
  207, 213
  management, 213–214
Cleidocranial dysostosis, 63
Clinical governance, 2
Clinical trials, 146
Clitoral hypertrophy, 229
Clonazepam, 157, **250**

Clothing, 81, 82
  sterilising, 85
Clotrimazole, 167
Clotting disorders, 150, 168, 187
Clotting factors, 186
Cloxacillin, **252**
Coarctation of aorta, 68, 209, 225
Cocaine addiction, 18–19, 96
Cochrane Foundation, 2
Coeliac disease, maternal, 15
Colostomy, 218
Colostrum, 97, 98, 118
  constituents, 94
  protection from infection, 116, 164
Community neonatal nurses, 123
Complement, 164
Complementary therapy in pregnancy,
  27
Computerised tomography (CT) scan,
  153, 156
Confidential Enquiry into Stillbirths
  and Deaths in Infancy (CESDI),
  89
Congenital adrenal hyperplasia, 69,
  205, 206, 229
Congenital anomalies and
  malformations
  and breast feeding, 96
  causes, 202–203
  diabetes mellitus, 53
  drug addiction, 18
  epilepsy in mother, 27
  prescribed drugs, 23
  developmental delay, associated
  conditions, 207–213
  early diagnosis, 8, 240
  genetic disorders, 204–207
  incidence, 202
  intrauterine treatment, 21
  life-threatening, 203–204
  parental reactions to, 204
  and perinatal mortality, 4, 5, 7
  prevention, 203
  structural malformations, 213–236
  alimentary tract, 213–219
  central nervous system, 230–233
  eyes, 233
  genitourinary tract, 226–230
  heart and great vessels, 221–226
  limbs and joints, 233–236
  lymphatic system, 236
  respiratory tract, 219–222
  support groups, 247–248
  twins, 56
Congenital heart disease, 41, 144, 203,
  207
  common malformations, 223–226
  investigations, 221–223
  presentation, 221
Conjunctivitis, 166
Containment, 114
Continuous positive airways pressure
  (CPAP), 120, 135–136,
  138–139

Convulsions *see* Seizures
Coombs' test, 193, 194
Cordocentesis, 23
Corneal injury, 66
Cornification, 111
Coroner, consulting, 246
Cot death *see* Sudden infant death
    syndrome (SIDS)
Cotinine in breast milk, 96
Cotrimoxazole, 173
Cough reflex, preterm infants, 111
Counselling parents
    birth of abnormal baby, 75,
        243–244
    breaking bad news, 242–243
    genetic counselling, 8, 9, 21–22
    perinatal death, 245–246
    stillbirth, 247
Cow's milk
    formulae, 101, 102
        allergens in, 94
    intolerance, 104
Coxsackie virus infection, 164, 169,
        176, 177, 199, 202, 213
Crack cocaine addiction, 18–19
Cranial nerve responses, 74–75
Craniosynostosis, 64, 233
Craniotabes, 63
Creatine phosphokinase levels,
        muscular dystrophy, 158
Cross-infection, reducing risk, 85,
    115
Crossed extension reflex, 74
Crown-rump length, 20, 108
Crying, 72
    in cerebral irritation, 151
    preterm infants, 110, 113
Cryptorchidism, 159
Cultural aspects, 241, 244
Cup feeding, 100, 116
Cutis navel, 68
Cyanosis
    central, 61, 221
    malformations presenting with,
        223–224
    management, 224–225
    persistant, 41
    traumatic, 62, 187
Cystic fibrosis, 8, 105, 199, **205**, 206,
    210
Cystic hygromas, 21, 236
Cysts
    branchial, 67
    choledochal, 200
    choroid plexus, 21
    congenital lung, 220
    dermoid, 67
    of Gaertner's duct, 228
    thyroglossal, 67
Cytogenetic analysis, fetal cells,
    22
Cytomegalovirus, 96, 164, 175,
        176–177, 199, 233
    jaundice, 198
Cytotoxic drugs in pregnancy, 24

D

Dacrocystitis, 166
Danazol, effects on fetus, 24
Deafness, 76, 176
Death certificate, 246
Deformities, 203
Dehydration, signs of, 174
Delivery
    forceps, 61, 66, 149
    maternal HIV, 179
    preterm infants, 112
Denial, 241, 242
Dental enamel hypoplasia, 157
Depression, puerperal, 84–85
Dermatitis
    ammoniacal, 87–88
    monilial, 87
Dermoid cysts, 67
Developmental delay, 2, 155
    conditions associated with, 207–213
Developmental needs, preterm
        infants, 114
Dexamethasone, **250**
    in chronic lung disease (CLD), 143
    reducing RDS, 112
Dextrose
    in hypoglycaemia, 55
    intensive care infants, 128
    in resuscitation, **39**
Diabetes mellitus
    childhood, 94
    maternal
        effect on fetus, 27, 45
        effect on neonate, 52–53, 61
Diamorphine, 144, **250**
Diaphragmatic hernia, **42**, 144, 220
Diarrhoea, 92, 174
Diazepam, **250**
    neonates, 157
    in pregnancy, 26, 158
Diet
    during lactation, 97
    in pregnancy, 14, 15
Dietary sources, maternal infection,
    28–29
Digestion, 92
    preterm infants, 112
Digoxin, **250**
Disability *see* Handicap
Disseminated intravascular
        coagulation, 168, 187
Dizygotic twins, 56
DNA analysis, **22**, **205**
Dobutamine, **250**
'Doll's-eye phenomenon', 75
Dominant inheritance, 205, 206
Dopamine, **250**
Doppler blood flow studies, 21, 142,
        151, 154, 222
Down syndrome, 7, 8, 16, 64, 205,
        207–209
    antenatal diagnosis, 22–23
    chromosome pattern, **207**

congential malformations, 208, 218,
    221
    hypotonia, 158
    and maternal age, 14, 22, 202
    nuchal translucency, 21
    recognition, 208–209
    tongue darting, 66
Dribbling micturition, 86
Drip milk, 117
Drug addiction, 17
    infant problems after birth, 18–19,
        87
    nursing care of infants, 19
    social management in pregnancy,
        17, 18
Drug interactions, 252
Drugs in pregnancy, 23–26
    and congenital anomalies, 203
Dubowitz method, gestational age
        assessment, 108
Duchenne muscular dystrophy, 23,
        158–159, 207
Ductus arteriosus, 31, 32
    persistent (PDA), 111, 128, 131, 140,
        142, 225, 226
Duodenal atresia, 216–217
Duodenal stenosis, 217
Duvets, 82
Dying infants, 126, 145, 146, 244–247
Dysmorphic syndromes, 64, 209, **210**

E

Ears
    examination, 65
    preterm infants, 109
Ebstein's pearls, 66
Echocardiography
    congenital heart disease, 222
    persistent ductus arteriosus (PDA),
        142
Echovirus infection, 164, 169, 177–178,
    202
Ectodermal dysplasia, congenital,
    233
Ectopia vesicae, 227–228
Ectopic anus, 218
Ectopic ureters, 86, 227
Eczema and cow's milk protein, 94
Edrophonium, **250**
Edward's syndrome, 209
Elbow, congenital dislocation, 70–71
Electrocardiography (ECG), 222, **226**
Electroencephalography (EEG), 153,
    156
Electrolytes, measuring, 128
Elemental feeds, 119
Emotional care, 114, 144–145
Encephalocele, 230
Encephalopathy, 150–155
    bilirubin, 190–191
Endotracheal intubation, 38, 39, 136
    preterm infants, 40, 113

Enflurane, 26
Engorgement, breast, 95, 99–100
Enteral feeding, 116, 117, 119, 128
Enterocolitis, necrotising, 94, 140
Environment, preterm infants,
    113–114
Environmental factors, congenital
    anomalies, 203
Ephedrine, 101, 167
Epicanthic folds, 65
Epidural anaesthesia in labour, effect
    on neonate, 26
Epilepsy, 151, 155
    maternal, effect on fetus, 27
    see also Seizures
Epinephrine (adrenaline) in
    resuscitation, **39**
Epiphyseal dysplasia, punctate, 233
Epispadias, 228
Epoprostenol, 140
Epstein–Barr virus, 96
Epulis, 66
Equipment
    bacterial contamination, 165
    intensive care unit, 127
Erb's palsy, 53, 74, 159, **160**
Erythema toxicum, 62
Erythromycin, **252**
Erythropoietin, 122, **250**
Escherichia coli infections, 141, 163,
    164, 168
    eyes, 166
    meningitis, 169
    urinary tract, 172
Ethamsylate, 141
Ethical aspects
    perinatal care, 9–10
    resuscitation room dilemmas, 40–41
Ethnic group
    and congenital malformations, 202,
        204
    and infant mortality, 6, 7
    and preterm birth, 107
Examination, 8, 59
    abdomen, 68–69
    chest, 67
    general, 61
    genitalia, 69
    head and neck, 63–67
    hearing, 75–76
    heart and circulation, 67–68
    inspection at birth, 60–61, 84
    joint dislocation, 70–71
    limbs, 70
    neurological, 71–75
    purposes, **59**
    skin, 61–63
    spine, 69–70
Exchange transfusion, 194
Exomphalos, 23, 144, 219
Expressed milk, 117
External cardiac massage, 39
Extracorporeal membrane
        oxygenation (ECMO), 137
Eye contact, 84

Eye movements, 65, 75
Eyes
    examination, 65–66
    infection, 166
    preterm infants, 110
    'sticky', 66, 164, 166

F

Face
    dysmorphic features, **64**, **210**
    examination, 64
Facial nerve palsy, 66, 160
Failure to thrive, 46, 209
Fallot's tetralogy, 224
Fat covering, 61
Fat necrosis, subcutaneous, 62
Fatty acids, 92, 94, 117, 118
Fear of blame, 241
Feeding, 91–106
    artificial see Bottle feeding
    breast see Breast feeding
    cup, 100, 116
    physiology of, 91–92
    preterm infants, 116–119
    principles of nutrition, 92–93
    problems, 104–105
    supplementary feeds, 99
Feet
    examination, 70
    preterm infants, 109
    talipes, **21**, 70, 203, 235–236
Female pseudohermaphroditism, 229
Femoral pulse, 68
Femur, fractures of, 70
Fetus
    alcohol, effects on, 16
    antenatal diagnosis of disorders, 8,
        9, 21–23
    assessment of health, 20–21
    blood sampling, 23
    cardiac monitoring, 23, 33–34, 154
    circulation, 31–32
    development, 13, **14**
    distress, recognition, 33–34
    drug addiction, effects on, 17–19
    growth retardation, 14, 18, 20, 50,
        51, 61, 150, 151, 203
    haemorrhage, 185
    hydrops fetalis, 192, 194
    maternal age, effects of, 14, **15**, 22,
        202, 207
    maternal disease/illness, effects on,
        19–20, 27–28, 28–29, 164,
        175–178
    maternal nutrition and, 14, 15
    movements, 20
        breathing, 32
    prescribed drugs, effects on, 23–26
    radiation, effects on, 16, 203
    smoking, effects on, 8, 15–16
    withdrawal, 17
Fever, 168

'Fighting the ventilator', 138, 139
Fistula
    rectourethral, 218
    tracheo-oesophageal, 214
Fits see Seizures
Floppiness, 72
    see also Hypotonia
Flucloxacillin, 130, 165, 166, 167, **252**
Fluconazole, effect on fetus, 24
Fluids
    during phototherapy, 99
    in hypoxic-ischaemic
        encephalopathy, 154
    in intensive care, 128
5-Fluocytosine, **252**
Fluorescent in-situ hybridisation
        (FISH), **205**
Fluoxetine (Prozac) in pregnancy, 25
Focal fits, 156
Folic acid supplements
    in neonate, 119, **250**
    in pregnancy, 15, 21, 202
Fontanelles, 48, 63, 152, 232
Food thickeners, 105
Foramen ovale, 31, 32, 131, 140
Forceps delivery
    corneal injury, 66
    facial marks, 61
    head injury, 149
Fore-milk, 117
Foreskin, 69
Formula milks
    comparision with breast milk, **102**
    cow's milk, 94, 101, 102
    fatty acids, 92
    mineral levels, 87
    preterm follow-on milks, 119
    preterm formula milks, 117–118
    soya milks, 104, 119
Fractures
    long bones, 70, 160
    skull, 149–150
Fragile X chromosomes, 7, 205, 209
Fragile X syndrome, 207
Fresh frozen plasma, 186
Friedreich's ataxia, 206
Fructosaemia, 199
Fundus, examination, 66
Funerals, 246
Fungal infections, 141, 164, 167
Furosemide (frusemide), 121, 142, 226,
    250
Fusidic acid in pregnancy, 24

G

Gaertner's duct cyst, 228
Galactosaemia, 23, 101, 198, 199, 206,
    211
Gaseous exchange, preterm infants,
    111
Gastro-oesophageal reflux, 88, 105,
    121

Gastroenteritis, 174
Gastroschisis, 23, 144, 219
Gastrostomy, temporary, 215
Gaviscon, **250**
Genetic counselling, 8, 9, 21–22
Genetic disorders, 7, 22–23, 202, 204–207
  dominant inheritance, 205, 206
  recessive inheritance, 206
  X-linked inheritance, 207
Genetic testing, 8, 204, 205
Geneticist, referral to, 247
Genital herpes infection, maternal, 29, 180–181
Genitalia
  ambiguous, 69, 228–230
  examination, 69
  structural abnormalities, 228
Gentamicin, 76, 130, 169, 171, 173, 249, **252**
  and dosage, 175
Gestational age assessment, 20, 49, 108, **109**
Glabella tap, 75
Glaucoma, congenital, 66, 233
Glomerular filtration rate, 86
Glucagon, use of, 53, 55
Glucose level, maintenance of, 54
Glucose monitoring
  in hypothermia, 83
  in hypoxic-ischaemic encephalopathy, 154
  infants of diabetic mothers, 53
  light for dates infants, 51
  seizures, 156, 157
Glucose-6-dehydrogenase deficiency, 194–195, 202
Glucuronyl transferase, 189
Glutamine in formula milks, 118
Glycogen, 54, 92
Glycogen storage disease, 23
Goitre, congenital, 28, 212
Gonococcal infection, 164
  ophthalmia neonatorum, 166
Granulocyte colony stimulating factor, 168
Grasp responses, 74
Green stools, 105
Grey baby syndrome, 171
Grief, parents, 244, 245, 246, 247
Groins, examination, 68
Group B beta-haemolytic streptococcal infection, 29, 132, 164, 168, 169, 171, 174
Growth
  disorders of, 14, 18, 20, 49–57, 61, 150, 151, 203
  head cricumference, 47–48
  length, 46, 47, **48**
  weight, 45–46, **47**
Growth charts, **47**, 48–49
  preterm girls, **110**
Growth rate, 92
  preterm infants, 118

Grunting, 41, 67
Gut priming, 128
Guthrie test, 188, 211

H

Haemangiomas, 62, 236
Haematemesis, 185, 186
Haematological values, 183, **184**
Haemoglobin
  fetal, 183
  maternal in pregnancy, 15
  neonate
    normal values, 184
    preterm infants, 111
Haemoglobinopathies, 23, 188, 202, 213
Haemolytic anaemia, 119, 122, 192
Haemolytic disease
  due to ABO incompatibility, 194
  inherited causes, 194–195
  of the newborn, 191
Haemolytic jaundice, treatment, 195–197
Haemophilia, 23, 187, 207
Haemophilus influenzae infections, 163
  bone and joints, 174
  meningitis, 169
Haemorrhage
  antepartum, 5
  fetal, 185
  neonate, 185–186
    intracranial, 141, 143, 150, 152, 154, 186, 231
    orbital, 66
    pulmonary, 186
    subaponeurotic, 149
    subconjunctival, 65, 66
    umbilical, 185
  placental, 19
Haemorrhagic disease of the newborn, prevention, 84, 95, 186–187
Hair, 64, 65
Halothane, 26
Hand washing, 85, 115
Handicap, 7–8
  cerebral injury and, 155
  predicting, 75
  in preterm infants, 123
  respiratory distress syndrome and, 143
  spina bifida and, 230–231
Handling, preterm infants, 114
Harlequin change, 62
Head circumference, 47–48
  average, **49**
  in hydrocephalus, 232
  preterm infants, 108
Head injury at birth, 149–150
Head and neck, examination, 63–67
Head retraction, 151
Health visitors, 240

Hearing, testing, 75–76
Heart
  cardiac massage, 39
  examination, 67–68
  fetal monitoring, 23, 33–34, 154
  preterm infants, 111, 131
Heart failure, 226
Heart murmurs, 68, 221
Heart rate, neonatal, 67
Heat loss, neonates, 80–81
  preterm infants, 115
Heavy for dates infants, 56
Heelprick tests, 76, 77, 134
  reducing pain, 144
Heparin
  in neonate, **250**
  in pregnancy, 25
Hepatitis, 189, 198, 199
  diagnosis and management, 199–200
Hepatitis B virus, 17, 29, 164, 176, 180
  carriers, breast feeding contraindication, 96
  immunisation, 18, 180, **250**
Hepatitis C virus, 29, 96, 180
Hereditary clotting factor deficiencies, 187
Hereditary spherocytosis, 195
Hermaphroditism, 230
Herniae
  diaphragmatic, **42**, 144, 220
  groin, 68
  hiatus, 105, 215–216
  inguinal, **123**, 218
  umbilical, 68–69, 122
Herpes simplex virus, 29, 175, 180–181, 199
  encephalitis, 169
Hiatus hernia, 105, 215–216
High dependency, **126**
High-frequency oscillatory ventilation (HFOV), 135, 137
  weaning from, 139
High-frequency positive pressure ventilation, (HFPPV), 135, 136, 137
Hind milk, 98, 117
Hips, congenital dislocation, 71, 202, 233–235
  splintage, 234
  ultrasound, 234–235
Hirschsprung's disease, 218
Home deliveries, 8
  resuscitation at, 40
Homeopathic remedies in pregnancy, 27
Human chorionic gonadotrophin (bHCG), Down syndrome testing, 22
Human immunodeficiency virus (HIV), 17, 29, 164, 175–176, 178
  breast feeding contraindication, 96
  management, 178
  social aspects, 179–180

Humerus, fractures of, 70, 160
Huntington's chorea, 206
Hyaline membrane disease *see*
Respiratory distress syndrome
(RDS)
Hydralazine, effect on fetus, 24
Hydranencephaly, 232
Hydrocele, congenital, 69
Hydrocephalus
congenital, 231–232
in spina bifida, 230, 231
X-linked, **205**
Hydronephrosis, 227
Hydrops fetalis, 192, 194
Hymen, imperforate, 228
Hyperbilirubinaemia, 190, 192
investigations, 198
Hypercalcaemia, 92
Hyperinsulinism, 53, 54
Hyperparathyroidism, maternal, 28
Hypertension
persistent pulmonary hypertension
of the newborn (PPHN),
139–140
pregnancy-induced, 5, 19
Hyperthermia, 81, 82, 88
Hyperthyroidism, fetal, 27
Hypertonia, 72, 73
Hypocalcaemia, 73, 117, 128, 156,
233
seizures and management, 157
Hypocaloric feeding, 128
Hypoglycaemia, 54–56, 156
asymptomatic, 55
heavy for dates infants, 56
hypothermia-associated, 81, 82–83
infants of diabetic mothers, 53
jitteriness, 73
light for dates infants, 51, 52
outcome, 56
post-term infants, 52
prevention and treatment, 53,
54–55, 157
seizures, 156, 157
Hypolastic left heart syndrome, 225
Hyponatraemia, 112, 117
Hypoparathyroidism, maternal, 28
Hypoplasia of lungs, 220–221
Hypospadias, 69, 228
Hypotension, neonatal, 140
periventricular leucomalacia (PVL),
141
Hypotensive agents, effect on fetus,
19, 24
Hypothermia, 81, 82–83
in hypoxic-ischaemic
encephalopathy, 155
light for dates infants, 50, 51
preterm infants, 115
prevention, 81
Hypothyroidism, congenital, 66, 198,
212
Hypotonia, 152, 158–159
Hypovolaemic shock, 185

Hypoxia
fetal, 5, 33, 34, 50, 151
neonatal, 133, 134
Hypoxic-ischaemic encephalopathy,
50, 73, 151
investigations, 152–154
management, 154–155
mild, 151–152
prognosis, 155
severe, 152

I

Ibuprofen, effects on fetus, 26
Idiopathic thrombocytopenic purpura,
maternal, 28, 187–188
Ileal atresia, 217
Imipramine in pregnancy, 25
Immunisations
BCG, 178
hepatitis B, 18, 180, **250**
pertussis following neurological
illness, 157–158
preterm infants, 122
rubella, 21, 176
schedule for HIV-infected infants,
179
Immunoglobulins, 163
anti-D administration, 22, 192
IgG, placental transfer, 112, 163
in serious acute infection, 168
see also Antibodies
Imperforate anus, 218
Imperforate hymen, 228
Inborn errors of metabolism, 210–213
galactosaemia, 23, 101, 198, 199,
206, 211
hypothyroidism, 66, 198, 212
modes of presentation, **211**
phenylketonuria, 28, **76**, 77, 101,
156, 206, 211–212
Incubators, 115, 127
temperatures, **115**
transport, **81**, 113
Indomethacin, 142, **250**
Induction of labour, post-term infants,
52
Infancy, definition, **2**, 3
Infant mortality
definition, **2**
infant mortality rate, 4
in UK by country of birth, **6**
Infections, 81, 163–182
acute serious infection, 167–173
antenatal, 17, 28–29, 175–176
chronic infection, 178–182
and congenital anomalies, 202
in intensive care unit, 141
prevention and management, 130
and jaundice, 198
mechanisms of protection from,
163–164

minimising risk, 85–86, 115
umbilical cord, 88
minor infections, 165–167
preterm infants, 122
poor resistance to, 112
sources and routes of, 164–165
see also Bacterial infections;
Protozoal infections; Viral
infections
Informed consent, postmortem
examinations, 246
Inguinal hernias, **123**
incarcerated, 218
Insulin administration, **250**, 253
Intensive neonatal care, 125–147
dying babies, 145, 146
emotional care, 144–145
enteral nutrition, 128
fluids and nutrition, 128
infection, prevention and
management, 130
kangaroo care, 146, **146**
monitoring, 127–128
pain control, 144
requirements for, 126–127
respiratory care, 130–131
respiratory distress syndrome
(RDS), 131–143
surgical problems, 143–144
total parenteral nutrition,
128–130
Intermittent mandatory (or positive
pressure) ventilation
(IMV/IPPV), 135, 136
Internet, 2, 10
Interpreters, 240, 242
Intestinal obstruction, 105, 121
anomalies causing, 214–217
Intracranial haemorrhage, 141, 143,
150, 231
intraventricular, 150, 152, 186
periventricular, 141
subarachnoid, 150
subdural, 150, 154
Intracranial pressure, raised, 48, 152,
154
Intrauterine growth retardation, 14,
49–52, 51, 61, 150, 151, 203
causes, 50
chronic illness in pregnancy, 20
drug addiction, 18
Intrauterine transfusions, 193
Intravenous cannulae insertion,
129–130
Intraventricular haemorrhage, 150,
152, 186
Iodine deficiency, 212
Iron supplements
breast-fed infants, 119
in pregnancy, 15
Isolation, in infection, 86
Isoniazid, 178, **252**
Isotope scan in urinary tract infection,
173

J

Jaundice, 61, 95, 188–200
  ABO incompatibility, 194
  breast milk jaundice, 197, 198
  congenital hypothyroidism, 198
  congenital infection, 198
  galactosaemia, 198
  glucose-6-dehydrogenase deficiency,
    194–195
  haemolytic disease of the newborn,
    191
  hereditary spherocytosis, 195
  investigations, 189, 190
  obstructive, 198–200
  patterns of, 189, **190**
  preterm infants, 112, 121, 195
  rhesus haemolytic disease, 191–194
  sepsis-induced, 198
  severity, evaluation, 195
Jaw, underdevelopment, 100–101, 213
Jejunal atresia, 217
Jitteriness, 73
Joints
  dislocation, 70–71
    hips, 202, 233–235
  septic arthritis, 174

K

Kangaroo care, 145, **146**
Kasai procedure, 199
Kernicterus, 121, 190–191, 192, 194
'Kick counts', 20
Kidneys
  palpation, 68
  structural abnormalities, 226–227
Klumpke's palsy, 159
Knee, congenital dislocation, 70
Kyphosis, 69

L

Labetolol, effect on fetus, 19, 24
Labia majora, 69
Labia minora, 69
  adhesion, 228
  preterm infants, 109
Laboratory tests, 76–77, 126
  in urinary tract infection, 173
Lactation
  physiology of, 98
  suppression of, 101
  see also Breast feeding
Lactose intolerance, 101
Language difficulties, parents, 241,
    242
Lanugo, 64, 109
Laryngeal stridor, congenital, 43

Last menstrual period, 108
Learning disability, 155
  causes, 7, 151
    fragile X chromosomes, 209
    periventricular leucomalacia
      (PVL), 142
    preterm infants, 123
Lecithin-to-sphingomyelin ratio,
    131
Length, 46, 47, **48**
  average, **49**
  preterm infants, 108
Let-down reflex, 98
Leukaemia, childhood and vitamin K,
    186
Lidocaine (lignocaine)
  before chest drain insertion, 144
  in labour, effect on neonate, 26
Light for dates (LFD) infants, 49–52,
    107, 108
  clinical features, 51
  feeding, 51–52
  management, 51
  prognosis, 52
Lighting, neonatal unit, 113
Limbs
  examination, 70
  hyperextension, 151, 152
  structural deformities, 233–236
Lipid levels, monitoring during TPN,
    129
Lisinopril, effect on fetus, 24
Listeria monocytogenes infection, 28–29,
    164, 169, 176
Literature review, 2
Lithium, effect on fetus, 25
Live birth, definition, 2
Liver, palpation, 68
Local anaesthesia, 144
  amethocaine gel, 144
  in labour, effect on neonate, 26
Long-chain polyunsaturated fatty
    acids, 92, 94, 117, 118
Low birth weight infants, 49
  causes, 50
  definition, **2**, 3
  food requirements, 104
  health problems in later life, 8
  heat loss, 81
  mortality, 4, 5, 6
  prevalence, 5, 107
  teenage mothers, 14
  twins, 56
Lowe's oculorenal syndrome, 233
Lumbar puncture, 168
  technique, 170–171
Lungs
  abscess, 172
  at birth, 32
  malformations, 220–221
Lymphangiomas, 236
Lymphatic system abnormalities,
    236
Lymphocytes, 164

M

Macrocytic anaemia, 122
Macroglossia, 66
Macrophthalmia, 233
Magnesium sulphate, 155, **251**
Magnetic resonance imaging (MRI),
    153, 156
Magnetic resonance spectroscopy,
    154–155
Malaria, 181–182
Male pseudohermaphroditism,
    229–230
Malmo splint, 234
Malnutrition and congenital
    anomalies, 202
Malrotation of midgut, 217
Mannitol, **251**
Marijuana, 19
Massage, preterm infants, 144
Mastitis
  maternal, 99
  neonate, 165–166
Maternal mortality, 2
Mechanical ventilation
  in respiratory distress, 130, 132, **133**,
    134–139
  resuscitation, 38, 39, 40
Meckel's diverticulum, 217–218
Meconium, 86
  aspiration syndrome, 40, 43, 133
  failure to pass, 105
  ileus, 105, 210
  in liquor, 33, 40
  peritonitis, 219
  plug, 86, 105, 218–219
Mediastinal shift, 67
Medical staff, neonatal intensive care
    unit, 126–127
Medium-chain acyl coenzyme-A
    dehydrogenase (MCAD)
    deficiency, 212
Megacolon, 218
Melaena, 185, 186
Mementos, 244–245
Memorial services, 247
Meningitis, 167, 169–171
  organisms causing, 168
  treatment and outlook, 171
Meningocele, 231
Metabolic acidosis, 43, 112, 134
Metabolic disorders, 23
  see also Inborn errors of metabolism
Metachromatic leukodystrophy, 23
Methadone in pregnancy, 17
Methicillin-resistant *Staphylococcus
    aureus* (MRSA), 115, 165,
    169
Metopic suture, 63
Metronidazole, 169, **252**
Miconazole, 167, **252**
Microcephaly, 48, 232, 233
Micrognathia, 100–101, 213

Microphthalmia, 233
Micturating cystogram, 173
Mid-trimester abortions, 3
Midazolam, **251**
Milia, 62
Milk *see* Breast milk; Formula milks
Mitochondrial disease, 226
Mongolian blue spots, 62
Monilial dermatitis, 87
Monitoring equipment, 127
Monozygotic twins, 56
Moro reflex, 73, 74, 159
Morphine
  effects on neonate, 26, 253
  neonatal pain control, 136, 144,
    251
Mortality rates, 2, 3, 4
Mouth, examination, 66
Mouth-operated mucus extractors,
  80
Movements
  fetal, 20
  neonatal, 73
    hypoxic-ischaemic
      encephalopathy, 151
    preterm infants, 110
Mucopolysaccharidoses, 23
Multiple birth, 56–57
  congenital anomalies, 203
  see also Twins
Muscle tone
  abnormal
    hypotonia, 152, 158–159
    physiotherapy, 155
  assessment, 72
  preterm infants, 110
Muscular dystrophy, 23, 158–159
Mustard procedure, 223
Myasthenia gravis, 159
  maternal, 28
Mycoplasma hominis infection, 164
Myelomeningocele, 23, 158, 230, 231
Myocardial infarction, 226
Myocarditis, 226
Myoclonic twitching, 151
Myopathy, 158
Myotonic dystrophy, 159, **205**

N

Naevi, pigmented, 62
Naloxone, 38, 41, 144, **251**
  infants of opiate addicted mothers,
    18
Nappies, disposal, 85
Nappy rash, 87–88, 167
Nasal obstruction, 101, 167
Nasogastric feeding, 117
Neck, examination, 66–67
Necrotising enterocolitis, 94, 140
Need for special care, 9
Neisseria meningitidis, 169

Neomycin in pregnancy, 24
Neonatal abstinence syndrome, 18
Neonatal mortality, 4, 6
  causes, 5
  definition, **2**
  trends in causes, **4**
Neonatal period, definition, **2**, 3
Nephroblastoma, 227
Nerve injuries, 159–160
Nesidioblastosis, 56
Netilmicin, 130, 171, 249
  and dosage, 175
Neural tube defects, 5, 202, 230
  anencephaly, 202, 203, 230
  antenatal diagnosis, 23
  encephalocele, 230
  prevention, 15, 21
  spina bifida, 5, 7, 23, 70, 202,
    230–231
Neurofibromatosis, 62, 206
Neurological assessment, 71–75
  interpreting, 75
Neurological disorders, 149–161
  encephalopathy, 150–155
  head injury at birth, 149–150
  hypotonia, 158–159
  intracranial haemorrhage *see*
    Intracranial haemorrhage
  nerve injuries, 159–160
  and pertussis immunisation,
    157–158
  seizures, 152, 154, 155–158
  spinal injury, 159
Neuromuscular disease, 158
Neutral thermal environment, 115
Nifedipine in pregnancy, 24
Nipple shields, 100
Nipples
  care of, 99
  cracked, 99–100
  non-protractile, 95, 100
Nitric oxide (NO), inhaled, 26, 137,
  140
Noise, reducing, 113–114
Non-steroidal anti-inflammatory
    drugs (NSAIDS) in pregnancy,
    26
Normal care, definition, 125
Normal infants, caring for *see* Care,
    normal infants
Nose, examination, 65
Nuchal translucency, 21
Nucleotides, preterm formulae, 118
Nursing brassières, 99
Nursing staff, neonatal intensive care
    unit, 126–127
Nutrition
  maternal, 14, 15
    during lactation, 97
  neonatal, 92–93
  sick preterm infants, 128
Nuts, avoiding during lactation, 95
Nystagmus, 66, 75
Nystatin, 87, 167, **252**

O

Observations
  intensive care units, **127**, 128
    respiratory distress syndrome,
      133
  preterm infants, 113
  routine, 61
Obstructive jaundice, 198–200
Occipitofrontal circumference, 47, 48
Oedema, 121
  and weight gain, 16
Oesophageal atresia, 214–215
Oesophagitis, persistent, 215–216
Oestriol levels, Down syndrome
    testing, 22
Oligohydramnios, 203, 227
Ophthalmia neonatorum, 166
Ophthalmoscopy, 66
Opiates, 158
  addiction, 18, 96
  neonates, 144, 253
Optico-kinetic nystagmus, 75
Oral thrush, 167
Orbital haemorrhage, 66
Orchidopexy, 122
Organ donation, 146
Orogastric feeding, 117
Orogastric tube aspiration, 138
Ortolani's test, 71
Osteogenesis imperfecta, 63
Osteomyelitis, 160, 174
Otitis media, 167
Otoacoustic response, 76
Ovaries, absent, 209
Overfeeding, 100
Oxygen saturation, 133
  at birth, 32
  test, 222
  ventilated infants, 138
Oxygen, supplemental, 38
  preterm infants, 120
  in RDS, 133, 142
Oxytocin, 98

P

Packed cell volume, 184
Pain, neonates, 72, 144
Palatal prosthesis, 213
Pallor, 61
Palmar grasp responses, 74
Pancuronium, 138, **251**
Paracetamol, neonates, 144, **251**
Parathyroid dysfunction, maternal, 28
Parenting ability, factors affecting,
    84–85
Parents
  counselling *see* Counselling parents
  of infant in intensive care,
    144–145

Parents (*continued*)
  'Preparation for Parenthood classes', 97, 239, **240**
  of preterm infant, 113, 119
  reactions to abnormal baby, 204, 241–242
Parity, 14
Paronychia, 165
Paroxetine during pregnancy, 25
Paroxysmal supraventricular tachycardia, 226
Partial thromboplastin time, 186
Patau's syndrome, 209
Patient-triggered ventilation (PTV), 135, 137
Pavlik harness, 234, **235**
Peak inspiratory pressure (PIP), 136, 138
Peanut allergens, 95
Pelvis, maternal, 15
Pemphigus neonatorum, 165
Penicillin, 166, 169, 172
Penis, 69
Perianal excoriation, 87
Perinatal health, factors influencing, 4–5
Perinatal mortality, 2
  causes, 5–7
    treatable, 6–7
  definitions, **2**, 3–4
  incidence by maternal age, **15**
  trends in, **3**
Perinatal mortality rate, 3, 4
Periodic respiration, preterm infants, 120
Peritonitis, meconium, 219
Periventricular leucomalacia (PVL), 141, 143, 155
Persistent ductus arteriosus (PDA), 111, 128, 131, 140, 142, 225, 226
Persistent pulmonary hypertension of the newborn (PPHN), 139–140
Persistent truncus arteriosus, 224
Pertussis immunisation, 157–158
Pethidine
  effects on neonate, 26, 100
    naloxone reversal, 38
pH
  fetal blood, 34
  in respiratory distress, 133–134
Pharmacopoeia, 249–253
Phenobarbital, 154, 157, **251**
  in rhesus haemolytic disease, 193
Phenylketonuria, 101, 156, 206, 211
  heelprick tests, **76**, 77
  maternal, 28
  treatment, 211–212
Phenytoin, 157, **251**
Phosphate supplements, preterm infants, 119, **251**
Photographs, 145, 244
Phototherapy, 121, 195–197
  and nappy rash, 87
  in rhesus haemolytic disease, 193
Physiological anaemia, 184

Physiological jaundice, 189
Physiotherapy, 155
Pierre Robin syndrome, 213
Pigmented naevi, 62
Placenta, 13, 14, 31
Placenta praevia, 5, 19, 185
Placental insufficiency, 5, 7, 19, 21, 50, 151
Plagiocephaly, 64
Planning for birth, 79
Plantar grasp responses, 74
Plasmodium falciparum see Malaria
Platelets, **184**, 187
Pleural drain insertion, 139
Pneumomediastinum, 139
Pneumonia, 167, 171–172
  organisms causing, 168
  treatment, 172
Pneumothorax, 40, 42–43, 67, 139
pO$_2$/pCO$_2$ recorders, 133
Polycystic kidneys, 227
Polycythaemia, 183, 184, 224
  infants of diabetic mothers, 53
  light for dates infants, 51
  and twins, 56
Polyhydramnios, 56, 203, 214, 216, 220
Polymorphonuclear leucocytes, 164
Pompe's disease, 23
Port-wine stains, 63
Portoenterostomy, 199
Position for
  artifical feeding, 103, **104**
  breast feeding, 97–98
Positive end expiratory pressure (PEEP), 136, 138
Posseting, 105
Post-anal dimple, 69–70
Post-term infants, 52, 150
  antibiotic dosage, 175
  definition, **2**, 3
Postmortem examinations, 5, 146, 246
Postneonatal mortality, 4
  definition, **2**
Posture, 72–73
  limbs, 70
  preterm infant, 110
  sleeping, 4, 88–89
Potassium chloride, **251**
Potter's facies, 227
Prader-Willi syndrome, 159, **205**
Pre-eclampsia, 19, 45
Preauricular skin tags, 65
Prednisolone, effects on fetus, 24
Prelabour rupture of membranes, 5, 29
Premature beats, benign, 67
Pressure marks
  birthmarks, 62–63
  preterm infants, 114
Preterm follow-on formulae, **102**, 119
Preterm formulae, **102**
Preterm infants, 107–124
  antibiotic dosage, 175
  bathing, 87, 114–115
  breast feeding, 94, 96, 118
  bruising, 111, 187

causative factors, 108
cerebral palsy, 7–8
characteristics, 108, 109, **110**
common disorders, 120–123
definition, **2**, 3
effects of immaturity, 110–112
gastro-oesophageal reflux, 105
gestational age assessment, 108
immunisations, 122
jaundice, 112, 121, 195
lanugo, 64, 109
and low birth weight, 49
management, 112–119
  care in neonatal unit, 113–116
  delivery, 112–113
  prevention, 112
maternal smoking, 16
mortality, 4, 5
outlook, 123
prevalence, 107
resuscitation, 38, 40
  and tension pneumothorax, 43
sudden infant death syndrome (SIDS), 88, 89, 123
twins, 56
Preterm labour, delaying, 112
Primary apnoea, 33
Primitive reflexes, 73, 74
Progression responses, 74
Progressive infantile spinal muscular atrophy, 158
Prolactin, 98
Prolonged rupture of membranes, infection, 29, 164, 169
Prone posture, 72, 73
Propranolol, effect on fetus, 24
Proptosis, 66
Prostacyclin, **251**
Prostaglandin infusion, 225
Protease inhibitor (Pi) typing, 199
Protein requirement, 92
Prothrombin time, 186
Protozoal infections
  malaria, 181–182
  toxoplasmosis, 29, 164, 175, 177, 198, 199, 202, 233
Prozac in pregnancy, 25
'Prune belly' syndrome, 227
Pseudohermaphroditism
  female, 229
  male, 229–230
Pseudomonas aeruginosa, 165
Pseudoparalysis, 160, 174
Psychological factors
  perinatal care, 8–9
  well-being of mother, 84, 85
Psychosocial factors
  breast feeding advantages, 94, 95
  during pregnancy, 16–17
  and parenting ability, 84
Psychotropic drugs in pregnancy, 25, 26
Pudendal blocks, 26
Puerperium, 84
Pulmonary atresia, 223

Pulmonary haemorrhage, 186
Pulmonary interstitial emphysema, 139
Pulmonary perfusion, poor, 224
Pulmonary stenosis, critical, 223
Pulmonary venous drainage, total
    anomalous, 223
Pulse oximetry, transcutaneous, 222
Pulses, feeling, 68
Purpura, 187
Pyloric stenosis, 207, 216
Pyridoxine, 157

Q

Quadriplegia, 123, 159
Quality of life, 2, 7–8

R

Radial nerve injury, 159
Radiation, effect on fetus, 16, 203
Raised intracranial pressure, 48, 152,
    154
Ramstedt's pyloromyotomy, 216
Ranitidine, 105, **251**
Ranula, 66
Rashkind's procedure, 223
Recessive inheritance, 206
    associated conditions, 23, 209–213
Rectosigmoidectomy, 218
Rectourethral fistulae, 218
Red cells
    lifespan, 188
    normal count, **184**
Reflexes
    let-down, 98
    neonates, 73, 74
        loss of, 152
Registering birth and death, 246
Religious aspects
    birth customs, 79
    blood transfusion issues, 184–185
    discussing with parents, 241
    dying babies, 146, 244
    postmortem examinations, 246
Renal agenesis, 203
Renal failure, 128
Renal function, 86–87
    preterm infants, 112
Renal pelves, dilatation, 21
Research, clinical, 2
Respiration
    normal breathing, 41
    onset of, 32–33
    preterm infants, 111–112
        problems, 120–121
Respiration rates, 41
Respiratory acidosis, 134
Respiratory centre, 32, 41, 120
Respiratory depression, 18, 26, 144, 253
Respiratory distress, 41–43

Respiratory distress syndrome (RDS),
    5, 53, 113, 130, 131–143, 186
    blood gases, 133–134
    clinical features, 131–132
    complications of, 139–142, 150
        and prognosis, 142–143
    management, 132–133
    mechanical ventilation, 134–137
        complications, 138
        management, 137–138
        weaning off, 138–139
    oxygen therapy, 133
    pathogenesis, 131
    preterm infants, 120–121
    surfactant therapy, 133
Respiratory syncitial virus (RSV), 143,
    167
Respiratory tract
    infections, 166–167, 171–172
    structural malformations, 219–222
Response to environment, 72
Resuscitation, 34, 36–40
    apparatus required, 35–36
    care of baby after, 41
    drugs used, **39**
    ethical dilemmas, 40–41
    keeping infant warm during, 81
    mild asphyxia, 37–38
    predicting need, 34–35
    preterm infants, 113
    severe asphyxia, 38–40
    in special circumstances, 40
    teaching parents, 240
Resuscitation Council algorithm, 36, **37**
Retinopathy of prematurity (retrolental
    fibroplasia), 133, 142–143
Rewarming, hypothermic infants,
    82–83
Rh gene, inheritance, 191, **192**
Rhesus antibody formation, 22, 191
Rhesus haemolytic disease, 191–194
    antenatal management, 193
    exchange transfusion, 194
    management at birth, 193–194
    prevention, 192
Rickets, 63, 95, 117, 119
Rifampicin, 178
Ritodrine in pregnancy, 26
Ritter's disease, 165
Room temperature, 82
Rooting reflex, 72, 73, **74**
Rotavirus infection, 174
Rubella, 164, 175, 176, 199, 202, 233
    immunisation, 21, 176
    jaundice, 198
Rupture of membranes
    prelabour, 5, 29
    prolonged, 29, 164, 169

S

'Salmon patches', 62–63
Salmonella infection, 29, 174

Salt-losing adrenal crisis, 229
Scalded skin syndrome, 165
Scalp vein
    cannulation, neonates, 130
    sampling, fetal, 34
Scaphocephaly, 233
Sclerema, 121–122
Scoliosis, 69, 203, 238
Scrotum
    examination, 69
    pigmentation, 61
Sedatives in pregnancy, 25, 26
Seizures, 152, 155–158
    diagnosis, 156
    management, 154, 157
    prognosis, 158
    see also Epilepsy
Sensorineural deafness, 76
Separating mother and child, 83
Septic arthritis, 174
Septicaemia, 141, 167, 168, 169
Sequestration of lung, 220
'Setting sun' sign, 232
Sex chromosomes, 204
Sexually transmitted diseases, 17, 29,
    164, 166
    chlamydial infection, 164, 166
    gonorrhoea, 164, 166
    syphilis, 29, 164, 167, 175, 181, 198
    see also Human immunodeficiency
        virus (HIV)
Shigella infection, 174
Short stature, maternal, 15, 45
Shoulder dystocia, 53, 70, 159
Siblings, 86, 242, 247
Sickle cell disease, 188, 202, 213
Signs indicating sick infant, 60
Single umbilical artery, 88, 203
Single ventricle, 224
Skin
    care of, 87–88
    examination, 61–63
    infections, 165–166
    preterm infants, 109, 111, 114, 115
    role in temperature maintenance, 80
Skin tags, preauricular, 65
Skull
    examination, 63
    fracture, 149–150
    preterm infant, 109
Sleep, 72
Sleeping position and SIDS, 4, 88–89
Sliding hernia, 215
Smoking
    by-product secretion in breast milk,
        96
    in pregnancy, 8, 15–16
'Snuffles', 166–167
Social concern during pregnancy, 16–17
Social worker, help from, 243
Socioeconomic conditions
    identifying problems, 241
    inadequate diet in pregnancy, 15
    low birth weight, 5
    and perinatal death, 6

Sodium bicarbonate in resuscitation, **39**
Sodium chloride, **251**
Sodium valproate, 157, 203, **251**
Soya milks, 104, 119
Spastic diplegia, 123
Spastic quadriplegia, 123, 159
Special care, definition, 125, **126**
Spherocytosis, hereditary, 195
Spina bifida, 5, 7, 202, 230–231
    antenatal diagnosis, 23
    occulta, 70
Spinal dysraphism, 231
Spinal injury, 159
Spinal muscular atrophy, progressive infantile, 158
Spine, examination, 69–70
Spiramycin, 177
Spironolactone, 121, **251**
Spitz-Holter valve, 231, 232
Spontaneous movements, neonate, 73
Squint, 65, 66
Staff
    counselling parents *see* Counselling parents
    with infections, 86
    in intensive care unit, 126–127
Staphylococcal infections, 141, 164, 168, 169
    bone and joints, 174
    eyes, 166
    mastitis, neonatal, 166
    paronychia, 165
    pneumonia, 172
    skin, 165
    upper respiratory tract, 167
Status epilepticus in pregnancy, 27
Stepping response, 74, **75**
Sterilisation, feeding equipment, 85, 102–103
Sternal recession, 131, **132**
Sternomastoid tumour, 66–67
Steroids
    maternal
        in pregnancy, 24
        reducing RDS, 112, 131
    neonatal, in chronic lung disease (CLD), 143
Sticky eyes, 66, 164, 166
Stillbirth, 240, 244
    causes, 5
    definition, 2, 3
    gender differences, 6
    helping parents, 246–247
    unexpected, 40–41
Stimulation, 84
Stools
    blood in, 185, 186
    normal, 86, 94
    unusual, 105
Storing prepared feeds, 103
'Stork marks', 62–63
Strawberry marks, 63, 122

Streptococcal infections, 29, 132, 141, 163, 164, 168
    bone and joints, 174
    eyes, 166
    meningitis, 169
    pneumonia, 171
    upper respiratory tract, 167
Streptomycin, effects on fetus, 24
Stridor, 43
Sturge-Weber syndrome, 63
Subaponeurotic haemorrhage, 149
Subarachnoid haemorrhage, 150
Subconjunctival haemorrhages, 65, 66
Subcostal recession, 131, **132**
Subdural haemorrhage, 150, 154
Submucosal mucus retention cyst, 66
Sucking, 72, 91–92
    blisters, 66
    problems related to, 100–101
Sucrose, oral, 144
Suction
    at delivery, 80
    endotracheal tube, 138
Sudden infant death syndrome (SIDS), 4
    chronic lung disease (CLD), 143
    hyperthermia, 81
    maternal drug addiction, 18, 19
    maternal smoking, 16
    preterm infants, 88, 89, 123
    risk factors, **89**
    sleeping position, 4, 88–89
Supine posture, 72, **73**
Supplementary feeds, 99
Support organisations, 242, 243, 246, 247
Suprapubic aspiration of bladder, 172–173
Surfactant, 111, 131
    therapy, 36, 133, 143
Sutures
    examination, 63
    widened, 48
Swabs, bacterial culture, 168, 169
Sweat, testing in cystic fibrosis, 210
Sweating, 80
Synchronised intermittent mandatory ventilation (SIMV), 135, 137
Syndactyly, 70
Syphilis, 164, 175
    congenital, 167, 181
    jaundice, 198
    maternal, 29
Syringe pump delivery, breast milk, 118

T

Tachycardia
    fetal, 27, 33
    neonatal, 67
        paroxysmal supraventricular, 226

Tachypnoea, 67
    transient neonatal, 43, 132
Talipes, 70, 203
    calcaneovalgus, **70**, 236
    equinovarus, 235, 236
    prenatal ultrasound, **21**
Tay-Sachs disease, 23
Teats
    flanged for cleft lip/palate, 213
    milk flow through, 103
    sterilising, 102–103
Teenage mothers
    low birth weight infants, 14
    perinatal death, 6
Teeth, 66
Temperature, maintenance of, 80–83
    clothing infant, 81, 82
    hypothermia, 82–83
    regulation, 80–81
        preterm infants, 115
Temperature recording, 82
    preterm infants, 115
Tension pneumothorax, **42**, 43, 139
Term infants
    antibiotic dosage, 175
    definition, **2**, 3
    length, 46, 47
    weight, 45
Terminal apnoea, 33
Termination of pregnancy, 8
Test feeding, 100
Testes, 69
    preterm infants, 109
Testosterone insensitivity, 69
Tetany, hypocalcaemic, 157
Tetracyclines
    effects on fetus, 24
    eye ointment, 166
Thalassaemia, 23, 188, 202, 213
Thalidomide, 203
Theophylline, **251**
Thrombocytopenia, 28, 187, 188
Thrush
    gastrointestinal, 167
    perineal, 87
    see also Candida infections
Thyroglossal cysts, 67
Thyroid-stimulating hormone (TSH) screening test, 198, 212
Thyrotoxicosis
    fetal, 23
    maternal, 27–28
    neonatal, 28
Tissue necrosis, TPN solutions, 129
Tobramicin, 249, **252**
Tocolytic agents in pregnancy, 26
Tog values, clothing and bedding, 81, **82**
Tolazoline, 140, 224, **251**
Tongue darting, 66
Tongue tie, 66
Tonic seizures, 156
Torticollis, 67

Total anomalous pulmonary venous drainage, 223
Total parenteral nutrition (TPN), 128–130
  complications, 129, 141
Toxoplasmosis, 29, 164, 175, 177, 199, 202, 233
  jaundice, 198
Tracheo-oesophageal fistula, 214
Traction response, 74
Tranquillisers in pregnancy, 25, 26
Transillumination of head, 232
Transport incubators, 81, 113
Transposition of great arteries, 56, 223, **224**
Trauma during delivery, 53
  fractures, 70, 149–150, 160
  ruptured liver or spleen, 68
Traumatic cyanosis, 62, 187
Treponema pallidum see Syphilis
Tricuspid atresia, 223, **224**
Trimethoprim, 173
Triplets, 57
Trisomies, 205, 207–209
  trisomy 13, 209
  trisomy 18, 209
  trisomy 21, 205, 207–209
  see also Down syndrome
Trometamol (TRAM), 134
Trophic feeding, 116, 128
Truncus arteriosus, persistent, 224
Trypsin, immunoreactive, 210
Tuberculosis, 164, 176, 178
Tuberous sclerosis, 62, 206
Turner's syndrome, 66, 209
Turricephaly, 233
Twins, 56–57
  blood transfer between, 185

U

Ultrasound imaging, 20–21, 23, 108
  in cerebral injury, 152, 156
    intraventricular haemorrhage, 141
    periventricular leucomalacia (PVL), 141
  in congenital hydrocephalus, **232**
  in congential dislocation of hip, 234–235
  in urinary tract infection, 173
  see also Doppler blood flow studies
Umbilical artery
  catheterisation (UAC), 134, 140
  single, 88, 203
Umbilical cord
  bleeding from, 185
  clamping of, 80, 88, 184
    preterm infants, 113
  prolapse, 5
  stump care, 85, 88

Umbilical vein
  catheterisation, 130
  transfusions, 193
Umbilicus
  disorders of development, 219
  examination, 68–69
  hernia, 68–69, 122
  infection, periumbilical skin, 165
  polyp, 68
Underfeeding, 100
  stools, 105
Undescended testes, 69, 109, 122
UNICEF, successful breast feeding, 93, **94**
Upper respiratory tract infections, 166–167
Urachus, 68
Uraemia, 92
Urate crystals, 86
Ureters, ectopic, 86, 227
Urethra, congenital obstruction, 227
Urethral valves, 86
Urinary chromatography, 156
Urinary tract
  congenital malformations, 226–228
  infections, 167, 172–173
  obstruction, 69, 227
Urine
  collection, 114, 128, 172
  cultures, 168
  delay in passing, 227
  normal, 86–87
  suprapubic aspiration, 172–173
Urticaria neonatorum, 62, 165
Uterine contractions, 151
  fetal heart rate, 34
  placental function, 50
Uterus, size, 108

V

Vacuum extraction, injury, 149
Vaginal bleeding, neonate, 186
Vancomycin, 169, **252**
Varicella virus, 176, 178
Vegan diet in pregnancy, 15
Vegetarian diet in pregnancy, 15
Velamentous insertion, umbilical cord, 185
Velocardiofacial syndrome, **205**
Venereal Disease Research Laboratories (VDRL) test, 181
Ventilation
  bag and mask, 37–38
  mechanical
    in respiratory distress, 130, 132, **133**, 134–139
    resuscitation, 38, 39, 40
Ventilator
  types, 134–135
  weaning baby from, 138–139

Ventricles
  brain, haemorrhage into, 150, 152, 186
  heart
    septal defects, 221, 225, 226
    single, 224
    subendocardial fibroelastosis, 226
Ventriculoatrial/peritoneal shunt, 231
Ventrosuspension, 73
Very low birth weight infants, 3
  adapted artifical feeds, 117–118
Viability, 107
Viral infections, 175–176
  Coxsackie virus, 164, 169, 176, 177, 199, 202, 213
  cytomegalovirus, 96, 164, 175, 176–177, 198, 199, 233
  echovirus, 164, 169, 177–178, 202
  hepatitis B virus, 17, 18, 29, 96, 164, 176, 180, **250**
  hepatitis C virus, 29, 96, 180
  herpes simplex, 29, 169, 175, 180–181, 199
  HIV *see* Human immunodeficiency virus (HIV)
  rubella, 21, 164, 175, 176, 199, 202, 233
  varicella virus, 176, 178
Vision, 65, 74
Vitamins
  deficiency
    vitamin D in pregnancy, 15, 157
    vitamin E, preterm infants, 122
    vitamin K, 24, 95
  supplements
    breast fed infants, 95
    preterm infants, 119
    in total parental nutrition, 129
  vitamin K, routine administration, 84, 113, 186, 187, **251**
Volume expanders in resuscitation, **39**
Volume-guaranteed ventilators, 134
Volvulus, 217
Vomiting, 91, 105, 174
  bile in vomit, 105
  blood in vomit, 105, 185, 186
  in duodenal atresia, 216
  in hiatus hernia, 215
  in pyloric stenosis, 216
Von Rosen splint, 234

W

Wakefulness, 72
  in cerebral irritation, 151
Warfarin, effects on fetus, 24
Warming bottled feeds, 103
Water
  for making up feeds, 103
  supplementary, 99
Water filters, contamination, 103

Website addresses, 10, 11, 35, 44, 106, 147, 237, 253
Weighing baby, 89
  preterm infants, 116
Weight, 3, 45–46, **47**
  average, **49**
  preterm infants, 108
  weight gain
    average baby, 92
    infants of diabetic mothers, 53
    maternal in pregnancy and breast feeding, 95–96
    preterm infants, 116, 118
  weight loss, neonates, normal, 46, 98
  see also Light for dates (LFD) infants; Low birth weight infants
Werdnig-Hoffman disease, 158, **205**
Whey-based milks, 102
White cell count, **184**

Wiedemann-Beckwith syndrome, **205**
Williams syndrome, **205**
Wilms' tumour, 227
Wind, 104, 105
Withdrawal
  fetal, 17
  neonates
    maternal antidepressants, 25
    maternal benzodiazepines, 26
    maternal drug abuse, 18, 87
Wolff-Parkinson-White anomaly, 226
Wrist drop, 159

X

X-linked conditions
  antenatal diagnosis, 23
  fragile X syndrome, 207, 209

hydrocephalus, **205**
  pattern of inheritance, **206**, 207
X-rays *see* Abdominal X-ray; Chest X-ray

Z

Zoster immune globulin, 178